D0265248

theclinics.com

CLINICS IN GERIATRIC MEDICINE

Infectious Diseases in Older Adults

GUEST EDITOR
Kevin High, MD, MSc

August 2007 • Volume 23 • Number 3

SAUNDERS

An Imprint of Elsevier, Inc.
PHILADELPHIA   LONDON   TORONTO   MONTREAL   SYDNEY   TOKYO

W.B. SAUNDERS COMPANY
A Division of Elsevier Inc.

Elsevier, Inc. • 1600 John F. Kennedy Blvd., Suite 1800 • Philadelphia, PA 19103-2899

http://www.theclinics.com

CLINICS IN GERIATRIC MEDICINE	Volume 23, Number 3
August 2007	ISSN 0749-0690
Editor: Lisa Richman	ISBN-13: 978-1-4160-5048-3
	ISBN-10: 1-4160-5048-5

Clinics in Geriatric Medicine (ISSN 0749-0690) is published quarterly by Elsevier Inc., 360 Park Avenue South, New York, NY 10010-1710. Months of issue are February, May, August, and November. Business and Editorial Offices: 1600 John F. Kennedy Blvd., Suite 1800, Philadelphia, PA 191023-2899. Customer Service Office: 6277 Sea Harbor Drive, Orlando, FL 32887-4800. Periodicals postage paid at New York NY, and additional mailing offices. Subscription prices is $178.00 per year (US individuals), $297.00 per year (US institutions), $232.00 per year (Canadian individuals), $362.00 per year (Canadian institutions) $232.00 per year (foreign individuals) and $362.00 per year (foreign institutions). Foreign air speed delivery is included in all *Clinics* subscription prices. All prices are subject to change without notice. POSTMASTER Send address changes to *Clinics in Geriatric Medicine*, Elsevier Periodicals Customer Service, 6277 Sea Harbor Drive, Orlando, FL 32887-4800. **Customer Service: 1-800-654-2452 (US). From outside of the US, call 1-407-345-4000. E-mail: hhspcs@wbsaunder.com**.

Clinics in Geriatric Medicine is covered in *Index Medicus*, *EMBASE/Excerpta Medica*, *Current Contents Clinical Medicine (CC/CM)*, *and the Cumulative Index to Nursing & Allied Health Literature*.

Printed in the United States of America.

GUEST EDITOR

KEVIN HIGH, MD, MSc, Chief, Section on Infectious Diseases; Professor of Medicine, Sections on Infectious Diseases, Hematology/Oncology, and Molecular Medicine, Wake Forest University Health Sciences, Winston-Salem, North Carolina

CONTRIBUTORS

DEVERICK J. ANDERSON, MD, Clinical Associate in Medicine, Division of Infectious Diseases, Duke University Medical Center, Durham; Duke Infection Control Outreach Network, Durham, North Carolina

STEVEN C. CASTLE, MD, Geriatric Research Education and Clinical Center (GRECC), VA Greater Los Angeles Healthcare System, Professor, UCLA School of Medicine, Los Angeles, California

HEATHER L. COX, PharmD, Clinical Specialist, Infectious Diseases, Department of Pharmacy Services, University of Virginia Health System, Charlottesville, Virginia

GERALD R. DONOWITZ, MD, Professor of Medicine, Department of Medicine, Infectious Disease, University of Virginia Health System, University of Virginia, Charlottesville, Virginia

E. WESLEY ELY, MD, MPH, Associate Director for Research, VA Tennessee Valley Geriatric Research, Education, and Clinical Center (GRECC), VA Service, Department of Veterans Affairs Medical Center; Associate Professor of Medicine, Division of Allergy, Pulmonary, and Critical Care Medicine and Center for Health Services Research, Vanderbilt University School of Medicine, Nashville, Tennessee

ANN R. FALSEY, MD, Associate Professor of Medicine, Division of Infectious Diseases, Department of Medicine at Rochester General Hospital, Rochester; and Department of Medicine, University of Rochester School of Medicine and Dentistry, Rochester, New York

TAMAS FULOP, MD, Research Scholar, Research Center on Aging, Immunology Program, Geriatric Division, University of Sherbrooke, Quebec, Canada

TIMOTHY D. GIRARD, MD, MSCI, Instructor in Medicine, Division of Allergy, Pulmonary, and Critical Care Medicine, Center for Health Services Research, Vanderbilt University School of Medicine, Nashville, Tennessee

VLADIMIR GULLER, MD, Senior Physician, Subacute Department, Harzfeld Geriatric Hospital, Kaplan Medical Center, Gedera, Israel

ALEXANDER GUREVICH, MD, Senior Physician, Subacute Department, Harzfeld Geriatric Hospital, Kaplan Medical Center, Gedera, Israel

ASHLEY R. HERRING, PharmD, Specialty Resident, Infectious Diseases, Department of Pharmacy, Wake Forest University Baptist Medical Center, Winston-Salem, North Carolina

KEVIN HIGH, MD, MSc, Chief, Section on Infectious Diseases; Professor of Medicine, Sections on Infectious Diseases, Hematology/Oncology, and Molecular Medicine, Wake Forest University Health Sciences, Winston-Salem, North Carolina

MANISHA JUTHANI-MEHTA, MD, Assistant Professor, Yale University School of Medicine, Department of Internal Medicine, Section of Infectious Disease, New Haven, Connecticut

KEITH S. KAYE, MD, MPH, Associate Professor of Medicine, Division of Infectious Diseases, Duke University Medical Center, Durham; Duke Infection Control Outreach Network, Durham, North Carolina

VERA P. LUTHER, MD, Fellow in Infectious Diseases, Section on Infectious Diseases, Department of Internal Medicine, Wake Forest University Baptist Medical Center Health Sciences, Winston-Salem, North Carolina

TAKASHI MAKINODAN, PhD, Health Science Officer, Geriatric Research Education and Clinical Center (GRECC), VA Greater Los Angeles Healthcare System, Professor, UCLA School of Medicine, Los Angeles, California

LONA MODY, MD, MSc, Assistant Professor, Division of Geriatric Medicine, University of Michigan Medical School, Geriatrics Research, Education and Clinical Center, Veterans Affairs Ann Arbor Healthcare System, Ann Arbor, Michigan

JOSEPH M. MYLOTTE, MD, Professor of Medicine and Associate Professor of Microbiology, School of Medicine and Biomedical Sciences, State University of New York, Buffalo, New York

CHRISTIE M. REED, MD, MPH, Travelers' Health Team Lead, Division of Global Migration and Quarantine, Departments of Medicine and Microbiology, Centers for Disease Control and Prevention, Atlanta, Georgia

KENNETH SCHMADER, MD, Associate Professor, Center for the Study of Aging and Human Development and Division of Geriatrics, Department of Medicine, Duke University Medical Center; and Geriatric Research, Education and Clinical Center, Durham Veterans Affairs Medical Center, Durham, North Carolina

SARI TAL, MD, MHA, Head, Subacute Department, Harzfeld Geriatric Hospital, Kaplan Medical Center, Gedera, Israel

KOICHI UYEMURA, PhD, Geriatric Research Education and Clinical Center (GRECC), VA Greater Los Angeles Healthcare System, Research Immunologist, UCLA School of Medicine, Los Angeles, California

AIMEE M. WILKIN, MD, MPH, Assistant Professor, Section on Infectious Diseases, Department of Internal Medicine, Wake Forest University Baptist Medical Center Health Sciences, Winston-Salem, North Carolina

JOHN C. WILLIAMSON, PharmD, Adjunct Assistant Professor of Medicine, Clinical Coordinator, Infectious Diseases, Department of Pharmacy, Wake Forest University Baptist Medical Center, Winston-Salem, North Carolina

CONTENTS

Immunosenescence results in populating immune tissues with less functional T cells, and perhaps B cells dendritic cells, that do not function well and produce more type 2 cytokines and fewer type 1 cytokines. Impaired immunity, distinct from immunosenescence, correlates more with disease burden than chronologic age. Older adults who have chronic diseases or chronic infections are more susceptible to common infections and have poor vaccine responses. Understanding specific mechanisms and targeting interventions are dependent on research to resolve the relationship between frailty-associated impaired immunity and the role of chronic infection versus immunosenescence in developing impaired immunity.

The fundamental principles of treating infectious diseases apply to elderly patients, but certain aspects of therapy such as the selection of empiric regimens and risk stratification for severe or atypical disease are influenced by comorbidities, lifestyle, and immunosenescence. Knowledge of age-related changes in pharmacokinetic parameters and potential drug-drug interactions assists the clinician in determining appropriate dosing and monitoring parameters. Based on current evidence, the recommended approach includes careful selection and aggressive dosing of initial broad-spectrum antimicrobials followed by de-escalation to appropriate agents to maximize clinical outcomes and minimize toxicity and adverse effects. Greater enrollment of the elderly in therapeutic studies is needed to detect differences in the efficacy and safety of antimicrobials

one respiratory symptom usually is present and the presence of hypoxemia is a key finding. Treatment recommendations vary depending on the organisms believed the predominant cause of NHAP. Pneumococcal and influenza vaccination remain the most important methods for prevention of NHAP at present.

varicella-zoster virus (VZV) in sensory ganglia in the setting of age, disease, and drug-related decline in cellular immunity. VZV-induced neuronal destruction and inflammation cause the pain, interference with activities of daily living, and reduced quality of life. The optimal treatment of HZ requires early antiviral therapy and pain management. For PHN, evidence-based pharmacotherapy can reduce pain burden. The zoster vaccine is effective in reducing pain burden and preventing HZ and PHN in older adults.

Bacteremia and sepsis are common complications of infection in older patients. Comorbidities, institutionalization, instrumentation, and immunosenescence place older persons at high risk for bacteremia and sepsis, and clinicians must have a heightened suspicion for these infectious disorders in older patients because nonspecific clinical manifestations of infection are common in this vulnerable population. Although increasing age is associated with a high risk of death due to bacteremia and sepsis, recent evidence suggests that many older patients respond well to treatments of proven efficacy. This article discusses the epidemiology, pathophysiology, diagnosis, and prognosis of bacteremia and sepsis in older patients and provides evidence-based recommendations regarding the treatment of these infectious disorders in older persons.

Evaluation of elderly patients who have fever of unknown origin (FUO) requires a different perspective from that needed for young patients. Differential diagnosis often varies with age, and presentation of the disease frequently is nonspecific and symptoms difficult to interpret. Noninfectious diseases are the most frequent cause of FUO in the elderly and temporal arteritis the most frequent specific cause. Tuberculosis is the most common infectious disease associated with FUO in elderly patients. FUO often is associated with treatable conditions in the elderly. Therefore, intensive, accelerated evaluation is necessary, as the lack of physiologic reserve makes this population vulnerable to irreversible changes and functional deterioration.

Older adults disproportionately sustain morbidity and mortality due to vaccine-preventable illnesses. Despite this observation, adult immunization rates continue to lag behind national goals. Reduced vaccine efficacy in older adults leading to apathy regarding the need for vaccine administration, unrealistic expectations for disease prevention rather than reduced illness severity, and system issues that make vaccine administration and tracking difficult all contribute to this problem. In this review, the biologic and system-based causes for vaccine failure in aged adults are reviewed, issues of efficacy and cost-effectiveness in older adults are summarized for influenza and pneumococcal vaccine, and ways to improve vaccine effectiveness in older adults, now and in the future, are outlined.

Older age is an important factor in preparing travelers owing not only to physiologic changes and the increased probability of underlying medical conditions and prescription medications but also to immune status with regard to naturally acquired immunity versus immunization for vaccine-preventable diseases. Cardiovascular events (including myocardial infarctions and cerebrovascular accidents) account for most deaths abroad, followed by injuries. To plan for healthy travel, international travelers should be advised to seek care at least 4 to 6 weeks before departure. Travel medicine is a dynamic field because conditions worldwide are subject to rapid change. Clinicians must maintain a current base of knowledge if they will be regularly advising travelers or must set a threshold for referral to a travel medicine specialist.

FORTHCOMING ISSUES

PREVIOUS ISSUES

ELSEVIER
SAUNDERS

Clin Geriatr Med 23 (2007) xi–xii

CLINICS IN
GERIATRIC
MEDICINE

Preface

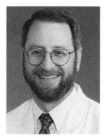

Kevin High, MD, MSc
Guest Editor

We are getting older; not just individually, but as a people. The increase in the percentage of the population in the oldest decades has been well documented in developed nations and is now a worldwide phenomenon. The average life expectancy is now over 80 years in some countries, and by 2020 the average "world" life expectancy is anticipated to be over 72 years. This dramatic increase in average life span is due in large measure to the conquering of infectious causes of death in childhood and early adulthood. Immunizations and sanitation/food safety efforts have undoubtedly contributed more to the increased life expectancy accomplished in the twentieth century than all other medical interventions combined. However, as we enter the twenty-first century, infectious diseases, particularly those related to HIV/AIDS, remain the most common causes of death in many parts of the developing world where life expectancy is under 50 years. No doubt there will be new and emerging challenges to meet in coming decades; pandemic influenza is but one example.

An interesting paradox of increased life expectancy is that we are now faced with a large number of older adults in whom the circle of life is evident. In this group, much like the neonate, infectious disease again becomes a severe, and common, malady. In this issue of the *Clinics in Geriatric Medicine*, authors who have focused much of their careers on the interface of aging and infectious diseases review the unique aspects of infectious diseases in older adults. Older adults experience biologic, social, and systems changes that increase their risk of infection, alter presentation of disease, complicate diagnosis and therapy, and present unique prevention and

doi:10.1016/j.cger.2007.05.002

treatment challenges. Our hope is that this series will increase awareness of the unique aspects of infection in older adults, assist clinicians with the management of these patients today, and serve as a call to action for investigators and the research enterprise to address the pressing needs of the most rapidly growing population in the developed world: adults over age 70.

Kevin High, MD, MSc
Wake Forest University Health Sciences
Internal Medicine/Infectious Diseases
100 Medical Center Blvd.
Winston Salem, NC 27157-1042

E-mail address: khigh@wfubmc.edu

CLINICS IN
GERIATRIC
MEDICINE

Clin Geriatr Med 23 (2007) 463–479

Host Resistance and Immune Responses in Advanced Age

Steven C. Castle, MD[a,*], Koichi Uyemura, PhD[a],
Tamas Fulop, MD[b], Takashi Makinodan, PhD[a]

[a]*Geriatric Research Education and Clinical Center (GRECC) (mail code 11G),
VA Greater Los Angeles Healthcare System, UCLA School of Medicine,
11301 Wilshire Boulevard, Los Angeles, CA 90073, USA*
[b]*Research Center on Aging, Immunology Program, Geriatric Division,
University of Sherbrooke, 2500, boulevard de l'Université Sherbrooke,
Quebec J1K 2R1, Canada*

Extensive studies suggest that although changes in immunity with healthy aging (termed immunosenescence) occur at the most rapid rate of any physiologic system, it is the compounding effects of age-related diseases and external conditions that result in an overall state of a dysfunctional immunity responsible for the increased risk for and severity of common infections in older adults. Hence, immunosenescence is a predisposing condition, but its contribution to infection risk likely is small until immunity is impaired further as a result of accumulating chronic illness, external conditions, or repeated or chronic infections. This is different from the changes related to immunosuppression that result from certain conditions, such as HIV infection, or immunosuppressive medications that result in unusual, opportunistic infections. Unfortunately, the challenge of studying a diverse population with multiple confounders and the focus of gerontologists on studying normal aging have limited research and understanding of why frail, older adults are so susceptible to common infections and outbreaks of infectious syndromes, including influenza, West Nile virus, and severe acute respiratory syndrome (SARS) and experience frequent vaccine nonresponse.

The high risk for infection in those of advanced age and who have multiple comorbidities is underscored by the high rates of health care–acquired infections in older adults residing in long-term care facilities (LTCF). In

U.S. Department of Veterans Affairs, Geriatric Research Education and Clinical Center (GRECC), and Research Service.

* Corresponding author.

E-mail address: steven.castle@med.va.gov (S.C. Castle).

1999, surveillance of LTCF-acquired infections by the National Nosocomial Infections Surveillance system reported an incidence of 3.82 infections per 1000 resident days of care but with significant variability depending on the type of facility, nature of the residents, definitions used for infections, and type of data analysis [1]. The prevalence of infection rates ranged from 1.6% to 32.7%, and overall incidence rates ranged from 1.8 to 13.5 infections per 1000 resident days of care, with equal variability for specific infections, such as urinary tract or pneumonia. Thus, in establishing infection control policies and vaccination protocols, addressing clear abnormalities in immunity in this varied population must be undertaken. Grouping individuals by disease severity or by level of impairment of specific components of immunity may assist in advancing the ability to identify predictors of impaired host resistance to infections and develop strategies to boost immune response in an at-risk population [2].

Conversely, there is much interest in how recurrent or chronic infections may result in progression of age-related "inflammatory" diseases, especially atherosclerosis. There is some evidence that the interaction of pathogenic burden with host genotype (eg, a mutation of Toll-like receptor (TLR) 4, a surface pathogen receptor on immune cells [discussed later]) may determine the character and enhanced and prolonged inflammatory responses known as "inflamm-aging" (discussed later) that may contribute to cardiovascular disease, autoimmunity, poor host resistance, tumor surveillance, and diminished longevity in the aged [3]. Additionally, factors often not considered immune mechanisms may compromise host resistance and increase infection risk, such as swallowing difficulty or inability to take oral medications [4]. In a vulnerable but less frail population, it is less clear why there remains increased risk for infection and poor vaccine response. The interaction of genetic predisposition for diseases, including susceptibility to certain infections, exposure to chronic pathogens, and other environmental/lifestyle factors, all interact to establish an increasingly impaired foundation of host resistance.

The role of chronic or recurrent infection has not been well studied but also is likely to impair immunity significantly. One study looked at the intraindividual variability on immune senescence markers and found that acute illness, both infectious and noninfectious illness, affected neutrophil (CD16) and T-cell (CD8+ CD28−) markers for up to 30 days but did not look at how this might have compromised host resistance further [5].

Overview of immunosenescence

Components of immune response as it relates to host resistance and aging

Innate immunity is the first line of host resistance against common microorganisms, with a cellular component, made up of neutrophils, macrophages, epithelial cells, eosinophils, basophils, natural killer cells, keratinocytes, and dendritic cells (DC), and a soluble component made up primarily of the complement cascade. This review focuses on neutrophils and macrophages that can kill pathogens and tumor cells either directly or through the release of proteins, and antigen-presenting cells (APCs) that are critical in regulating subsequent acquired immunity. All these innate immune cells are capable of responding directly and without prior exposure to pathogens via recognition of microbial products (lipids, DNA/RNA, and protein) that bind to surface receptors, including TLR. Toll, a German slang word for jazzy or cool, is the name of a receptor found in fruit fly that codes for dorsal-ventral patterning but also was found to have a role in host defense against fungal infections and has much homology with human immune cell receptors that are important in communication between innate and acquired immunity [6]. In addition to responding directly to pathogens, innate immune cells also provide a link to activation of acquired immunity. DC are the predominant innate immune cells to activate acquired immunity. In response to a pathogen, DC produce bursts of cytokines and other substances that not only kill the pathogen but also recruit and promote the differentiation of other immune cells, including additional DC. Acquired immunity is distinct from innate immunity because of its antigen specificity and the generation of memory responses. This requires activation of lymphocytes (T or B cells) that have specific cell-surface receptors to foreign antigens generated by random recombination of gene segments in the T-cell receptor. These recombinations of molecules and pairings of different variable chains produce a wide repertoire of lymphocytes with specific unique receptors that can recognize virtually any infectious organism or pathogen. Therefore, the acquired immune system has the unique characteristic of specificity of response to a given antigen, whereas the TLR of APC involves pattern recognition of families of proteins common to many pathogens. Because the specificity of the acquired immune response is generated in immune tissues at a distance from the site of infection, however, such as the thymus and lymph nodes, it is necessary to clonally expand antigen-specific lymphocytes to the novel pathogen to have efficacy at a distant site of infection. Acquired immunity requires 4 to 7 days to generate appropriate numbers of cells to counter the infection whereas innate immunity can act in minutes or even seconds.

Another unique feature of acquired immunity is establishment of memory cells, which enables a rapid response on subsequent rechallenge with the same antigen. Cells of the innate immune system interact to play a pivotal role in the initiation and subsequent direction of acquired immune responses. The specificity and regulation of the acquired immune response is dependent on the interaction of fully matured DC with T cells, cytokines and other signaling molecules, and, of course, T cells with the capacity to respond to such signals. Aging, illness, and chronic conditions clearly alter cytokine production and response, altering the integrity of the immune response, and may not only reduce host resistance but also potentiate inflammatory, age-related diseases, often referred to as "inflamm-aging" [3].

If the interaction of innate and acquired immune cells is ineffective and fails to result in clonal expansion of T cells, the acute immune response is shut off, which could result in impaired host resistance or could be a normal shutting off of the immune response that no longer is needed. Persistent activation of immune cells may result in autoimmune or inflammatory diseases. With aging, it seems the acquired immune cells once "fired" are not removed. This process normally is accomplished by a process called programmed cell death or apoptosis. Aging is associated with ineffective apoptosis of some cells that may populate immune tissues and either prevent fresh cells from being produced or impair activity of those cells (so called suppressor cells). Hence, both premature apoptosis (failing to sufficiently activate an immune response) or inability of immune cells to undergo apoptosis (populate immune tissues with ineffective cells) can result in impaired host resistance [7]. The interface between innate and acquired immunity, that regulation of turning on or off of an immune response occurs, may be particularly vulnerable to the effects of aging and the interaction of age- or comorbidity-related inflammation. It seems this critical interface is where the major age-associated impairment in host resistance occurs and results in increased risk for common infections and poor vaccine responses [7–12].

In summary, studies to date have shown that (1) age-related studies of immunity largely have been limited to the T cells of acquired immunity, with a presumption of essentially intact APC function in healthy older adults; (2) healthy aging changes in immunity, termed immunosenescence, may not have significant clinical relevance in host defense; but (3) rates of common infections and susceptibility to epidemics are increased in chronically ill older adults, and the contribution on immunosenscence in that population may be greater as a result of loss of other redundant host defense mechanisms. Innate immunity is critical to the number of immunocompetent units and the magnitude of the immunologic burst on activation of the adaptive immune system [2].

Cytokines orchestrate the immune response, and specific cytokines are classified as pro- or anti-inflammatory cytokines, depending on their effects on immune function, but the distinction depends on the setting [8,10,11]. Interaction between the different immune constituent cell types of host defense is performed by the strength and balance of cytokine signals. The ultimate signal received and the response and differentiation of effector cells to specific signals likely are affected by aging and chronic illness. In general, activation of acquired immunity that involves cell-mediated immune response is described as a T helper 1 (Th1 or type 1) response and is associated with production of high levels of the cytokines interleukin (IL) 2 and interferon-γ (IFN-γ). In contrast, a T helper 2 (Th2 or type 2) response, which is associated with allergic or parasitic infections but not associated with clearance of most bacterial or viral infections, is associated with production of high levels of IL-10, IL-4, and IL-5 [7]. The relative concentrations of proinflammatory cytokines, defined as those that up-regulate a Th1 response, or anti-inflammatory cytokines that are important in turning off a Th1 response, are influenced by gene activation of effector immune cells and allow further specificity of the eventual outcome of an inflammatory response. These distinctions of pro- and anti-inflammatory are from immunologists' perspective and often are confused with the discussion of inflammatory mediators that increase with aging and age-related diseases, which is particularly true of IL-6, which has pro- and anti-inflammatory characteristics (discussed later). With aging, therefore, it is the interaction of genetic predisposition and environmental exposure that dictates proinflammatory status, cardiovascular disease, autoimmunity, host resistance, tumor surveillance, and longevity versus increased morbidity and mortality resulting from susceptibility to common infections [3].

Changes in innate immunity with healthy aging

Neutrophils first, then macrophages, use chemotaxis, phagocytosis, and killing via secreted proteins to control invading pathogens and to alert other lines of immune defense. This requires cells to follow a gradient of chemokines by receptor binding to cell adhesion molecules and cellular activation primarily through TLRs by pattern recognition of common microbial peptides. With healthy aging, evidence suggests innate immunity remains intact or is up-regulated in very healthy aging. The frequently reported increase in activated monocytes [8] and nonspecific increase of proinflammatory substances, primarily IL-1 and IL-6, produced by the innate immune system and down-regulation of acquired immunity may reflect a compensatory event by either component, but their causality is unclear [2,10,13].

Changes in phagocytic cells with aging

For many years, no age-associated decline in neutrophil function was demonstrated, but this may have been because of the challenge of studying neutrophil functions. Studies have been focused on possible alterations in their ability to seek out and migrate toward pathogens, phagocytize, and kill the invading organisms in older adults. Cytoskeletal and membrane changes have an impact on key neutrophil functions, including adherence and membrane fluidity, and are vulnerable to changes in the microenvironment that occur with aging and especially in age-related diseases [14]. More recent studies also demonstrate a decline in the phagocytic ability of neutrophils in older adults [15]. Other studies report that tumor necrosis factor α (TNF-α), in particular, causes a higher suppression of CD18-mediated, fibronectin-primed, superoxide release in neutrophils from older adults. In addition, neutrophils from healthy older adults are more susceptible to oxidative stress and apoptosis [14]. In looking for a central theme for these age-related changes in neutrophils, impaired signaling elicited by TLR (although number of TLR seems unaltered) and changes in fluidity and the presence of lipid rafts important in forming an immune synapse to facilitate cell-to-cell communication are found in healthy older adults. In advanced age, activation of TLR2, which recognizes primarily gram-positive bacteria, or TLR4, the predominant recognition protein for gram-negative bacteria, results in altered second messenger integrity leading to altered nuclear transcription factor function, such as nuclear factor κB (NF-κB) when compared with younger adults [16]. Altered aspects with aging of second messenger pathways include shifts in activation of p42/p44 mitogen-activated protein kinase (MAPK), resulting in a shift in cytokine patterns (discussed later) [14].

Neutrophils undergo spontaneous programmed cell death (apoptosis) without the support of proinflammatory stimulation in vitro. Neutrophils from older adults cannot be rescued from apoptosis with proinflammatory cytokines, as can be demonstrated with neutrophils from younger adults, as multiple apoptotic pathways are favored in the aged neutrophils [17,18]. This suggests that although older adults may have adequate numbers of neutrophils, they likely have functional impairments and an inability to sustain activity at the site of infection.

Changes in antigen presentation with aging

The transition from innate to acquired immunity requires APCs to take up, process, and present specific antigen to T cells expressed in conjunction with the immmunohistocompatibility complex II (major histocompatibility complex) molecule that recognizes self–T-cell receptor. DC are the most significant APC, but monocytes, macrophages, B cells, and possibly neutrophils all can function in this capacity. Increased numbers of DC generated in vitro from circulating monocytes of very healthy older adults in comparison to younger adults are reported [19]. Processing of the antigen so that it eventually can be presented on the surface of the APC is a complex process, and the proteosomes that are required seem to be altered with aging. There has been study of proteosome activity in the induction of NF-κB in T cells with regard to age that identified impaired degradation of IκB-α, shifting the cytokine response [20]. Protesosome activity also is known to be crucial in antigen processing, and because altered proteosome activity is found in T cells, aging quite likely also could have an impact on antigen processing. In a small study on DC generated in vitro from healthy older adults, processing and presentation of antigen seemed intact, and the DC from healthy older adults actually were capable of restoring the proliferative capacity of T cells from older adults and prevented the development of apoptosis in T cells grown to senescence (no longer able to proliferate) in culture [21,22]. In mixing experiments using superantigen, it has been shown that the antigen-presenting capacity of circulating APCs (including DC) actually is greater in APC from healthy older adults in comparison with younger adult controls and is associated with increased production of IL-12 and IL-10 [23].

Effect of aging and the environment on dendritic cells regulation of the immune response

DC are the most potent APC and have a direct role in the priming of T-cell immune responses. There are distinct DC subsets, more pronounced in murine models, with myeloid (DC1) that supports T-cell Th1 response and lymphoid (DC2) that supports T cells differentiating toward a Th2 response. DC1 from old mice (21–24 months) were 4 times less effective than DC1 from young mice (3–6 months) in stimulating syngenic CD4+ T-cell proliferation, stimulating less tumor regression and less DC-specific intercellular adhesion molecule (ICAM)-grabbing nonintegrin expression (important in differentiation to macrophage) but producing more IL-10, which shuts off a Th1 response [24]. The small studies (discussed previously) on monocyte-derived DC (monocytes from peripheral blood, stimulated with granulocyte-macrophage colony-stimulating factor and IL-4) from healthy older adults have not identified differences in number, phenotype, or functional ability to support T-cell proliferation, and DC from healthy older adults are shown to reinduce proliferation of aged T cells [16,21]. This could represent either an in vitro artifact (only responsive cells are selected in culture conditions) or be related to the study of very healthy older adults.

DC regulate immunity as DC sense pathogens through a variety of pattern recognition receptors, such as TLRs, including by lipopolysaccharide, which stimulates TLR4. Different TLRs differentially induce expression of costimulatory or inhibitory surface receptors and the production of proinflammatory (primarily IL-12 and TNF-α) versus anti-inflammatory (especially IL-10) cytokines [25]. TLR stimulation on DC also results in a direct antimicrobial response, including generation of nitric oxide and vitamin D–dependent antimicrobial peptides, such as cathelicidin [26]. Although there has been little study of potential changes in TLR activation in aging, there is evidence that genetic and environmental factors may alter this signaling between innate and acquired immunity at the level of DC that may alter the host resistance. For example, DC activation by double-stranded DNA, a major constituent of many viruses, to support a Th1 response is enhanced in the presence of keratinocytes and dependent on keratinocyte-derived IFN-α/β and IL-18 [27]. Likewise, stimulation of DC by *Mycobacterium tuberculosis* was associated with up-regulation of vitamin D–receptor and the vitamin D-1-hydroxylase genes that leads to induction of the antimicrobial peptide cathelicidin and killing of intracellular *M tuberculosis*, whereas sera from African American individuals, known to have increased susceptibility to *M tuberculosis*, had low levels of 25-hydroxyvitamin D and less induction of cathelicidin messenger RNA, suggesting a link between TLRs, vitamin D–mediated innate immunity, and host resistance that could have relevance to older adults, especially frail older adults who likely have lower levels of vitamin D [26]. TLRs also seem to play a key role at the subcellular phagosome level that allows DC to discriminate self-antigens from phagocytized apoptotic cells from nonself-antigens from phagocytized microbial cells, and dictate DC maturation, costimulatory molecule expression, and antigen presentation; what effect aging or chronic inflammatory states has on this TLR signaling pathway is unknown [28]. Further, impaired TLR1/2 signaling has been demonstrated in DC isolated from older humans [29].

These data support the hypothesis that genetic predisposition, microenvironment, and aging impair host resistance to infection and response to vaccination by influencing the effect of innate immunity on the development of adaptive immune responses.

Summary of changes in acquired immunity from aging (immuosenescence)

Changes in T-cell function in healthy older adults
The overall impact of normal aging on host immunity is believed to occur primarily along two linked mechanisms. The first is replicative senescence that limits T-cell clonal expansion (resulting from a Hayflick's phenomenon, loss of telomerase activity/telomere length, or a decrease in CD28 costimulatory molecule expression that could be related more to repeated exposure to antigen than age). The second is the developmental changes associated with involution of the thymus that precedes dysfunction of the T-cell component of acquired immunity, resulting in shifts in peripheral T-cell subsets, with expansion of memory T cells with the impaired proliferative capacity (discussed previously) [30]. Studies show a decrease in telomere length with age in T cells and B cells; however, it is demonstrated that there is no significant change in telomerase activity [31]. The loss of CD28 that is seen in age-related shifts in T-cell subpopulations, however, occurs predominately in the CD8 subset, suggesting repeated exposure to antigen characteristic of chronic illness, and these CD8 memory cells with shortened telomeres accumulate as a result of ineffective apoptosis [30]. The age-related decline in T-cell function is preceded by involution of the thymus gland, with dramatic decline in thymic hormone levels. In addition, changes in bone marrow stem cells are described that are distinct from thymic changes. These changes are believed to result in a shift in the phenotype of circulating T cells, with a decrease in the number of naïve T cells and a relative accumulation of memory T cells. As a result of the combination of thymic involution, repeated antigenic exposure, and alteration in susceptibility to apoptosis (increased for CD4+, decreased for CD8+), thymic and lymphoid tissues become populated by anergic (nonresponsive) memory CD8+ CD28− T cells [7]. Likewise, there are significant age-related changes in the CD4+ subset. CD4+ T cells have decreased, but not absent, levels of CD28, which correlate with delay in reaction time to in vitro stimulation and accumulation of suppressive T regulatory cells

that have low CD4+ expression with CD25+ expression [32]. The delay in activation is related to impaired costimulatory pathways and significant postreceptor changes that can be elicited after cell-to-cell interaction of T cells with APC, likely the result of physical changes in the cell membrane lipid rafts and an impaired ability to form efficient immune synapses during cell-to-cell interaction. Surface receptors seem to be organized in structures called lipid rafts, and alteration in cholesterol and sphingolipid composition associated with aging may be associated with impaired polarization of lipid rafts on the T-cell surface, resulting in an impaired ability to interact with APC, with the effect more pronounced on CD4+ T cells [7]. These membrane changes could be a result of changes in the microenviroment, including the hormonal milieu, exposure to free radicals, and other inflammatory mediators (discussed later). As a result of, and in addition to, abnormal surface signaling, there are altered second messenger functions, including autophosphorylation of Lck and activation of ZAP-70 and linker of activated T cells [33–35], resulting in decreased activation of transcription factors, especially NF-κB that is pivotal in regulation of cytokine production, with the most important finding being a decline in IL-2 and impaired proliferation [20,36,37]. These altered second messenger functions may be related to age-related changes in phosphatases' activity related to shifts in the lipid content of the cells that can be mimicked by cholesterol repletion in young T cells [18,38]. So, with aging, there is an accumulation of dysfunctional, clonally expanded, memory T cells that should be removed from immune tissue but also have impaired apoptosis that prevents the efficient removal [14,17,39]. There is a fine balance between anti- and proapoptotic pathways in T cells, including the Bcl-2 family, and caspases that act either as initiators or executioners (beyond the scope of this review) [40,41]. With aging, altered regulation of apoptosis may be tied to decline in CD28; hence, there is more susceptibility of apoptosis in CD4+ and less in CD8+ T cells [30,42–44].

The CD28− T cells usually are anergic—they do not respond despite exposure to the antigen that would be expected to trigger responses in the T cell. Chronic disease and external factors, such as malnutrition, increased propensity for autoimmune disorders, or repeated, chronic infection (eg, lifelong cycles of reactivation or suppression and reactivation of cytomegalovirus [CMV] and other herpes viruses), are associated with a shift in cytokine propensity toward a Th2 anti-inflammatory response, as evidenced by an increase in IL-10 production and expansion of the CD28− cells [7,8,10,21,23]. The presence of CD28− T cells either has direct effects on other parts of immunity or is a marker of impaired immunity. One study of 153 residents of assisted living facilities in Rochester, Minnesota, demonstrated that nearly half of the residents failed to generate an antibody response to any of the trivalent components of influenza vaccine, and this correlated with age and the expansion of CD8+ CD28− T cells [45].

This combination of increase in CD8+ but decrease in CD4+ T cells, with impaired proliferative response, is called the immune risk phenotype

(IRP). IRP is described as an increase in CD8+ CD28−CD57+ cells, with a CD4:CD8 ratio of less than 1, decreased mitogen-stimulated proliferative response of T cells, and CMV seropositivity, suggesting chronic CMV antigenic stimulation is causative to the aging changes [46]. IRP was found to be associated with increased IL-6 and, together with the presence of cognitive impairment, predicted 58% of deaths in adults over age 85 in a 4-year longitudinal study in Sweden and is linked to frailty [46,47]. Measurement of C-reactive protein (CRP) may be useful particularly in identifying chronic infections, because CRP synthesis is dependent on IL-6 [48]. Despite the universal changes in T-cell response with age, the relevance is unclear, as impaired proliferative response to specific antigen or a mitogen, even after adjusting for relative sensitivity to mitogen, failed to correlate with impaired antibody response to influenza immunization [22].

Changes in B cells in healthy older adults

Primary and secondary antibody responses to vaccination are found to be impaired, and whereas much is due to altered T-cell support, age-related changes in B cells seem to have similarities to T-cell changes. B cells from older individuals show impaired activation and proliferation that also could be related to changes in costimulatory molecule expression [10]. In addition, the specificity and affinity of antibodies produced in older adults is lower than in younger populations, and there also is alteration in isotype [10,31,49]. A longitudinal study of young and older adults demonstrated that the proliferative responses to influenza antigen on yearly immunization were lower in older adults, as was the percentage of older adults who had protective antibody titers [22]. In parallel with changes in the T-cell compartment of immune tissue, there seems to be an accumulation of antigen-experienced B cells in the immunologic space that have a shrunken immunoglobulin repertoire that makes less quantity and decreased specificity of antibody to new antigen [50]. These accumulated memory B cells are CD27+ CD19+, a marker associated with differentiation of B cells to immunoglobulin-producing cells, and as in the T-cell compartment, also may have impaired apoptosis [51–53]. At the same time, as a result of alteration in self-antigens due to oxidative damage and glycation, there is an increase in autoantibody production.

The impact of chronic illness on adapative immune function in the aged

Despite nearly 90% involution of the T-cell generating thymus by age 40, true opportunistic infections are not seen among older adult patients, even those who have significant chronic disease. This suggests that there likely is compensation for lost immunologic tissue of the thymus gland. Typical bacterial infections (ie, pneumonia, urinary tract, and skin and soft tissue infections), however, are a common problem in older adults. Other age-related infections include viral infections (ie, reactivation of *Herpes zoster*) and significantly increased morbidity and mortality associated with influenza virus and infections that are related to microbial colonization of *Clostridium difficile* or methicillin-resistant *Staphylococcus aureus* in severely ill individuals treated with antibiotics [31]. In addition, changes in immunity create difficulty in detecting active (primary and reactivation) and inactive tuberculosis. Response to vaccination, which requires intact cell-mediated immunity to drive the humoral response, clearly is diminished in many different older adult populations and in aged laboratory animals. Underlying chronic illness increases the risk for influenza infection dramatically and impairs the response to vaccination. The presence of one or two chronic illnesses (such as emphysema, diabetes, or chronic renal insufficiency) is associated with a 40- to 150-fold increase in the incidence rate for influenza pneumonia [10]. Whether or not chronic illness, medication, or other related external conditions compromise immune competence further is not elucidated definitively but is likely. One study on vaccine response in nursing home residents demonstrated that only 50% of residents had an adequate response (ie, a fourfold increase in antibody titers), but the response to vaccination failed to correlate with nutritional status or dehydroepiandosterone levels [10]. Another study in a nursing home setting reported that although only 36% of 137 vaccinated residents demonstrated a rise in antibody titer, there was no correlation with age, body mass index, or functional status, as measured by the Barthel index [54]. Another study of 154 individuals found that nonresponders to influenza vaccine were characterized by higher levels of anti-CMV IgG, a higher percentage of CD57+ CD28− T cells (exposure to CMV), and increased serum levels of TNF-α and IL-6 [55]. Understanding how age-related inflammatory diseases and altered immunity resulting from chronic infections will be extremely difficult to unravel as it represents a chicken-versus-the-egg story.

Another example of how chronic illness impairs immunity further is that aging and impaired renal function reduce the response to hepatitis B vaccine in renal failure patients. Findings showed that 86% of patients who had creatinine at or below 4 mg/dL had a protective antibody titer after hepatitis B immunization, in comparison to only 37% of individuals who had a serum creatinine above 4 mg/dL. Likewise, age independently was inversely associated with antibody response. Immunization of patients who have chronic renal insufficiency before serum creatinine exceeds 4 mg/dL, therefore, is recommended [56].

It is known that T cell–dependent immune response declines gradually with age. In a review of more than 200 scientific articles that evaluated healthy older adults who were selected by the SENIEUR protocol [57], the magnitude of decline in T-cell–dependent immune response with age is modest (ie, ∼25% decline versus healthy older adults) [23] relative to that of the aging mouse model [8,9]. In contrast, the T-cell–dependent immune response of frail older adults is impaired 2 to 3 times more than that of healthy older adults of ages comparable to those of frail older adults, [23]. Moreover, the greater impairment in immunity in vulnerable older adults is associated with a decline in induction of proinflammatory IL-12 response and increased anti-inflammatory IL-10 [2,23]. These results suggest that changes in the immune tissue microenvironment may play an important role in age-related decline in T-cell–dependent immune response in humans. This is not unexpected, for the aging mouse model had shown previously that the age-related decline in T-cell–dependent immune response is caused by changes occurring in the immune cells (intrinsic changes) and in immune tissue microenvironment (extrinsic changes) [58]. Also consistent with this is a review that analyzed changes in various physiologic functions with age from 469 studies involving more than 54,000 older adults. The comprehensive review included 43 immunologic studies of 372 individuals. They found that the mean annual rate of decline with age in immune functions is greater than the average rate of decline of all other physiologic functions that were assessed. The investigators concluded that the deterioration in immune function in older adults is the result not only of biologic aging but also of the presence of chronic disease [59]. To address this hypothesis directly, a study analyzed the influence of chronic disease burden on T-cell immunity using the Cumulative Illness Rating Scale (CIRS). CIRS is an instrument that measures disease burden in individuals who have various chronic diseases but no evidence of acute deterioration or infection. T-cell immunity was related inversely to disease burden (increasing CIRS), with impaired proliferation to phytohemagglutinin, increased production of immunoinhibitory IL-10, and trends toward decreased immunoenhancing IL-12 but no correlation with chronologic age between 51 and 95 years [2].

Inflammatory mediators and immunity

The finding that impaired immunity is correlated more with comorbidity than age in older adults suggests that changes in the composition of inflammatory mediators that occur in the immune tissue microenvironment of older adults could play an important role in accelerating the gradual age-related decline in type 1 immune response caused by changes in T cells. The fact that excessive production of inflammation actually could be immunosuppressive is counterintuitive, and the effects of this increase in inflammatory mediators as a part of inflamm-aging on the acute immune response largely has not been studied. Part of this seeming contradiction is that many of the large epidemiologic studies measure serum cytokine levels and fail to address what effect IL-6 (perhaps the most recent studied of the inflammatory mediators) in particular has on acute immunity to infection or vaccination.

Many studies have shown an increase in plasma or serum levels of IL-6, IL-8, IL-10, and TNF-α and a decrease in IL-1 [8,10]. An earlier study defined markers of "inflammation" as albumin less than 3.8 g/dL, cholesterol less than 170 mg/dL (bottom decile), IL-6 greater than 3.8 pg/mL (top tertile), and CRP greater than 2.65 mg/L (top tertile). The study found a strong association with mortality in subjects who had three or four markers of inflammation, with the adjusted odds ratios for 3- and 7-year mortality 6.6 and 3.2, respectively, compared with those who had no abnormal markers. Subjects who had one or two markers were at more moderate and statistically insignificant increased risk for 3- and 7-year mortality with adjusted odd ratios of 1.5 and 1.3, respectively [60]. Clearly, these markers are nonspecific and have many causes in addition to inflammation. Longitudinal studies suggest that higher circulating levels of IL-6 and other inflammatory mediators are associated with and are predictive of functional disability and increased mortality in older adults who had no functional impairment at entry into these longitudinal studies [61]. An association also exists between physical activity and lower levels of serum IL-6. Moreover, higher serum IL-6 levels are reported in many chronic diseases, with slight (27% to 72%) increase in relative risk for mortality but significant increase in coronary heart disease, stroke, and congestive heart failure in subjects 70 to 79 years of age who do not have evidence of cardiovascular disease at baseline [60,62].

It remains unclear, however, what increased serum IL-6 levels represent. The association with disease more likely is from a hormonal effect of IL-6, secreted by adipose tissue, and mediated by catabolic changes in somatic muscle, rather than on an immunologic basis. Few studies have been done comparing how circulating levels of IL-6 or other markers of inflammation correlate with traditional measures of cell-mediated immunity. One mouse study using a cecal ligation infection model demonstrated that high inflammation, including plasma IL-6 levels, were associated with high mortality during acute infection, but mortality in the chronic phase of the infection was correlated with immunosuppression and very low IL-6 levels [63]. In one study, only one out of 32 patients who had Alzheimer's disease demonstrated a decline in production of IL-6 and TNF-α associated with severe dementia in comparison to IL-6 and TNF-α levels among patients who had mild to moderate dementia [62]. A recent review describes 14 studies that report increases in IL-6 with aging but IL-6 itself is shown inhibitory to mycobacteriostatic activities in macrophages, suggesting a causative role for the increased susceptibility to tuberculosis in advanced age [62]. Chronic illness likely contributes further to dysregulation of immune response. A study comparing IL-2 and IL-6 levels in young adults, healthy older adults, and "almost-healthy" older adults (individuals who do not meet the SENIEUR protocol because of no history of regular exercise or the use of medications for conditions, such as hypertension or osteoarthritis) reported lower levels of IL-2 and higher levels of IL-6 in the "almost-healthy" older adult population [57,64]. Another study assessed the association between prior CMV infection, proinflammatory status, and effectiveness of the anti-influenza vaccination in 154 individuals during the influenza season and analyzed associations age and/or inclusion by the SENIEUR protocol, with response to the vaccine as determined by antihemagglutinins (HI), TNF-α, IL-1β, IL-6, IL-10, corticotropin/cortisol axis, anti-CMV antibodies, and CD28+CD57− lymphocytes. Nonresponders of younger and older ages (not specified) were characterized by having higher levels of anti-CMV IgG and higher percentages of CD57+ CD28− lymphocytes (known to be associated with CMV carrier status) together with increased concentrations of TNF-α and IL-6 and decreased levels of cortisol. Influenza vaccine induced increases in TNF-α and IL-10 in all nonresponders, whereas cortisol increased only in the young. It was concluded that CMV carrier status was eliciting elevated proinflammatory potential that could contribute to unresponsiveness to influenza vaccine [55].

Preliminary studies of acute infections in humans have suggested an association of increases in inflammatory mediators, especially increases in IL-6 and IL-10, with poor outcome, including severe community-acquired pneumonia and Q fever [65,66]. In addition, association of IL-10 polymorphism is found associated with severity of illness in community-acquired pneumonia [67] and persistent increased levels of IL-10 and soluble TNF receptor I 1 week after development of pneumococcal pneumonia correlated with older age [62]. Clearance of inflammatory mediators in the sputum (IFN-γ, TNF-α, IL-6, and IL-8) is reported an early marker of clearance of pulmonary tuberculosis [68]. Finally, there is evidence that proinflammatory cytokines can be modulated with medication, as IL-6 levels were attenuated in severe pneumonia requiring mechanical ventilation by the addition of glucocorticoids, and IL-6 and CRP were reduced by the addition of aspirin in subjects who had chronic stable angina [69,70].

The relationship between aging, inflammatory mediators, response to infection, and the progression of chronic inflammatory diseases is important but complicated. There likely is a final common pathway interaction of these factors that alters the microenvironment of an acute response to infection that, together with accumulation of anergic/nonresponse T and B cells, results in crossing the threshold of host resistance, resulting in the marked increase in common infections, susceptibility to epidemics, and the poor vaccine response in chronically ill, older adults. Despite these challenges, there are many opportunities to intervene.

References

[1] Stevenson KB. Regional data set of infection rates for long-term care facilities: description of a valuable benchmarking tool. Am J Infect Control 1999;27:20–6.
[2] Castle S, Uemura K, Rafi A, et al. Reduced immunity of elders with chronic illness correlates with cumulative illness rating scale, but not age. J Am Geriatr Soc 2005;53: 1565–9.
[3] Candore G, Aquino A, Balistreri CR, et al. Inflammation, longevity, and cardiovascular diseases: role of polymorphisms of TLR4. Ann N Y Acad Sci 2006;1067:282–7.

[4] Loeb M, McGeer A, McArthur M, et al. Risk factors for pneumonia and other lower respiratory tract infections in elderly residents of long-term care facilities. Arch Intern Med 1999; 159:2058–64.

[5] High KP, Trader M, Pahor M, et al. Intraindividual variability and the effect of acute illness on immune senescence markers. J Am Geriatr Soc 2005;53:1761–6.

[6] Lemaitre B, Nicolas E, Michaut L, et al. The dorsoventral regulatory gene cassette spatzle/Toll/cactus controls the potent antifungal response in Drosophila adults. Cell 1996;86(6): 973–83.

[7] Fulop T, Larbi A, Wikby A, et al. Dysregulation of T cell function in the elderly: Scientific basis and clinical implications. Drugs Aging 2005;22:589–603.

[8] Pawelec G. Immunosenescence: impact in the young as well as the old? Mech Ageing Dev 1999;108:1–7.

[9] Wick G, Grubeck-Loebenstein B. The aging immune system: primary and secondary alterations of immune reactivity in the elderly. Exp Gerontol 1997;32:401–13.

[10] Burns EA, Goodwin JS. Immunodeficiency of aging. Drugs Aging 1997;11:374–97.

[11] Banchereau J, Steinman RM. Dendritic cells and the control of immunity. Nature 1998;392: 245–52.

[12] Sudeghi HM, Schnelle JF, Thoma JK, et al. Phenotypic and functional characteristics of circulating monocytes of elderly persons. Exp Gerontol 1999;34:959–65.

[13] Orme I. Mechanisms underlying the increased susceptibility of aged mice to tuberculosis. Nutr Rev 1995;53(S4):S35–40.

[14] Larbi A, Douziech N, Fortin C, et al. The role of MAPK pathway alterations in GM-CSF-modulated human neutrophil apoptosis with aging. Immun Ageing 2005;2(1):6.

[15] Lord JM, Butcher S, Killampali V, et al. Neutrophil ageing and immunosenescence. Mech Ageing Dev 2001;122:1521–35.

[16] Agrawal A, Agrawal S, Gupta S. Dendritic cells in human aging. Exp Gerontol 2006.

[17] Fulop T, Larbi A, Douziech N, et al. Signal transduction and functional changes in neutrophils with aging. Aging Cell 2004;3:217–26.

[18] Fortin CF, Larbi A, Lesur O, et al. Impairment of SHP-1 down-regulation in the lipid rafts of human neutrophils under GM-CSF stimulation contributes to their age-related, altered functions. J Leukoc Biol 2006;79:1061–72.

[19] Steger MM, Maczek C, Grubeck-Loebenstein B. Morphologically intact dendritic cells can be derived from peripheral blood of aged individuals. Clin Exp Immunol 1996;105: 544–50.

[20] Ponnapan U, Zhong M, Trebilcock GU. Decreased proteosome-mediated degradation in T cells from the elderly: a role in immune senescence. Cell Immunol 1999;192:167–74.

[21] Steger MM, Maczek C, Grubeck-Loebenstein B. Peripheral blood dendritic cells reinduce proliferation in in vitro aged T cell populations. Mech Ageing Dev 1997;93:125–30.

[22] Murasko DM, Bernstein ED, Gardner EM, et al. Role of humoral and cell-mediated immunity in protection from influenza disease after immunization of healthy elderly. Exp Gerontol 2002;37:427–39.

[23] Castle S, Uyemura K, Crawford WW, et al. Age-related impaired proliferation of peripheral blood mononuclear cells is associated with an increase in both IL-10 and IL-12. Exp Gerontol 1999;34:243–52.

[24] Grolleau-Julius A, Garg MR, Mo RR, et al. Effect of aging on bone marrow-derived murine CD11c+CD4-CD8- dendritic cell function. J Gerontol A Biol Sci Med Sci 2006;61(10): 1039–47.

[25] Thoma-Usynski S, Kiertscher SM, Ochoa MT, et al. Activation of toll-like receptor 2 on human dendritic cells triggers induction of IL-12, but not IL-10. J Immunol 2000;165:3804–10.

[26] Liu PT, Stenger S, Li H, et al. Toll-like receptor triggering of a vitamin D-mediated human antimicrobial response. Science 2006;311:1770–3.

[27] Lebre MC, Antons JC, Kalinski P, et al. Double-stranded RNA-exposed human keratinocytes promote Th1 responses by inducing a Type-1 polarizing phenotype in dendritic cells:

roll of keratinocyte-derived tumor necrosis factor alpha, type I interferons, and interleukin-18. J Invest Dermatol 2003;120(6):990–7.

[28] Blander JM, Medzhitov R. Toll-dependent selection of microbial antigens for presentation by dendritic cells. Nature 2006;440:808–12.

[29] van Duin D, Mohanty S, Thomas V, et al. Age-associated defect in human TLR-1/2 function. J Immunol 2007;178:970–5.

[30] Effros RB. Replicative senescence of CD8 T cells: effect of human aging. Exp Gerontol 2004; 39:517–24.

[31] Hodes RJ, Fauci AS, editors. Report of task force on immunology and aging. National Institutes of Aging and Allergy and Infectious Disease. Bethesda (MD): US Department of Health and Human Services; 1996.

[32] Gregg RK, Jain R, Schoenleber SJ, et al. A sudden decline in active membrane-bound TGF-beta impairs T regulatory function and protection against diabetes. J Immunol 2004;173: 7308–16.

[33] Simons K, Ikonen E. Functional rafts in cell membranes. Nature 1997;387:569–72.

[34] Simons K, Ikonen E. How cells handle cholesterol. Science 2000;290:1721–6.

[35] He HT, Lellouch A, Marguet D. Lipid rafts and the initiation of T cell signaling. Semin Immunol 2005;17:23–33.

[36] Schindowski K, Frohlich L, Maurer L, et al. Age-related impairment of human T lymphocytes' activation: specific differences between CD4(+) and CD8(+) subsets. Mech Ageing Dev 2002;123:375–90.

[37] Ponnapan U, Trebilcock GU, Zheng MZ. Studies into the effect of tyrosine phosphatase inhibitor phenylarsine oxide on NfkappaB activation in T lymphocytes during aging: evidence for altered IkappaB-alpha phosphorylation and degradation. Exp Gerontol 1999;34:95–107.

[38] Hermiston ML, Xu Z, Majeti R, et al. Reciprocal regulation of lymphocyte activation by tyrosine kinases and phosphatases. J Clin Invest 2002;109:9–14.

[39] Gupta S. Molecular and biochemical pathways of apoptosis in lymphocytes and aged humans. Vaccine 2000;18:1596–601.

[40] Werner AB, de Vries E, Tait SW, et al. TRAIL receptor and CD95 signal to mitochondria via FADD, caspase-8/10, Bid, and BAX but differentially regulate events downstream from truncated Bid. J Biol Chem 2002;277:40760–70.

[41] Fas SC, Fritzsching B, Suri-Payer E, et al. Death receptor signaling and its function in the immune system. Curr Dir Autoimmun 2006;9:1–17.

[42] Kirchoff S, Muller WW, Li-Webber M, et al. Up-regulation of c-FLIPshort and reduction of activation-induced cell death in CD28-costimulated T cell. Eur J Immunol 2000;30:2765–74.

[43] Gupta S, Kim C, Yel L, et al. A role of fas-associated death domain (FADD) in increased apoptosis in aged humans. Clin Immunol 2004;242:4–9.

[44] Larbi A, Douzeich N, Fortin C, et al. Differential role of lipid rafts in the functions of CD4+ and CD8+ human T lymphocytes with aging. Cell Signal 2006;18:1017–30.

[45] Goronzy JJ, Fulbright JW, Crowson CS, et al. Value of immunological markers in predicting responsiveness to influenza vaccination in elderly individuals. J Virol 2001;75:12182–7.

[46] Wikby A, Ferguson F, Forsey R, et al. An immune risk phenotype, congnitive impairment, and survival in very late life: impact of allostatic load in Swedish octogenarian and nonagenerian humans. J Gerontol A Biol Sci Med Sci 2005;60:556–65.

[47] Ferrucci L, Cavazzini C, Corsi A, et al. Biomarkers of frailty in older persons. J Endocrinol Invest 2002;25:10–5.

[48] Park HS, Park JY, Yu R. Relationship of obesity and visceral adiposity with serum concentrations of CRP, TNF-alpha, and IL-6. Diabetes Res Clin Pract 2005;69:29–35.

[49] Daily RW, Eun SY, Russell CE, et al. B cells of aged mice show decreased expansion in response to antigen, but are normal in effector function. Cell Immunol 2001;214:99–109.

[50] Johnson SA, Cambier JC. Ageing, autoimmunity, and arthritis: senescence of the B cell compartment—implications for humoral immunity. Arthritis Res 2004;6:131–9.

[51] Agematsu K, Hokibara S, Nagumo H, et al. CD27: a memory B-cell marker. Immunol Today 2000;21:204–6.

[52] Gupta S, Su H, Bi R, et al. Life and death of lymphocytes: a role in immunosenescence. Immun Ageing 2005;23:2–12.

[53] Montes CL, Maletto BA, Acosta Rodriquez EV, et al. B cells from aged mice exhibit reduced apoptosis upon B-cell antigen receptor stimulation and differential ability to up-regulate survival signals. Clin Exp Immunol 2006;143:30–40.

[54] Potter JM, O'Donnel B, Carman WF, et al. Serological response to influenza vaccination and nutritional and functional status of patients in geriatric medical long term care. Age Ageing 1999;28:141–5.

[55] Trzonkowski P, Mysliwska J, Szmit E, et al. Association between cytomegalovirus infection, enhanced proinflammatory resonse and low level of anti-hemagglutins during the anti-influenza vaccination: an impact of immunosenescence. Vaccine 2003;21(25–26):3826–36.

[56] Fraser GM, Ochana N, Fenyves D, et al. Increasing serum creatinine and age reduce the response to hepatitis B vaccine in renal failure patients. J Hepatol 1994;21:450–4.

[57] Ligthart GJ, Corberand JX, Fournier C, et al. Admission criteria for immunogerontological studies in man: the SENIEUR Protocol. Mech Ageing Dev 1984;28:47–55.

[58] Price GB, Makinodan T. Immunologic deficiencies in senescence II. Characterization of extrinsic deficiencies. J Immunol 1972;108:41–7.

[59] Sehl ME. Yates FE kinetics of human aging: I. Rates of senescence between ages 30 and 70 years in healthy people. J Gerontol A Biol Sci Med Sci 2001;56:B198–208.

[60] Reuben DB, Cheh AI, Harris TB, et al. Peripheral blood markers of inflammation predict mortality and functional decline in high-functioning community-dwelling older persons. J Am Geriatr Soc 2002;50(4):638–44.

[61] Elousa R, Bartali B, Ordovas JM, et al. Association between physical activity, physical performance and inflammatory biomarkers in an elderly population: the InCHIANTI study. J Gerontol A Biol Sci Med Sci 2005;60:760–7.

[62] Bruunsgaard H, Pedersen BK. Age-related inflammatory cytokines and disease. Immunol Allergy Clin North Am 2003;23:15–39.

[63] Xial H, Siddiqui J, Remick DG. Mechanisms of mortality in early and late sepsis. Infect Immun 2006;74(9):5227–35.

[64] Mysliwska J, Bryl E, Foerster J, et al. The upregulation of TNFa production is not a generalised phenomenon in the elderly between their sixth and seventh decades of life. Mech Ageing Dev 1999;107:1–14.

[65] Fernandez-Serrano S, Dorca J, Coromines M, et al. Molecular inflammatory responses measured in blood of patients with severe community-acquired pneumonia. Clin Diagn Lab Immunol 2003;10:813–20.

[66] Glynn P, Coakley R, Kilgallen I, et al. Circulating interleukin 6 and interleukin 10 in community acquired pneumonia. Thorax 1999;54:51–5.

[67] Gallagher PM, Lowe G, Fitzgerald T, et al. Association of IL-10 polymorphism with severity of illness in community acquired pneumonia. Thorax 2003;58:154–6.

[68] Ribeiro-Rodrigues R, Co TR, Johnson JL, et al. Sputum cytokine levels in patients with pulmonary tuberculosis as early markers of Mycobacterial clearance. Clin Diagn Lab Immunol 2002;9:818–23.

[69] Monton C, Ewig S, Torres A, et al. Role of glucocorticoids on inflammatory response in nonimmunosuppressed patients with pneumonia: a pilot study. Eur Respir J 1999;14(1):218–20.

[70] Ikonomidis I, Andreotti F, Economou E, et al. Increased proinflammatory cytokines in patients with chronic stable angina and their reduction by aspirin. Circulation 1999;100(8):793–8.

ELSEVIER
SAUNDERS

CLINICS IN
GERIATRIC
MEDICINE

Clin Geriatr Med 23 (2007) 481–497

Principles of Antimicrobial Use in Older Adults

Ashley R. Herring, PharmD,
John C. Williamson, PharmD*

*Department of Pharmacy, Wake Forest University Baptist Medical Center,
Medical Center Boulevard, Winston-Salem, NC 27157, USA*

Older adults, generally considered persons over age 65 years, comprise a distinct population that often provides diagnostic and therapeutic challenges to clinicians. Due to the presence of various age-related comorbid conditions and dysfunction of the body's host defense mechanisms, older adults may have a relatively atypical disease presentation and may not respond to antimicrobial therapy in the same manner as their younger counterparts. Differences in pharmacokinetic and pharmacodynamic parameters and the lack of clinical data in the elderly complicate effective dosing strategies. The purpose of this review is to provide guiding principles for antimicrobial use in older adults to optimize patient outcomes. A summary of these principles is provided in Box 1.

Many principles of antimicrobial therapy pertain to all age groups. These principles include the critical nature of early and adequate empiric coverage of pathogens followed by de-escalation based on clinical status and identification of the pathogens. Early antimicrobial therapy (within 8 and 4 hours of admission, respectively) was found to significantly decrease 30-day mortality in two large retrospective studies of Medicare patients aged greater than 65 years with pneumonia [1,2]. Other studies have found reduced mortality rates in patients with ventilator-associated pneumonia and sepsis when appropriate antibiotics were administered earlier in the course of infection [3–6].

Elderly patients with community-acquired pneumonia treated according to national guidelines obtained survival benefit at 3 days and 30 days when compared with patients treated with other regimens [7,8]. Although no

---

* Corresponding author.
E-mail address: johnwill@wfubmc.edu (J.C. Williamson).

0749-0690/07/$ - see front matter © 2007 Elsevier Inc. All rights reserved.
doi:10.1016/j.cger.2007.03.009
geriatric.theclinics.com

Box 1. Guiding principles for appropriate use of antimicrobials in older adults

Risk stratify patients for severe infections and multidrug-resistant pathogens based on lifestyle and functional status.

Provide early and broad empiric therapy using national guidelines and local antibiogram information when available.

Obtain a complete medication history and carefully select antimicrobials to avoid severe drug-drug interactions and drug-disease interactions.

Dosing of antimicrobials should account for age-related changes in pharmacokinetic and pharmacodynamic parameters, but maximal therapeutic dosing should not be sacrificed to avoid potential adverse effects.

De-escalate antimicrobial therapy based on the patient's clinical status and identified pathogen.

Consider participation in studies of antimicrobial agents in elderly populations and report adverse drug events when they occur to augment clinical information.

---

age-stratified data were included, adult patients with hospital-acquired pneumonia treated with guideline-concordant therapy also demonstrated decreased mortality at 14 days and 30 days [9]. The use of national guidelines for determining appropriate antimicrobial therapy must be balanced with the necessity of incorporating regional or hospital-specific antibiogram information. Adequate empiric coverage, defined as a regimen including an antimicrobial active against the causative organism, has been shown to decrease mortality in patients with pneumonia, bacteremia, and severe sepsis [10–13]. The use of institutional clinical pathways for ventilator- and hospital-acquired pneumonia has resulted in increased proportions of patients receiving adequate initial empiric therapy [14,15].

De-escalation, the narrowing of broad empiric agents once a pathogen is identified, and the use of shorter durations of therapy are practices aimed at reducing antibiotic exposure while not adversely impacting clinical outcomes. In a study of ventilator-associated pneumonia, an institutional guideline that required re-evaluation of antibiotic therapy after 2 to 3 days resulted in high rates of adequate empiric coverage, reduced duration of therapy, and decreased overall antibiotic use. No difference in mortality or length of hospital stay was noted in this study [14]. Discontinuing antibiotics when noninfectious etiologies are determined and in patients with a low probability of pulmonary infection is another effective de-escalation strategy [14,16]. Although no age-stratified data on de-escalation have been published to date, elderly groups are expected to obtain similar benefit as the wider adult population.

A critical and fundamental principle that directly impacts the care of older adults is risk stratification for specific infections or pathogens based on lifestyle and functional status. For example, older adults who reside in long-term care facilities are known to be at higher risk for multidrug resistant pathogens. Greater exposure to the health care system, cumulative exposure to a number of antimicrobials, and a decreased ability to perform activities of daily life, including regular personal hygiene, may contribute to colonization with a variety of resistant organisms. Recent guidelines for the treatment of pneumonia have reinforced this tenet, recommending broader empiric coverage and consideration of atypical and multidrug resistant pathogens in patients who reside in long-term care facilities [17,18].

In contrast to these common principles which may be applied to members of all age groups, several nuances in the interactions between age, disease, and environment should be considered for optimal care of the older adult. These nuances include an assessment of infectious etiology and the potential for severe or atypical disease, changes in pharmacokinetic and pharmacodynamic parameters, the risk of adverse drug events and drug interactions, and the availability of therapeutic studies in this population.

Risk of infection and disease severity

The clinical presentation of infections can be different in the elderly. Signs and symptoms may be more subtle, atypical, or absent [19]. Despite this appearance, elderly individuals may be at higher risk for severe infection and poorer outcomes. Fever is a nonspecific sign of inflammation that is diminished in older adults. One group found a linear inverse relationship between the decade of life and maximal body temperature during the first 2 days of hospitalization for moderate-to-severe pneumonia, suggesting a decrease of 0.15°C in body temperature for each decade of life. This difference persisted at hospital discharge, which was considered a surrogate for basal body temperature [20]. The maximal sensitivity and positive predictive value for infection is achieved when body temperature is greater than 99°F (orally) or 100°F (rectally), and a decline in functional status is present in elderly patients and long-term care facility residents [21,22]. The presence of fever, leukocytosis, or bandemia may be used as a screening tool, because only 6% of infected patients aged 70 to 99 years presenting to a community emergency department fail to demonstrate any of these signs [23]. Early antibiotic therapy may be beneficial in cases in which infection cannot be excluded, because a delay in therapy may adversely affect clinical outcomes.

When older adults are infected, they are at risk for more severe disease or greater morbidity and mortality due to the same disease. Recent accounts of a clonal outbreak of a binary toxin-producing strain of *Clostridium difficile* in Canada described a dramatically greater incidence and attributable mortality with increasing age [24]. When the incidence and severity of *C difficile*–associated diarrhea were compared between the years 1991 and 2003, the incidence among adults aged more than 65 years increased approximately tenfold. In addition, 19.1% of these patients sustained complicated infection [25].

The elderly suffer greater morbidity and mortality from other ailments such as influenza and pneumonia. The rate of hospitalization due to influenza rises incrementally with each additional 5 years of age over 65 years. The duration of hospital stay also increases with increasing age over 65 years [26]. Underlying respiratory and cardiac conditions likely contribute to the need for hospitalization and prolonged inpatient stays in this population. Approximately 90% of influenza-related mortality occurs in persons older than 65 years. The old-old ($\geq$ 85 years) with influenza carry a 16-fold higher risk of death from any cause when compared with infected persons aged 65 to 69 years [27]. The National Vital Statistics Reports has cited influenza or pneumonia as the leading infectious cause of mortality in persons aged more than 75 years [28]. Due to the high burden of morbidity and mortality among this group, clinicians should not be discouraged from using aggressive antibiotic dosing regimens. Persons older than 65 years should receive influenza and pneumococcal vaccinations according to Centers for Disease Control schedules to prevent these illnesses (see the article by High elsewhere in this issue).

It is possible that a disproportionate risk for multidrug-resistant pathogens affects appropriate care and survival of the elderly. A review of bacterial isolates obtained from patients treated at 32 hematology and oncology centers in the United States and Canada revealed age-related trends in pathogen occurrence and susceptibility. Rates of methicillin-resistant *Staphylococcus aureus* and vancomycin-resistant enterococci increased with age, as did fluoroquinolone resistance among isolates of *S aureus*, coagulase-negative *Staphylococcus*, enterococci, and viridans group streptococci. *Klebsiella* species with extended-spectrum beta-lactamase phenotyes were found to be highest among patients older than 65 years and younger than 14 years [29]. Greater exposure to the health care system and cumulative antibiotic exposure may explain these trends in resistance, although studies of other age-stratified patient groups are necessary to verify these findings.

Several factors may account for the disparate outcomes observed in older populations. Immunosenescence decreases the individual's ability to respond to infections, comorbidities such as diabetes or vascular insufficiency derange host defense mechanisms, and there is decreased recognition by clinicians of blunted clinical presentations of infectious diseases. Less aggressive dosing of antimicrobials due to the fear of adverse drug events or the misunderstanding of certain pharmacokinetic and pharmacodynamic parameters specific to the elderly population may also contribute to poor outcomes. Although for many chronic disease states less aggressive dosing is preferred when initiating therapy in the elderly patient, treatment of acute infectious processes requires providers to consider the need to rapidly achieve therapeutic targets to optimize outcomes. Clinicians often prescribe reduced doses of antimicrobials due to age-related renal dysfunction; however, the first dose or loading dose should not be adjusted. By maintaining the "usual" first dose, therapeutic concentrations will be achieved rapidly to ensure optimal clinical response, especially in the setting of serious infections.

The need for a different dosing strategy: pharmacokinetic and pharmacodynamic differences in the elderly

Several age-related physiologic changes may impact the pharmacokinetics and pharmacodynamics of medications. Table 1 lists these physiologic changes and potential clinical implications. Increased pH of the stomach due to atrophy of the acid-producing parietal cells has long been implicated in decreased absorption of certain medications dependent on acidic conditions for solubility, such as ketoconazole, itraconazole, cefuroxime,

Table 1
Age-related changes in pharmacokinetic parameters and potential effects on antimicrobial dosing

	Physiologic change	Potential clinical implication
Absorption	Increase in gastric pH	Decreased absorption of pH-dependent drugs; increased absorption of acid-labile drugs
	Decreased absorptive surface	Decreased absorption
	Decreased splanchnic blood flow	Decreased absorption
	Decreased gastrointestinal motility	Decreased or delayed absorption
Distribution	Increased body fat composition	Increased half-life of lipophilic drugs
	Decreased total body water	Increased concentrations of hydrophilic drugs
	Decreased serum albumin	Increased free concentrations of acidic drugs
Metabolism	Decreased hepatic blood flow	Decreased first-pass metabolism
	Decreased phase I (CYP450) activity	Increased half-life of drugs undergoing phase I metabolism
Elimination	Decreased renal blood flow and glomerular filtration rate	Increased half-life of renally eliminated drugs

dapsone, atazanavir, tipranavir, and delavirdine. Acid-labile drugs that would be expected to exhibit increased absorption in this environment are penicillins, erythromycin, and clarithromycin; however, recent studies of gastric function have demonstrated similar rates of achlorhydria in older adults and younger populations, which means the observed reduction in absorption may be attributable to underlying pathology and concomitant medications (such as proton-pump inhibitors) rather than the process of aging [30,31]. Regardless, care should be taken during the medication history to elicit the use of acid-suppressing therapies (prescription and non-prescription) when antibiotics affected by gastric pH are concurrently prescribed.

Delayed gastric emptying time that limits the rate of absorption and thus peak concentrations has been described as another age-related phenomenon. A study of oral and intravenous ciprofloxacin in patients with diabetic gastroparesis found a decrease in area under the curve ratios in this group in comparison with ratios previously reported in healthy populations [32]. Other factors associated with age, such as decreased surface area of intestinal mucosa and reduced blood flow to the small intestine, may impact the rate and extent of absorption. It remains unclear how often these changes reach clinical significance [33].

Changes in body composition impact the distribution and half-life of several compounds. With age, lean muscle mass is lost and body fat increases. Men may double their body fat from 18% to 36% on average, whereas in women body fat may rise from 33% to 45% [34]. In addition, total body water from intracellular and extracellular spaces decreases 10% to 15% from the third to the ninth decade of life [35]; therefore, the volume of distribution and half-life of lipophilic drugs are substantially increased in the elderly, whereas those parameters decrease for water-soluble medications including aminoglycosides, vancomycin, beta-lactams, and daptomycin. Decreased or altered concentrations of serum-binding proteins such as albumin or alpha$_1$-acid glycoprotein can impact the distribution of highly protein-bound drugs, but these changes are rarely clinically relevant because increased unbound concentrations result in increased drug clearance.

The most significant change in pharmacokinetics in the elderly is due to renal insufficiency. The glomerular filtration rate (GFR), tubular secretion, and renal blood flow decrease with age. The GFR, as measured by excreted creatinine and inulin, exhibits an almost linear decline from the age of 20 to 80 years, whereas serum creatinine increases little until very advanced age [35] owing to reduced creatinine production corresponding to the loss of muscle mass in aging. The Cockcroft-Gault (CG) formula, the most commonly used method of estimating renal function, adjusts for serum creatinine, age, gender, and lean body weight [36]. The more recently developed Modification of Diet in Renal Disease (MDRD) equation estimates GFR based on age, gender, race (black or non-black), serum creatinine, serum albumin, and blood urea nitrogen. Neither an abbreviated version of the

MDRD equation, which eliminates serum albumin and blood urea nitrogen, nor the CG formula has shown good correlation with actual renal clearance in elderly populations (Box 2).

One prospective study of 380 subjects aged 18 to 88 years compared estimates with directly measured inulin clearance and found that both the CG and abbreviated MDRD formulas underestimated GFR in older patients [37]. The abbreviated MDRD estimate was more accurate in patients with low GFRs; therefore, it showed better correlation with measured GFR in the older subjects. Another study determined that the CG formula overestimates renal function in elderly patients who are deconditioned or malnourished with abnormally low serum creatinine [38]. Accordingly, one must not only consider the accuracy of a renal function estimate with respect to age but also with respect to nutritional and functional status. In elderly patients with low serum creatinine (less than 1.0 mg/dL), a common practice is to replace the serum creatinine with a value of 1.0 mg/dL to prevent overestimation of renal function in either equation. Nevertheless, the only study to evaluate this practice has found that it still overestimates creatinine clearance [39].

Liver metabolism is not significantly altered with age. Interindividual variation in activity of cytochrome P-450s and other phase I metabolizing enzymes is likely greater than any age-related change [40]; however, as cardiac output decreases due to age and comorbidities such as heart failure

---

Box 2. Formulas used to estimate glomerular filtration rate [36–38]

Cockcroft and Gault
Creatine Clearance (mL/min) = $[(140 - \text{age}) \times \text{IBW(kg)}]/ (S_{Cr} \times 72) \times 0.85$ for females

Modification of Diet in Renal Disease
GFR (mL/min) = $170 \times S_{Cr}^{-0.999} \times \text{Age}^{-0.176} \times \text{BUN}^{-0.170} \times \text{Albumin}^{0.318} \times 0.762$ (if female) $\times 1.180$ (if black)

Abbreviated Modification of Diet in Renal Disease
GFR (mL/min) = $170 \times S_{Cr}^{-0.999} \times \text{Age}^{-0.176} \times 0.762$ (if female) $\times 1.180$ (if black)

Ideal Body Weight
IBW for Males = $50 + (2.3 \times \text{inches} > 60)$
IBW for Females = $45.5 + (2.3 \times \text{inches} > 60)$

Abbreviations: BUN, blood urea nitrogen; IBW, ideal body weight; S_{Cr}, serum creatinine.

and chronic obstructive pulmonary disease, the blood flow to the liver is reduced, thereby extending the half-life of hepatically cleared drugs.

There is limited information regarding age-related pharmacodynamic changes that impact antimicrobial therapy; however, a study of levofloxacin in patients with hospital-acquired pneumonia determined that age and the area under the curve (AUC) to minimum inhibitory concentration (MIC) ratio are significant factors in the eradication of known bacterial pathogens. No patient greater than age 67 years who failed to achieve the target AUC to MIC ratio of 87 experienced pathogen eradication, indicating that, in this population, special pharmacodynamic considerations may be necessary to achieve an optimal clinical response [41].

Risk for adverse drug events

Older adults are typically more sensitive to the adverse effects associated with drug therapies. One study of emergency department visits revealed that one third of patients suffering an adverse drug event were elderly; 24.4% of this elderly cohort required hospitalization. In that study, anti-infectives were the most common drug class associated with an adverse event [42]. A 10-year surveillance of hospital adverse event reporting found antibiotics to be the second most frequent class of medications associated with adverse events, causing 20.1% of all events and 16.9% of severe events [43]. Generally, the frequency of adverse drug events increases with age; however, age has not been identified as a consistent independent risk factor [43,44]. It is possible that age-related factors such as comorbidity and polypharmacy confound or even overshadow the age-specific risk of adverse effects.

A large percentage of preventable adverse events may be due to inappropriate dosing based on an inaccurate assessment of renal function. The rate of adverse events associated with inappropriate dosing was 15% in one study conducted in France [45]. Making a distinction between adverse events due to inappropriate renal dosing and those due to aging itself is problematic in the case of aminoglycoside-related nephrotoxicity and ototoxicity. Older adults are at greater risk for developing renal, auditory, and vestibular toxicity with longer durations of therapy, elevated baseline serum creatinine, and concomitant use of nephrotoxic and ototoxic medications [46,47]. Nephrotoxicity occurs more commonly than ototoxicity, but when either of these events occurs, quality of life of the older adult can be severely reduced. For this reason, careful monitoring of serum markers of renal function is warranted. Similarly, authorities recommend baseline and serial (eg, weekly) audiometry during aminoglycoside therapy. This follow-up may be especially important during prolonged courses, such as treatment of enterococcal endocarditis [48]. Unfortunately, no routine tests can be performed to detect or monitor vestibular toxicity; therefore, patients should be counseled about the signs and symptoms and encouraged to report them immediately after onset.

The fluoroquinolones are generally perceived to be safe antibacterial agents and are prescribed frequently in the elderly, usually for urinary tract infection or pneumonia. Nevertheless, rare cardiac toxicity can occur. Prolongation of the QT interval by fluoroquinolones increases the risk for torsades de pointes, a life-threatening arrhythmia. The QT interval generally increases with age, potentially putting elderly groups at greater risk, but studies have found other genetic determinants of susceptible populations [49]. For renally eliminated fluoroquinolones, dose adjustment may be required to prevent excessive concentrations that may lead to exhaustion of corrective mechanisms in heart muscle. Fluoroquinolones should also be avoided in patients with an underlying cardiac arrhythmia, prolonged QT interval, depletion of magnesium or potassium, and those taking class IA or III antiarrhythmics.

Hepatotoxicity has been reported with increased frequency with isoniazid and other antitubercular agents in elderly patients. One study of patients treated for latent tuberculosis found that patients aged more than 50 years suffered a toxic event five times as often as persons between the ages of 24 and 34 years (event rate of 20.83 per 1000 patients) [50]. Advanced age, chronic liver disease, alcoholism, abuse of illicit drugs, and malnutrition increase the probability of experiencing a significant elevation in transaminases (more than three times the upper limits of normal) during treatment with isoniazid, rifampin, and pyrazinamide [51]. Adherence to Centers of Disease Control guidelines on drug selection, dosing, and monitoring is essential to ensure safe use of these medications.

Hepatotoxicity has also been linked to use of amoxicillin-clavulanate in the elderly. A recent review of all patients with idiopathic liver injury registered between 1995 and 2005 by the Spanish National Health System produced a cohort of 69 "definite" or "probable" cases attributed to amoxicillin-clavulanate. Persons greater than 55 years of age were more likely to exhibit cholestatic or mixed type liver injury and to develop liver damage later in the course of therapy than their younger counterparts [52]. Several series have found an increased incidence of amoxicillin-clavulanate hepatotoxicity with age [52–54]. The highest numbers of reported cases have been among patients between 61 and 80 years of age [54]. Careful stratification based on other underlying risk factors for liver disease may be beneficial in reducing this adverse effect. Periodic liver function tests may also be warranted when prolonged courses of amoxicillin-clavulanate are prescribed.

Potential drug-drug or drug-disease interactions

Polypharmacy is prevalent in older adults, with 23% of non-institutionalized women and 19% of non-institutionalized men greater than 65 years of age using more than five prescription medications [55]. Among these chronic prescription medications are some with narrow therapeutic indices, such as warfarin and digoxin. When warfarin is combined with metronidazole, trimethoprim/sulfamethoxazole, or voriconazole, the international normalized ratio (INR) may be increased several-fold, leading to a higher risk of major and minor bleeds. Many other antibiotics have the potential to increase the INR to a lesser extent via interaction with metabolic pathways (eg, azole antifungals, ciprofloxacin, and erythromycin) or through suppression of vitamin K production by gut bacterial flora (eg, beta-lactams, fluoroquinolones, and clindamycin). Use of rifampin, nafcillin, or griseofulvin with warfarin may lead to enhanced metabolism and a decreased INR, posing a risk for thromboembolism. More frequent monitoring of the INR during antibiotic therapy is recommended.

Digoxin concentrations may be increased by concomitant administration of erythromycin, clarithromycin, and tetracyclines. More dramatic increases in digoxin concentrations leading to digitalis toxicity have been observed when used with itraconazole, which inhibits elimination of digoxin. Close monitoring of digoxin serum concentrations and a query of patient symptoms consistent with digoxin toxicity are recommended when itraconazole must be co-administered. Well-known interactions of antimicrobials with other cardiac medications include voriconazole- or erythromycin-associated increases in verapamil or diltiazem concentrations; therefore, concomitant use of these agents is not recommended. Interactions between antimicrobials and these calcium channel blockers are driven primarily by inhibition of cytochrome P-450 (CYP450) enzymes.

In addition to cardiac medications, antimicrobials interact with many "statins," such as simvastatin and lovastatin, prescribed for hyperlipidemia. Serum concentrations of these statins are dramatically increased during co-administration with potent inhibitors of the CYP450 3A4 enzyme, such as macrolides (erythromycin and clarithromycin), azole antifungals (itraconazole, voriconazole, ketoconazole, and fluconazole), and telithromycin. When these agents are combined, the risk of rhabdomyolysis from the statin is increased. Product labeling for telithromycin recommends suspending use of simvastatin, lovastatin, or atorvastatin during the course of antibiotic therapy [56]. Through a similar mechanism, voriconazole, itraconazole, and fluconazole inhibit the metabolism of glipizide and other sulfonylureas via CYP450 2C8/9, which may lead to hypoglycemic events. Information regarding additional drug-drug interactions may be found in Table 2.

The elderly are more likely to have other noninfectious chronic diseases or multiple comorbidities. As such, drug-disease interactions pose challenges for the clinician, as demonstrated by recent reports of hypo- and hyperglycemia with the use of gatifloxacin. Age-related renal dysfunction or borderline diabetes likely contributes to the risk of glucose dysregulation. In another example, high-dose beta-lactam antibiotics have the potential to lower the seizure threshold in patients with a history of seizure disorder.

Lastly, clinicians should consider the potential additive effects of linezolid in patients with uncontrolled hypertension.

Assessment of potential drug-drug and drug-disease interactions is an essential step in selecting appropriate antimicrobial agents for the elderly patient. Better recognition of these interactions by clinicians is necessary to maximize benefit and reduce adverse events associated with therapy.

Efficacy of therapy in the elderly

Few pre-marketing clinical studies have included sufficient numbers of the elderly to determine optimal dosing and any potential differences in therapeutic efficacy when compared with younger patients. Pre-marketing study populations are skewed toward younger and healthier individuals. Many investigators exclude subjects with multiple comorbidities, concomitant medications, or those in the very aged group (greater than 80 years); however, as the population becomes increasingly old and ill, it is important to tease out the differences in safety and efficacy before widespread use.

Two post-marketing studies of fluoroquinolones have included elderly patients. One was a retrospective review of age-stratified safety data of phase II/III moxifloxacin studies. The second study reviewed data on gatifloxacin for community-acquired respiratory tract infections. Interestingly, of the 12,231 patients enrolled in the analyzed moxifloxacin studies, only 13.4% were 65 to 74 years old, and 7.6% were aged greater than 75 years [57]. Since its release, moxifloxacin has been used extensively in elderly groups; therefore, it is important that this safety analysis did not find any significant age-related differences in the rate of adverse events and study terminations. In contrast, the study of gatifloxacin found significantly higher reports of hyperglycemia among non-diabetic patients aged 65 to 79 and ≥ 80 years [58].

Pneumonia in the Japanese elderly has been examined in two studies. One comparison of ampicillin/sulbactam versus imipenem/cilastatin for the treatment of moderate-to-severe community-acquired pneumonia found these therapies to be equivalent in clinical and bacteriologic efficacy in patients older than 65 years [59]. Clindamycin monotherapy was found to be efficacious in mild-to-moderate aspiration pneumonia in adults aged 71 to 94 years [60]. These studies have been prompted, in part, by concerns over the increasingly aging Japanese population, not unlike that of the United States. Although the US Food and Drug Administration has recognized the need for more drug studies in pediatric groups, there seems to be an increasing need for similar studies in geriatric subjects.

Low enrollment of the elderly in clinical studies is not due solely to investigator bias; most clinicians instinctively protect their most fragile patients from the potential hazards of new drugs. Also, those involved in recruitment may have limited access to subjects with advanced age, who are more likely to be institutionalized or reside in assisted-living facilities.

Table 2
Selected drug-drug interactions of antimicrobial agents with medications commonly used in elderly populations

Chronic medication/class		Interacting antimicrobial	Potential effect
Acid suppressant	PPIs, H$_2$ antagonists, antacids	Rifampin Tetracyclines Ketoconazole Itraconazole Cefuroxime Dapsone	Decreased absorption of antimicrobial
Anticoagulant	Warfarin	Metronidazole Trimethoprim/ sulfamethoxazole Ciprofloxacin Erythromycin Azole antifungals: fluconazole, ketoconazole, itraconazole, voriconazole	Increase in INR, potential bleed
		Rifampin Nafcillin Griseofulvin	Decrease in INR, potential clot
Cardiac medications	Antiarrhythmics	Erythromycin, clarithromycin Fluoroquinolones Foscarnet Telithromycin Trimethoprim/ sulfamethoxazole Voriconazole	Additive QT prolongation
	Digoxin	Erythromycin, clarithromycin Tetracyclines Itraconazole Telithromycin	Increased digoxin concentration, potential toxicity
		Amphotericin B	Digoxin toxicity if potassium depleted
	Verapamil or diltiazem	Erythromycin, clarithromycin Itraconazole, voriconazole Telithromycin	Increased calcium channel blocker concentration
		Rifampin, quinupristin/ dalfopristin	Decreased calcium blocker concentration
Endocrine agents	Sulfonylureas	Trimethoprim/ sulfamethoxazole Azole antifungals: fluconazole, ketoconazole, itraconazole, voriconazole	Increased sulfonylurea concentration, potential hypoglycemia

(*continued on next page*)

Table 2 (*continued*)

Chronic medication/class		Interacting antimicrobial	Potential effect
	Allopurinol	Ampicillin Amoxicillin	Additive risk of rash
	Colchicine	Clarithromycin	Increased level of colchicine
Lipid agents	Simvastatin or lovastatin	Erythromycin, clarithromycin Telithromycin Azole antifungals: fluconazole, ketoconazole, itraconazole, voriconazole	Increased statin concentration, potential rhabdomyolysis
	All statins	Daptomycin	Additive risk of rhabdomyolysis
Neurologic/ psychiatric medications	Phenytoin	Acyclovir Ciprofloxacin Rifampin	Decreased level phenytoin, potential seizure
		Fluconazole Metronidazole Trimethoprim/ sulfamethoxazole	Increased level of phenytoin, potential toxicity
		Caspofungin Doxycycline Itraconazole, ketoconazole Metronidazole	Decreased level of antimicrobial
	Carbamazepine	Voriconazole	Decreased level of voriconazole
		Itraconazole Caspofungin Doxycycline	Decreased level of antimicrobial
		Erythromycin Rifampin Fluconazole Ketoconazole Isoniazid Metronidazole	Increased level of carbamazepine
	SSRIs, TCAs, MAOIs	Linezolid	Increased risk of serotonin syndrome
Vitamins, minerals, and medications containing cations	Calcium, iron, magnesium supplements, sucralfate	Fluoroquinolones Tetracyclines	Decreased absorption of antimicrobial

Abbreviations: INR, international normalized ratio; MAOIs; monoamine oxidase inhibitors; PPIs, proton pump inhibitors; SSRIs, selective serotonin reuptake inhibitors; TCAs, tricyclic antidepressants.

While antimicrobial therapy focuses on pharmacokinetic and pharmacodynamic targets, inclusion of more elderly subjects could elucidate other factors that impact clinical resolution of illness. Elderly patients enrolled in long-term follow-up of 3- versus 8-day amoxicillin therapy for uncomplicated mild-to-moderate community-acquired pneumonia recovered as well as other study subsets based on pre-pneumonia scores from quality-of-life and symptom questionnaires [61]. Indeed, the optimal duration of therapy for many infectious diseases is uncertain. Studies might be especially helpful for illnesses from which elderly patients demonstrate delayed clinical resolution, such as community- and hospital-acquired pneumonia and *C difficile*–associated diarrhea.

Summary

Optimal use of antibiotics in elderly patients requires special considerations from health care providers. Many fundamental principles of treating infectious diseases apply. Patients benefit from early and adequate empiric therapy followed by de-escalation and shorter courses of therapy when appropriate. Empiric regimens should be selected based on consideration of patient-specific factors such as comorbidities and the living environment that may increase the likelihood of particular pathogens. Unlike other groups, the probability that the elderly patient will suffer severe or atypical disease is increased. Although the risk for and consequence of adverse effects and drug interactions have traditionally led to less aggressive use of medications, the best strategy appears to be careful drug selection followed by aggressive dosing to rapidly achieve pharmacokinetic and pharmacodynamic targets. Knowledge of the age-related changes in pharmacokinetic and pharmacodynamic parameters will aid the clinician in determining appropriate dosing and monitoring parameters. Greater enrollment of the elderly in therapeutic studies, especially of subjects greater than 70 to 80 years of age and with comorbid illnesses, will augment our ability to treat infections effectively and maximize clinical outcomes.

References

[1] Meehan TP, Fine MJ, Krumholz HM, et al. Quality of care, process, and outcomes in elderly patients with pneumonia. JAMA 1997;278:2080–4.
[2] Houck PM, Bratzler DW, Nsa W, et al. Timing of antibiotic administration and outcomes for Medicare patients hospitalized with community-acquired pneumonia. Arch Intern Med 2004;164:637–44.
[3] Luna CM, Aruj P, Niederman NS, et al. Appropriateness and delay to initiate therapy in ventilator-associated pneumonia. Eur Respir J 2006;27:158–64.
[4] Iregui M, Ward S, Sherman G, et al. Clinical importance of delays in the initiation of appropriate antibiotic treatment for ventilator-associated pneumonia. Chest 2002;122:262–8.
[5] Valles J, Rello J, Ochagavia A, et al. Community-acquired bloodstream infection in critically ill adult patients: impact of shock and inappropriate antibiotic therapy on survival. Chest 2003;123:1615–24.

[6] Kang CI, Kim SH, Park WG, et al. Bloodstream infections caused by antibiotic-resistant gram-negative bacilli: risk factors for mortality and impact of inappropriate initial antimicrobial therapy on outcome. Antimicrob Agents Chemother 2005;49:760–6.

[7] Frei CR, Restrepo MI, Mortensen EM, et al. Impact of guideline-concordant empiric antibiotic therapy in community-acquired pneumonia. Am J Med 2006;119:865–71.

[8] Mortensen EM, Restrepo M, Anzueto A, et al. Effects of guideline-concordant antimicrobial therapy on mortality among patients with community-acquired pneumonia. Am J Med 2004;117:726–31.

[9] Soo Hoo GW, Wen YE, Nguyen TV, et al. Impact of clinical guidelines in the management of severe hospital-acquired pneumonia. Chest 2005;128:2778–87.

[10] Fraser A, Paul M, Almanasreh N, et al. Benefit of appropriate empirical antibiotic treatment: thirty-day mortality and duration of hospital stay. Am J Med 2006;119:970–6.

[11] Ibrahim EH, Sherman G, Ward S, et al. The influence of inadequate antimicrobial treatment of bloodstream infections on patient outcomes in the ICU setting. Chest 2000;118:146–55.

[12] Schramm GE, Johnson JA, Doherty JA, et al. Methicillin-resistant *Staphylococcus aureus* sterile-site infection: the importance of appropriate initial antimicrobial treatment. Crit Care Med 2006;34:2069–74.

[13] MacArthur RD, Miller M, Albertson T, et al. Adequacy of early empiric antibiotic treatment and survival in severe sepsis: experience from the MONARCS Trial. Clin Infect Dis 2004;38: 284–8.

[14] Ibrahim EH, Ward S, Sherman G, et al. Experience with a clinical guideline for the treatment of ventilator-associated pneumonia. Crit Care Med 2001;21:1109–15.

[15] Beardsley JR, Williamson JC, Johnson JW, et al. Using local microbiologic data to develop institution-specific guidelines for the treatment of hospital-acquired pneumonia. Chest 2006; 130:787–93.

[16] Singh N, Rogers P, Atwood CW, et al. Short-course empiric antibiotic therapy for patients with pulmonary infiltrates in the intensive care unit. Am J Respir Crit Care Med 2000;162: 505–11.

[17] ATS Board of Directors and IDSA Guideline Committee. Guidelines for the management of adults with hospital-acquired, ventilator-associated and healthcare-associated pneumonia. Am J Respir Crit Care Med 2005;171:388–416.

[18] Mandell LA, Bartlett JG, Dowell SF, et al. Update of practice guidelines for the management of community-acquired pneumonia in immunocompetent adults. Clin Infect Dis 2003; 37(11):1405–33.

[19] Bentley DW, Bradley S, High K, et al. Practice guideline for evaluation of fever and infection in long-term care facilities. Clin Infect Dis 2000;31:640–53.

[20] Roghmann MC, Warner J, Mackowiak PA. The relationship between age and fever magnitude. Am J Med Sci 2001;322:68–70.

[21] Castle SC, Yeh M, Toledo S, et al. Lowering the temperature criterion improves detection of infections in nursing home residents. Aging Immunol Infect Dis 1993;4:67–76.

[22] Norman DC, Yoshikawa TT. Fever in the elderly. Infect Dis Clin North Am 1996;10:93–9.

[23] Wasserman M, Levinstein M, Keller E, et al. Utility of fever, white blood cells, and differential count in predicting bacterial infections in the elderly. J Am Geriatr Soc 1989; 37:537–43.

[24] Loo VG, Poirier L, Miller MA, et al. A predominantly clonal multi-institutional outbreak of *Clostridium difficile*–associated diarrhea with high morbidity and mortality. N Engl J Med 2005;353:2442–9.

[25] Pepin J, Valiquette L, Alary ME, et al. *Clostridium difficile* associated diarrhea in a region of Quebec from 1991 to 2003: a changing pattern of disease severity. CMAJ 2004;171:466–72.

[26] Thompson WW, Shay DK, Weintraub E, et al. Influenza-associated hospitalizations in the United States. JAMA 2004;292:1333–40.

[27] Thompson WW, Shay DK, Weintraub E, et al. Mortality associated with influenza and respiratory syncytial virus in the United States. JAMA 2003;289:179–86.

[28] Hoyert DL, Heron MP, Murphy SL, et al. Deaths: final data for 2003. Natl Vital Stat Rep 2006;54:1–120.

[29] Kirby JT, Fritsche TR, Jones RN. Influence of patient age on the frequency of occurrence and antimicrobial resistance patterns of isolates from hematology/oncology patients: report from the Chemotherapy Alliance for Neutropenics and the Control of Emerging Resistance Program (North America). Diagn Microbiol Infect Dis 2006;56:75–82.

[30] Hurwitz A, Ruhl CE, Kimler BF, et al. Gastric function in the elderly: effects on absorption of ketoconazole. J Clin Pharmacol 2003;43:996–1002.

[31] Feldman M, Cryer B, McArthur KE, et al. Effects of aging and gastritis on gastric acid and pepsin secretion in humans: a prospective study. Gastroenterology 1996;110:1043–52.

[32] Marangos MN, Skoutelis AT, Nightingale CH, et al. Absorption of ciprofloxacin in patients with diabetic gastroparesis. Antimicrob Agents Chemother 1995;39:2161–3.

[33] Beyth RJ, Shorr RI. Medication use. In: Duthie EH, Katz PR, editors. Practice of geriatrics. 3rd edition. Philadelphia: W.B. Saunders; 1998. p. 38–47.

[34] Vestal RE. Aging and pharmacology. Cancer 1977;80:1302–10.

[35] Turnheim K. Drug dosage in the elderly: Is it rational? Drugs Aging 1998;13:357–79.

[36] Cockcroft DW, Gault MH. Prediction of creatinine clearance from serum creatinine. Nephron 1976;16:31–41.

[37] Cirillo M, Anastasio P, De Santo NG. Relationship of gender, age, and body mass index to errors in predicted kidney function. Nephrol Dial Transplant 2005;20:1791–8.

[38] Drusano GL, Munice HL, Hoopes JM, et al. Commonly used methods of estimating creatinine clearance are inadequate for elderly debilitated nursing home patients. J Am Geriatr Soc 1988;36:437–41.

[39] Smythe M, Hoffman J, Kizy K, et al. Estimating creatinine clearance in elderly patients with low serum creatinine concentrations. Am J Hosp Pharm 1994;51:198–204.

[40] Turnheim K. Drug therapy in the elderly. Exp Gerontol 2004;39:1731–8.

[41] Drusano GL, Preston SL, Fowler C, et al. Relationship between fluoroquinolone area under the curve:minimum inhibitory concentration ratio and the probability of eradication of the infecting pathogen, in patients with nosocomial pneumonia. J Infect Dis 2004;189:1590–7.

[42] Schneitman-McIntire O, Farnen TA, Gordon N, et al. Medication misadventures resulting in emergency department visits at an HMO medical center. Am J Hosp Pharm 1996;53:1416–22.

[43] Evans RS, Lloyd JF, Stoddard GJ, et al. Risk factors for adverse drug events: a 10-year analysis. Ann Pharmacother 2005;39:1161–8.

[44] Bates DW, Miller EB, Cullen DJ, et al. Patient risk factors for adverse drug events in hospitalized patients. Arch Intern Med 1999;159:2553–9.

[45] Peyriere H, Cassan S, Floutard E, et al. Adverse drug events associated with hospital admission. Ann Pharmacother 2003;37:5–11.

[46] Baciewicz AM, Sokos DR, Cowan RI. Aminoglycoside-associated nephrotoxicity in the elderly. Ann Pharmacother 2003;37:182–6.

[47] Paterson DL, Robson JM, Wagener MM. Risk factors for toxicity in elderly patients given aminoglycosides once daily. J Gen Intern Med 1998;13:735–9.

[48] Baddour LM, Wilson WR, Bayer AS, et al. Infective endocarditis: diagnosis, antimicrobial therapy, and management of complications. A statement for healthcare professionals from the Committee on Rheumatic Fever, Endocarditis, and Kawasaki Disease, Council on Cardiovascular Disease in the Young, and the Councils on Clinical Cardiology, Stroke, and Cardiovascular Surgery and Anesthesia, American Heart Association: endorsed by the Infectious Diseases Society of America. Circulation 2005;111:394–434.

[49] Owens RC Jr, Ambrose PG. Antimicrobial safety: focus on fluoroquinolones. Clin Infect Dis 2005;41(Suppl 2):S144–57.

[50] Fountain FF, Tolley E, Chrisman CR, et al. Isoniazid hepatotoxicity associated with treatment of latent tuberculosis infection. Chest 2005;128:116–23.

[51] Fernandez-Villar A, Sopena B, Fernandez-Villar J, et al. The influence of risk factors on the severity of anti-tuberculosis drug-induced hepatotoxicity. Int J Tuberc Lung Dis 2004;8: 1499–505.

[52] Lucena MI, Andrade RJ, Fernandez MC, et al. Determinants of the clinical expression of amoxicillin-clavulanate hepatotoxicity: a prospective series from Spain. Hepatology 2006; 44:850–6.

[53] Larrey D, Vial T, Pauwels A, et al. Hepatitis associated with amoxicillin-clavulanic acid combination: report of 15 cases. Gut 1992;33:368–71.

[54] Garcia Rodriguez LA, Stricker BH, Zimmerman HJ. Risk of acute liver injury associated with the combination of amoxicillin and clavulanic acid. Arch Intern Med 1996;156: 1327–32.

[55] Kaufman DW, Kelly JP, Rosenberg L, et al. Recent patterns of medication use in the ambulatory adult population of the United States: the Slone Survey. JAMA 2002;287:337–44.

[56] Ketek (telithromycin) [package insert]. Bridgewater (NJ): Sanofi-Aventis; 2006.

[57] Andriole VT, Haverstock DC, Choudhri SH. Retrospective analysis of the safety profile of oral moxifloxacin in elderly patients enrolled in clinical trials. Drug Saf 2005;28:443–52.

[58] Nicholson SC, High KP, Gothelf S, et al. Gatifloxacin in community-based treatment of acute respiratory tract infections in the elderly. Diagn Microbiol Infect Dis 2002;44:109–16.

[59] Yanagihara K, Fukuda Y, Seki M, et al. Clinical comparative study of sulbactam/ampicillin and imipenem/cilastatin in elderly patients with community-acquired pneumonia. Intern Med 2006;45:995–9.

[60] Kadowaki M, Demura Y, Mizuno S, et al. Reappraisal of clindamycin IV monotherapy for treatment of mild-to-moderate aspiration pneumonia in elderly patients. Chest 2005;127: 1276–82.

[61] El Moussaoui R, Opmeer BC, de Borgie CA, et al. Long-term symptom recovery and health-related quality of life in patients with mild-to-moderate-severe community-acquired pneumonia. Chest 2006;130:1165–72.

ELSEVIER
SAUNDERS

Clin Geriatr Med 23 (2007) 499–514

CLINICS IN
GERIATRIC
MEDICINE

Infection Control Issues in Older Adults

Lona Mody, MD, MSc

*Division of Geriatric Medicine, University of Michigan Medical School, Geriatrics Research,
Education and Clinical Center, Veterans Affairs Ann Arbor Healthcare System,
11-G GRECC, AAVAMC, 2215 Fuller Drive, Ann Arbor, MI 48105, USA*

Health care delivery in the United States changed significantly during the latter part of the twentieth century. In the past, health care delivery occurred mainly in acute care facilities. Today, health care is delivered in hospital, subacute care, long-term care or nursing home (NH), rehabilitation, assisted living, home, and outpatient settings. Measures to reduce health care costs have led to a reduced number of hospitalizations and shorter lengths of stay (with an increase in severity of illness and ICU admissions), along with increased outpatient, home care, and NH stays for older adults [1].

There are approximately 36.57 million (projected to be 63.5 million by 2025) adults over 65 years of age in the United States; of these, 4.9 million are over 85 years of age (projected to be 8 million by 2025). Approximately 1.43 million older adults reside in NHs certified by the Centers for Medicare and Medicaid [2]. About 3%–15% of such patients acquire an infection in these facilities. In 1 year, approximately 2.1 million patients are discharged from NHs with the primary reasons of death or transfers to hospitals. These numbers are expected to grow as the population ages [2].

Infections in NHs increase the mortality and morbidity of residents and generate additional costs for the facilities and hospitals. This article focuses on infection control issues pertaining to older adults in various health care settings. It also discusses the elements of infection control programs with a focus on the NH setting.

Infection control challenges in older adults

Older adults in the United States have many different options on where to reside, ranging from independent single-family homes to senior apartments,

Supported by National Institute on Aging K23 AG028943 and ASP/AGS T. Franklin Williams Research Scholarship.

E-mail address: lonamody@umich.edu

0749-0690/07/$ - see front matter. Published by Elsevier Inc.
doi:10.1016/j.cger.2007.02.001

assisted living, group homes, and traditional NHs or long-term care facilities. Older adults also undergo several care transitions—home to acute care hospital, acute care hospital to rehabilitation facility, acute care hospital to NH, NH to home, and acute care hospital to home [3]. This section focuses on infection control issues pertaining to older adults in various health care settings.

Acute care hospitals

Traditionally, acute care hospitals have been the major center for infection control research and activities, since most health care has been delivered in the acute care setting. However, during the 1990s, there was a reduction in the number of acute care hospital beds, along with reduced length of stay and greater severity of illness in the hospitalized population. Hospitals are downsizing their infection control operations, compelling the infection control departments to focus surveillance activities on those at highest risk of infection, and antimicrobial resistance. Older adults, particularly those admitted from NHs, with multi-morbid conditions and poor functional status, form one such high-risk group.

There are several issues pertaining to infection control in older adults admitted to acute care. It is common for acute care facilities to receive frail older adults from NHs without a patient assessment from a physician before the transfer, with poor documentation of their comorbidities and medications, with resistant pathogens. Older adults typically present with atypical clinical findings of infection [4]. For example, a NH resident with pneumonia is more likely to present with confusion and deteriorating functional status than shortness of breath or new cough. This can lead to delayed diagnosis resulting in delayed administration of appropriate treatment.

Recently, several investigations have shown the value of surveillance cultures in controlling hospital acquired methicillin-resistant *Staphylococcus aureus* (MRSA) and vancomycin-resistant enterococci (VRE) colonization and infection. The Society for Healthcare Epidemiology of America (SHEA) recommends active surveillance culture programs for these resistant pathogens [5]. Patients colonized with these pathogens are to be placed under surveillance conditions to prevent the spread of these organisms to other susceptible patients. Whether all new admissions should be subjected to a surveillance program or only those at high risk, such as ICU admissions or NH transfers, is a matter of active debate. Several recent investigations also have challenged the quality of care provided to patients in isolation. One study found that isolated patients were twice as likely as control patients to experience adverse events during hospitalization [6,7]. Isolated patients also were more likely to complain about their care, not having their vital signs recorded as ordered, and have days with no physician progress notes [6]. The effects of isolation practices in older adults (in terms of depression, delirium, and functional decline) has not been evaluated, but they are likely to be deleterious. These debates and controversies highlight the need for further data on infection control and isolation practices in older adults admitted to acute care hospitals.

Nursing homes

Older adults, especially those in NHs, have unique characteristics that create special challenges to implementing an effective infection control program. These characteristics include diagnostic uncertainty, time and resource limitations, rapid staff turnover, high staff/patient ratios, limited and intermittent physician coverage, increasing acuity of care, and frequent care transitions. These characteristics can be divided into in three categories: host factors, structural concerns, and process factors.

Host factors

NH residents are susceptible to infections because of an increased prevalence of chronic diseases, increasing severity of illness, medications that affect resistance to infection (eg, steroids and frequent antibiotic usage), level of debility, impaired mental status (predisposing to aspiration and pressure ulcers), incontinence and resultant indwelling catheter usage, and the institutional environment in which they live [8]. Most infections found in NH residents are thought to be endogenous in nature and often result from the resident's flora.

NH residents also may serve as host reservoirs for antimicrobial-resistant pathogens, such as MRSA and VRE. With a reduction in the length of hospital stay, the severity of illness among residents of the subacute care nursing unit has increased with resultant inherent rapid transfers to a hospital and increased polypharmacy. All of these factors combine to create a vulnerable resident who is prone to develop infections and transmit resistant pathogens.

Structural concerns

Structural concerns affecting infection control relate to a facility's capacity to provide care, whereas an assessment of the process of care is an evaluation of the actual delivery of service. Structural factors of concern in implementing an effective infection control program within a NH include suboptimal full-time equivalents for registered nurses, nursing aides and therapists; high staff turnover; a changing case mix; limited availability of information systems; and variable availability of laboratory and radiologic services.

The number of staff per resident varies considerably among facilities [9]. Hospital based NHs and skilled NHs for residents covered by Medicare have almost twice the nursing staff of other community nursing facilities. The relationship between nursing care intensity and health outcomes for NH patients has been examined for years, and associations between increased nursing hours per patient and improved health outcomes have been reported [10]. For example, in a sample of Maryland NHs, registered nurse turnover has been associated with increased risk of infection and a higher risk of hospitalization caused by infection [11]. Potential explanations for these findings include difficulties in establishing and maintaining effective infection control practices, reduced familiarity between staff and residents to detect minor changes in residents' health, and inconsistent supervision and training.

To reduce the length of acute hospital stay, NHs now are accepting patients who are sicker and have more severe illnesses. This change in case mix has led to increased care transitions between hospitals and NHs, which has led to increased lapses in information exchange. These care transitions also lead to increased risk of pathogen transmission between the hospital and NHs.

Process factors

The processes of care in NHs pertain to health care service delivery. Process factors affecting infection control in NHs include variable staff education, availability and use of diagnostic specimens, and use of quality improvement tools, such as regional databases, quality indicators, and minimum datasets.

Whereas the effectiveness of staff education alone is controversial, the value of education as part of a comprehensive quality control program has been recognized in all health care settings for a long time. The importance of staff education is accentuated further by considerable turnover in NH personnel. However, there are currently no standard guidelines regarding curriculum or frequency of staff education in NHs, which includes education in infection control measures. Nursing aides, who are the frontline personnel in recognizing any change in clinical status of NH residents, may receive little or no formal educational training in various infection control issues, such as hand hygiene, antimicrobial resistance, early signs and symptoms of common infections, and infection control measures to reduce infections related to indwelling devices. However, NHs can overcome these barriers by scheduling monthly in-service training for staff members. However, the content, frequency, and attendance of these in-services will vary among facilities.

Diagnostic specimens have limited usefulness in the NH setting for two reasons (1) they cannot be or are not obtained, or (2) if they are obtained, the results may not be communicated to the appropriate health care provider in a timely fashion, or in the case of radiologic investigations, may not be interpreted accurately. The onsite availability of diagnostic or radiologic services is lacking in many NHs. In addition, patients may not be able or willing to cooperate in the collection of valid specimens. Thus, diagnostic tests may be requested infrequently, resulting in initiation of therapy without appropriate clinical information. On the other hand, whereas urine specimens are obtained more frequently than other types of specimens, the prevalence of bacteriuria in 30%–50% of urine specimens means that without an assessment of symptoms, a positive culture has a low predictive value for appropriate diagnosis of infection. Often, these specimens are not collected or handled appropriately before delivery to the laboratory. These diagnostic dilemmas can lead to further delay in initiation of care, inappropriate or unnecessary use of antibiotics, and delayed transfers for sicker patients to acute care.

Home health care

With a move toward reduced hospital stay, home health care delivery remains the fastest growing segment in health care. Established in the 1880s, the home care industry grew from 1,100 home health care organizations in 1963 to over 20,000 in 2004 [12]. Per the 2000 Home and Hospice Care Survey, about 7.2 million individuals received home health care (5 million or 69% over 65 years of age) [12]. This number represents an increase of nearly 90% in 15 years. Home health care agencies, home care aide organizations, and hospices are known collectively as *home health care organizations.* Durable medical equipment and supply companies, while not included under the traditional home health care umbrella, are ancillary to home health care and provide products ranging from respirators and sleep apnea machines to walkers, catheters, and wound care supplies.

These home health care organizations provide care for elderly adults, who frequently have multiple medical problems including diabetes, congestive heart failure, cancer, chronic obstructive pulmonary disease, and chronic wounds. Coupled with the use of indwelling devices, such as urinary catheters, intravascular catheters, and feeding tubes, their infection risk increases tremendously. Data on the epidemiology of infections in this group are limited, albeit several outbreaks of bloodstream infections have been documented [13,14].

Although attempts have been made to standardize surveillance definitions, several challenges remain [15,16]. These include the fact that few dedicated infection control personnel are employed by home health care agencies, the role of informal caregiving in the spread of infections and adherence to infection control recommendations, and the paucity of data to understand the epidemiology of infections among patients receiving home health care.

Infection control and care transitions

Transitional health care is defined as "a set of actions designed to ensure the coordination and continuity of health care as patients transfer between different locations or different levels of care in the same location" [3]. These locations can include acute care hospitals, NHs, skilled nursing facilities, rehabilitation units, home care, and outpatient primary and specialty clinics. During care transitions, older adults are susceptible to care fragmentation, which may lead to medical errors and poor quality care. These transitions also provide an opportunity for pathogens to be transferred from one setting to another. Different financing and contractual agreements with pharmaceutical companies also may impede these transitions. For example, as patients are transferred across settings, each facility has incentives to substitute medications according to their own formulary.

Thus, these care transitions have implications for the spread of pathogens and the appropriateness of antimicrobial usage, including choice of antibiotics, dosage, and duration. In addition, care transitions can cause confusion for the patient, caregiver, and clinicians providing care at different settings. These care transitions also can cause confusion in exercising isolation practices. A patient with MRSA colonization could be confined to his/her room during the acute care stay, but he/she may not be isolated in the skilled nursing facility to undergo rehabilitation, which leads to confusion among health care workers (HCWs), patients, and families.

In summary, infection control issues in older adults vary as they move through various health care settings caused by the type of care provided, patient characteristics, the unique need for social and personal contact, and staff and facility resources.

Infection control and prevention: functions and elements

Infection prevention and control is important for continuum of care across various health care settings. The main functions are (1) to obtain and manage critical data, including surveillance information for endemic and epidemic infections; (2) to develop and recommend policies and procedures; (3) to intervene directly to prevent infections; and (4) to educate and train HCWs, patients, and nonmedical caregivers [1]. The next section focuses on the requirements and scope of infection control committees with specific focus on the NH setting.

Elements of infection control

Infection control program

An effective infection control program includes a method of surveillance for infections and antimicrobial-resistant pathogens, an outbreak control plan for epidemics, isolation and standard precautions, hand hygiene, staff education, an employee health program, a resident health program, policy formation and periodic review with audits, and a policy to communicate reportable diseases to public health authorities (Fig. 1).

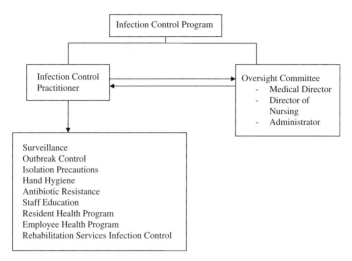

Fig. 1. Components of infection control program in long-term care facilities.

Surveillance

Infection surveillance in NHs involves collection of data on NH acquired infections. Surveillance is defined as "ongoing, systematic collection, analysis, and interpretation of health data essential to the planning, implementation, and evaluation of public health practice, closely integrated with timely dissemination of these data to those who need to know" [13]. Surveillance can be limited to a particular objective or may be a facility-wide goal. Surveillance often is based on individual patient risk factors, focused on a unit, or based on a particular pathogen or infection type.

Surveillance can be either passive or active. In passive surveillance, also known as routine surveillance, an infection control professional uses data collected for routine patient care. Although less costly in terms of resources, passive surveillance is inherently biased. It may also underestimate the magnitude of the outcomes measured and delay detection of outbreaks. The feasibility of passive surveillance has been demonstrated and has led to continuing education opportunities. On the other hand, active surveillance uses multiple data sources to detect infections and antimicrobial resistance early. It requires routine infection control practitioner (ICP) rounds to detect infections early and may involve patient screening for resistant pathogens. Active surveillance for antimicrobial-resistant pathogens in acute care has created significant debate in recent years, but data in NHs are lacking.

For surveillance to be conducted correctly, objective valid definitions of infections are crucial. Hospital surveillance definitions are based on the National Nosocomial Infection Surveillance (NNIS) criteria, which depend rather extensively on laboratory investigations. Radiology and microbiology data are less available, and if available, are delayed; therefore, these criteria may not be applicable in NH settings. Modified NH specific criteria were developed by a Canadian consensus conference, which took into account the unique limitations of the NH setting [17]. The criteria have been used widely, but not uniformly [14].

In addition to using valid surveillance definitions, a facility must have clear goals and aims for setting up a surveillance program. These goals, like other elements of an infection control program, have to be reviewed periodically to reflect changes in the facility's population, pathogens of interest, and changing antimicrobial resistance patterns. In addition, plans to analyze the data and use them to design and implement proven preventive measures must be made in advance.

The analysis and reporting of infection rates in NHs typically are conducted monthly, quarterly, and annually to detect trends. Because the length of stay at a NH is typically long, and each resident is at risk for a prolonged duration, an analysis of absolute numbers of infections can be misleading. Infection rates (preferably reported as infections/1,000 resident days) can be calculated by using resident days or average resident census for the surveillance period as the denominator.

These data can be used to establish endemic baseline rates and recognize variations from the baseline that could represent an outbreak. Feedback to the nursing staff, physicians, and appropriate quality control and review committees is critical to the success of any surveillance program. This information eventually should lead to specific, targeted infection control initiatives and follow-up surveillance to evaluate the success of the changes.

Furthermore, surveillance data can be combined at a regional or a national level, and individual facility rates can be compared with an aggregate of other facilities using visual and simplified statistical methods (Table 1). The success in the reduction of nosocomial infection rates in acute care hospitals that participate in an NNIS system has been demonstrated. While one study among 17 NHs has demonstrated the feasibility of using interfacility comparisons, it needs to be studied further at other sites [18].

Outbreak control

An illness in a community or region is considered an outbreak when it clearly exceeds the normal rate of expectancy. Thus the existence of an outbreak is always relative to the number of cases that are expected to occur in a specific population in a specific time period.

The main objectives of an outbreak investigation are control and elimination of the source, prevention of new cases, prevention of future outbreaks, research to gain additional knowledge about the infectious agent and its mode of transmission, program evaluation and strategies for improvement, and epidemiologic training to conduct outbreak investigations.

It is vital that the ICP know the following (1) appropriate data collection methods; (2) methods of interpreting the data using simple epidemiologic measures; (3) effective study designs to conduct an effective and efficient

Table 1
Summary of results from surveillance for infection from 17 regional nursing homes

| Facility | Total UTIs[b] | Catheter UTIs[c] | Infection rates[a] | | | | | |
			Respiratory	GI	Skin	Bloodstream	Febrile	Total
A	0.61	0.00	2.55	0.12	2.67	0.00	0.00	5.95
B	0.69	3.70	1.56	0.09	1.26	0.00	0.00	3.60
C	0.63	3.70	1.77	0.14	1.12	0.00	0.03	3.69
D	0.66	3.15	1.12	0.03	0.66	0.03	0.00	2.50
E	0.53	5.14	0.23	0.00	0.69	0.00	0.00	1.45
F	0.30	2.92	2.11	0.08	0.83	0.00	0.00	3.31
G	0.40	1.80	1.76	0.09	0.97	0.00	0.00	3.21
H	0.68	4.56	2.02	0.09	0.68	0.02	0.00	3.49
I	0.21	1.33	1.65	0.15	0.72	0.00	0.05	2.78
J	0.27	1.66	1.06	0.64	0.77	0.00	0.00	2.75
K	0.69	4.74	2.36	0.25	1.16	0.04	0.00	4.50
L	2.28	6.90	2.88	0.22	1.54	0.00	0.04	6.96
M	0.00	0.00	1.90	0.38	1.43	0.10	0.10	3.91
N	0.28	7.43	2.24	0.09	0.75	0.00	0.00	3.36
O	0.29	2.99	0.79	0.13	2.30	0.00	0.00	3.51
P	0.67	1.32	2.88	0.15	1.83	0.00	0.04	5.58
Q	0.44	3.04	1.54	0.00	0.83	0.00	0.00	2.81
Mean infection rates[d]	0.57	3.20	1.79	0.16	1.19	0.01	0.01	3.73
SD	0.49	2.12	0.72	0.16	0.60	0.02	0.03	1.36
Total infections	282	130	828	77	520	4	6	1,717

Abbreviations: GI, gastrointestinal; SD, standard deviation; UTIs, urinary tract infections.
[a] Expressed as number of infections per 1000 resident or device days.
[b] Catheter-associated and non–catheter-associated UTIs combined.
[c] Catheter-associated UTIs.
[d] Interfacility mean of the number of infections per 1000 resident days.
Data from Stevenson KB, Moore J, Colwell H, et al. Standardized infection surveillance in long-term care: interfacility comparisons from a regional cohort of facilities. Infect Control Hosp Epidemiol 2005;26(3):234.

outbreak investigation; and (4) effective and appropriate infection control measures. Local health departments are available for counsel, but it also may be beneficial for the ICP to have access to a hospital epidemiologist for consultation.

Antibiotic resistance

Infection and colonization with antimicrobial-resistant pathogens are important concerns in NHs and develop primarily because of widespread use of empiric antibiotics, functional impairment, use of indwelling devices, mediocre adherence to hand hygiene programs among HCWs, and cross-transmission during group activities. A NH can reduce infections and colonization with resistant pathogens by emphasizing hand hygiene compliance, developing an antimicrobial use program, encouraging evidence-based clinical evaluation and management of infections, and ensuring that the facility has a well established individualized infection control program. Guidelines to control MRSA and VRE have been published by SHEA and provide a good base for developing facility specific policies [19].

Isolation precautions

The Centers for Disease Control and Prevention's Healthcare Infection Control and Prevention Advisory Committee (HICPAC) has proposed a two-tiered structure for isolation precautions. In the first tier, HICPAC proposes use of "Standard Precautions," which have been designed for the care of all patients in hospitals, regardless of the diagnosis, infectious or otherwise. In the second tier are "Transmission-based Precautions," which have been designed for the care of patients suspected of or known to be infected with epidemiologically important pathogens that have been acquired by physical contact or airborne or droplet transmission [20].

Standard precautions apply to blood, all body fluids, secretions and excretions regardless of whether they contain visible blood, skin that is not intact, or mucous membrane material. Designed to reduce the risk of transmission of pathogens from apparent and ambiguous sources of infection, these precautions include hand hygiene compliance, glove use, masks, eye protection, gowns, and avoidance of injuries from sharp materials. Transmission-based precautions are intended for use with patients who may be infected with highly transmissible or epidemiologically significant pathogens. These include airborne precautions (eg, for tuberculosis), droplet precautions (eg, for influenza), and contact precautions (eg, for *Clostridium difficile*). Although these guidelines were designed for acute care settings, several of them, especially the universal precautions, apply to NHs as well. These recommendations have to be adapted to the needs of the individual facility.

There has been some debate on the role of active surveillance cultures and their impact on isolation policies in acute care hospitals. The SHEA guideline for preventing nosocomial transmission of multidrug resistant organisms advocates for aggressive active surveillance cultures [5], whereas the recent draft of HICPAC guidelines calls for individual facilities to assess their own needs and conduct surveillance cultures as necessary [20]. These guidelines refer to studies from acute care hospitals serving a sicker, shorter stay population. Facilities should evaluate these guidelines and individualize the plan to obtain active surveillance cultures based on the population it serves, baseline rates of MRSA and VRE, and any recent outbreaks.

Hand hygiene compliance

Contamination of the hands of HCWs has been recognized as playing a role in the transmission of pathogenic bacteria to patients since the observations of Holmes, Semmelweis, and others more than 100 years ago [21]. Hand antisepsis remains the most effective and least expensive measure to prevent transmission of nosocomial infections. However, compliance with hand washing recommendations among HCWs averages only 30%–50% and improves only modestly following educational interventions [22]. HCWs frequently reported poor compliance with hand hygiene measures because of skin irritation from frequent washing, too little time because of a heavy workload, and simply forgetting.

The use of waterless, alcohol-based hand rub in addition to washing hands with soap and water has become a routine practice by HCWs in many acute care facilities. Introduction of alcohol-based hand rubs has been shown to significantly improve hand hygiene compliance among HCWs in acute care hospitals and to decrease overall nosocomial infection rates and transmission of MRSA infections. Alcohol-based hand rubs also have been shown to enhance compliance with hand hygiene in the NH setting and should be used to complement educational initiatives [22]. While the cost of introducing alcohol-based hand rubs could be a concern of NHs, recent data in acute care have shown that the total costs of a hand hygiene promotion campaign, including alcohol-based hand rubs, corresponded to less than 1% of costs that could be attributed to nosocomial infections [23].

Although introducing the alcohol-based hand rub in health care settings is a prudent, cost-effective measure, several issues need to be considered. Alcohol-based hand rubs should not be used if hands are visibly soiled, in which case hand hygiene with antimicrobial soap and water is recommended. Alcohol-based hand rubs can cause dry skin; however, recent data on rubs containing emollients have shown to cause significantly less skin irritation and dryness [24]. Facilities should be aware that alcohols are flammable. Facilities have reported difficulties in implementing the current hand hygiene guidelines and use of alcohol-based hand rubs because of fire safety concerns. Existing national fire codes permit use of alcohol-based hand rub dispensers in patient rooms, but they cannot be used in egress or exit corridors. Because state and local fire codes may differ from national codes, facilities should work with their local fire marshals to ensure that installation of alcohol-based hand rub containers is consistent with local fire codes.

Staff education

Ongoing staff education is critical in health care settings because of the plethora of literature published every year, advancements in technology, and regulatory demands. The Joint Commission on Accreditation of Healthcare Organizations expects new employee orientation to include the facility's infection control program and the employee's responsibility to prevent infections. In addition, the Occupational Safety and Health Administration (OSHA) requires training for bloodborne pathogens and tuberculosis for any employee expected to come into contact with potentially infectious agents.

The ICP plays a vital role in meeting these requirements and educating NH personnel on various infection control measures, particularly in view of rapid staff turnover. Informal education during infection control and quality improvement meetings and during infection control walking rounds should be complemented with in-service education on various topics including hand hygiene compliance, antimicrobial usage and antimicrobial resistance, appropriate and early diagnosis of infections, infection control and prevention measures, and isolation precautions and policies.

Resident health program

The resident health program should focus on immunizations, tuberculin testing, and infection control policies to prevent specific infections, include areas such as skin care, oral hygiene, prevention of aspiration, and catheter care to prevent urinary tract infections. Adults over the age of 65 should receive pneumococcal vaccination at least once, influenza vaccination every year, and a tetanus booster every 10 years. Despite proven effectiveness, compliance with these measures remains low. Average influenza and pneumococcal vaccination rates among NH residents are 60% and 40%, respectively [25]. In addition to poor documentation, reasons for lower immunization rates include lack of physician emphasis, patient concerns about the side effects of vaccinations, and the inability to obtain consent [26]. Adopting a standing order policy for immunization could eliminate implementation delays caused by the consent process.

Employee health program

The employee health program mainly applies to employees with potentially communicable diseases, policies for sick leave, immunizations, and OSHA regulations to protect them from blood-borne pathogens. NH bar employees who have known communicable diseases or infected skin lesions from direct contact with the residents, and who have infected skin lesions or infectious diarrhea are prevented from having direct contact with residents' food. Moreover, when hiring new employees, an initial medical history and a physical examination and screening for tuberculosis must be obtained. Infection control education also must be provided to staff members.

Infection control policies and measures in NHs must be in place to address postexposure prophylaxis for infections such as HIV and hepatitis B. Varicella vaccine should be given to employees who are not immune to the virus. Employees are expected to be up-to-date with their tetanus boosters and to receive influenza vaccinations every year. The vaccine is effective not only in preventing influenza and reducing absenteeism in HCWs, but it also has been associated with a decrease in influenza mortality in patients [26]. Annual influenza vaccination campaigns play a central role in deterring and preventing nosocomial transmission of the influenza virus and should be promoted by ICP and NH leadership.

Rehabilitation services

NHs increasingly are responsible for postacute care rehabilitation, including physical therapy (PT), occupational therapy (OT), and wound care with or without hydrotherapy. These therapists, like other clinical staff such as nurses and nurses' aides, provide many opportunities for the transmission of pathogens. In an NH, PT and OT services can be provided either at the bedside or in a central therapy unit. For bedside therapy, therapists move between rooms and units and do not routinely wear gloves and gowns. For care at a central therapy unit, residents are transported to an open unit, where hand washing sinks may not be readily available. While these therapists have not been implicated in any major outbreaks, hydrotherapy for wounds has been shown to facilitate outbreaks with resistant pathogens [27].

A detailed infection control program for rehabilitation services should be prepared and should focus on facility design to promote hand hygiene compliance, which includes convenient and easy access to sinks and the use of alcohol based hand rubs. Patients who are infectious should not be treated at the central facility. Facilities providing hydrotherapy should consider providing the service in a separate room with a separate resident entrance.

Infection control practitioner

An ICP, usually a staff nurse, is assigned the responsibility of directing infection control activities in an NH. The ICP is responsible for implementing, monitoring, and evaluating the infection control program. Because of financial constraints, an ICP usually functions as an assistant director of nursing, or is involved in staff recruitment and education. Need for a full time ICP usually depends on the number of beds, the acuity level of residents, and the level of care provided at the facility. Nonetheless, for an infection control program to succeed, the ICP should be guaranteed sufficient time and resources to carry out infection control activities. A basic background is advisable in infectious disease, microbiology, geriatrics, and educational methods. The ICP also should be familiar with the federal, state, and local regulations regarding infection control.

Additionally, an alliance with and access to an infectious disease epidemiologist should be encouraged. Such collaborations also could provide assistance with outbreak investigations, emergency preparedness in the events of bioterrorism and vaccine shortages, and the use of microbiologic and molecular methods for infection control.

Oversight committee

The Federal Nursing Home Reform Act from the Omnibus Budget Reconciliation Act (OBRA) of 1987 mandated the formation of a formal infection control committee to evaluate infection rates, implement infection control programs, and review policies and procedures. However, this mandate has been dropped by OBRA at the federal level, although some states still may require them. A small subcommittee or a working group comprised of a physician/medical director, an administrator, and an ICP should evaluate the NH infection rates on a regular basis, present the data at quality control meetings, review policies and any research in the area, and make decisions to implement infection control changes. This subcommittee can review and analyze the surveillance data, assure this data is presented to the nursing and physician staff, and approve targeted recommendations to reduce infections. Records pertaining to these activities and infection data should be kept and filed for future reference.

Principles guiding infection control practices also provide a model for enhancing quality of care and patient safety for other noninfectious adverse outcomes such as falls, delirium, inappropriate medication usage, and adverse drug events.

Appendix: Resources for infection control practitioners

1. Society for Healthcare Epidemiology of America (SHEA) and the Association for Professionals in Infection Control (APIC) have long-term care committees that publish and approve NH infection guidelines and publish periodic position papers related to pertinent infection control issues. Their websites have several educational resources for staff education and in-services. In addition, APIC also publishes a quarterly long-term care newsletter.
2. Local APIC chapters provide a network for ICPs to socialize, discuss infection control challenges and practical solutions to overcome them, and provide access to educational resources and services. ICPs should become members of APIC at the local and national level to remain up-to-date with practice guidelines, position statements, information technology resources, and changes in policies and regulations.
3. Mayhall CG. Hospital Epidemiology and Infection Control. 3rd edition. Philadelphia: Lippincott Williams & Wilkins; 2004.
4. Selected internet websites:
   a. Centers for Disease Control and Prevention: http://www.cdc.gov.
   b. Society for Healthcare Epidemiology of America: http://www.shea-online.org/.
   c. Association for Professionals in Infection Control: http://www.apic.org.
   d. Occupational Health and Safety Administration: http://www.osha.gov.
   e. Joint Commission on Accreditation of Healthcare Organizations-Infection Control Initiatives: http://www.jcaho.org/accredited± organizations/patient±safety/infection±control/ic±index.htm.

References

[1] Friedman C, Barnette M, Buck AS, et al. Requirement for infrastructure and essential activities of infection control and epidemiology in out-of-hospital settings: a consensus panel report. Infect Control Hosp Epidemiol 1999;20:695–705.

[2] Jarvis WR. Infection control and changing health-care delivery systems. Emerg Infect Dis 2001;7:170–3.

[3] Coleman EA. Falling through cracks: challenges and opportunities for improving transitional care for persons with continuous complex care needs. J Am Geriatr Soc 2003;51:549–55.

[4] Marrie TJ. Community-acquired pneumonia in the elderly. Clin Infect Dis 2000;31:1066–78.

[5] Muto CA, Jernigan JA, Ostrowsky BE, et al. SHEA guideline for preventing nosocomial transmission of multidrug-resistant strains of staphylococcus aureus and enterococcus. Infect Control Hosp Epidemiol 2003;24:362–86.

[6] Stelfox HT, Bates DW, Redelmeier DA. Safety of patients isolated for infection control. JAMA 2003;14:1899–905.

[7] Kirkland K, Weinstein J. Adverse effects of contact isolation. Lancet 1999;354:1177–8.

[8] Nicolle LE. Infection control in long-term care facilities. Clin Infect Dis 2000;31:752–6.

[9] Mody L, Langa KM, Saint S, et al. Preventing infections in nursing homes: A survey of infection control practices in Southeast Michigan. Am J Infect Control 2005;33:489–92.

[10] Loeb MB, Craven S, McGeer AJ, et al. Risk factors for resistance to antimicrobial agents among nursing home residents. Am J Epidemiol 2003;157:40–7.

[11] Zimmerman S, Gruber-baldini AL, Hebel JR, et al. Nursing home facility risk factors for infection and hospitalization: importance of registered nurse turnover, administration and social factors. J Am Geriatr Soc 2002;50:1987–9.

[12] National Association for Home Care and Hospice. Basic statistics about home care. Available at: www.nahc.org. Accessed January 25, 2007.

[13] Do AN, Ray BJ, Banerjee SN, et al. Bloodstream infection associated with needleless device use and importance of infection control practices in the home health setting. J Infect Dis 1999;179:442–8.

[14] Danzig LE, Short LJ, Collins K, et al. Bloodstream infections associated with a needleless intravenous infusion system in patients receiving home infusion therapy. JAMA 1995;273:1862–4.

[15] Schantz M. Infection control comes home. Home Healthcare Management & Practice 2001;13:126–33.

[16] Horan TC, Gaynes RP. Surveillance of nosocomial infections. In: Glen Mayhall C, editor. Hospital epidemiology and infection control. 3rd edition. Philadelphia: Lippincott Williams & Wilkins; 2004. p. 1661–702.

[17] McGeer A, Campbell B, Emori TG, et al. Definitions of infection for surveillance in long-term care facilities. Am J Infect Control 1991;19:1–7.

[18] Stevenson KB, Moore J, Colwell H, et al. Standardized infection surveillance in long-term care: interfacility comparisons from a regional cohort of facilities. Infect Control Hosp Epidemiol 2005;26:231–8.

[19] Strausbaugh LJ, Crossley KB, Nurse BA, et al. Antimicrobial resistance in long-term care facilities. Infect Control Hosp Epidemiol 1996;17:129–40.

[20] Garner JS. The Hospital Infection Control Practices Advisory Committee, guideline for isolation precautions in hospitals. Infect Control Hosp Epidemiol 1996;17:53–80.

[21] Otherson MJ, Otherson HB. A history of handwashing: seven hundred years at a snail's pace. The Pharos 1987;50:23–7.

[22] Mody L, McNeil SA, Sun R, et al. Introduction of a waterless alcohol-based hand rub in a long-term care facility. Infect Control Hosp Epidemiol 2003;24:165–71.

[23] Pittet D, Sax H, Hugonnet S, et al. Cost implications of successful hand hygiene promotion. Infect Control Hosp Epidemiol 2004;25:264–6.

[24] Centers for Disease Control and Prevention. Guideline for hand hygiene in healthcare settings: recommendations of the healthcare infection control practices advisory committee and the HICPAC/SHEA/APIC/IDSA hand hygiene task force. MMWR Recomm Rep 2002;51:S3–40.

[25] Mody L, Langa K, Malani P. Impact of the 2004–05 influenza vaccine shortage on immunization practices in long-term care facilities. Infect Control Hosp Epidemiol 2006;27:383–7.

[26] Carman WF, Elder AG, Wallace LA, et al. Effects of influenza vaccination of health-care workers on mortality of elderly people in long-term care: a randomised controlled trial. Lancet 2000;355:93–7.

[27] Embril JM, McLeod JA, AL-Barrak AM, et al. An outbreak of methicillin-resistant Staphylococcus aureus on a burn unit: potential role of contaminated hydrotherapy equipment. Burns 2001;27:681–8.

CLINICS IN
GERIATRIC
MEDICINE

ELSEVIER
SAUNDERS

Clin Geriatr Med 23 (2007) 515–534

Bacterial Community-Acquired Pneumonia in Older Patients

Gerald R. Donowitz, MD[a],*, Heather L. Cox, PharmD[b]

[a]Department of Medicine, Infectious Disease, University of Virginia Health System,
University of Virginia, Box 800466, Charlottesville, VA 22908, USA
[b]Department of Pharmacy Services, University of Virginia Health System,
Box 800674, Charlottesville, VA 22908, USA

In 1888, Sir William Osler [1] noted that "Pneumonia remains now, as then, the most serious acute disease with which physicians have to deal; serious because it attacks the old, the feeble...persons who are not able to withstand the sudden sharp onset of the malady." Over a century later, pneumonia in the elderly remains a major clinical challenge. Influenza and pneumonia are the eighth leading causes of death in all age groups in the United States, the sixth leading cause of death in those 65 years of age or older, and the leading cause of infection-related mortality for all age groups [2]. The incidence of community-acquired pneumonia increases dramatically with age from 18.2 cases per 1000 person years for patients aged 65 to 69 years to 52.3 cases per 1000 patient years for those aged greater than 85 years [3]. For persons aged greater than 65 years, pneumonia is the third most common reason for hospitalization [4]. These numbers become even more important when one considers that it is estimated that 20% of the world's population (over 2.9 million people) will be over the age of 65 years by 2050 [5].

As the study of the epidemiology of pneumonia has become more developed and diagnostic techniques more sophisticated, pneumonia in the elderly has been categorized demographically as well as microbiologically. Viral pneumonia, nursing home–associated, and health care–associated pneumonia are discussed elsewhere in this issue. This review will center on community-acquired, bacterial pneumonia in the elderly.

---

* Corresponding author.
E-mail address: grd@virginia.edu (G.R. Donowitz).

0749-0690/07/$ - see front matter © 2007 Elsevier Inc. All rights reserved.
doi:10.1016/j.cger.2007.03.006   *geriatric.theclinics.com*

Pathogenesis and predisposing factors

As a general rule, pneumonia develops when the usual host defenses are in someway undermined, by-passed, or overwhelmed. The reasons for an increased incidence of pneumonia in older populations remain unclear. Although multiple factors appear to have a role, the direct effect of aging on host defenses remains an area of great interest.

Pulmonary host defenses include anatomic and mechanical barriers, humoral immunity, T-cell immunity, and phagocytic activity. Age-related effects have been documented in animal models and humans to involve many of these host defense systems [6–8].

Key elements of basic lung mechanics are affected by age, leading to a decrease in elastic recoil, a decrease in expiratory flow, and an increase in air trapping. Chest wall compliance decreases owing to changes in costovertebral joint mobility and anatomic changes in the spine. Respiratory muscles undergo loss of mass and efficiency. The overall effect of these changes is to increase the work of breathing. Although these changes by themselves have not been shown to increase the incidence of pneumonia in the elderly, they may serve to increase the morbidity and mortality once pneumonia develops.

Clearance of potential pathogens from the oropharynx involves flow of saliva, sloughing of epithelial cells, local humoral immunity, and bacterial interference by resident flora. Decreased clearance of organisms in the oropharynx has been observed in elderly patients [9]. Because the study population involved consisted of patients institutionalized at a Veterans' home or hospitalized at a university medical center, it is difficult to know whether the observations noted were primary or occurred as a result of some other condition or comorbidity other than age. Similarly, silent aspiration has been noted to occur in elderly patients with pneumonia but not in aged-match controls [10]. Why this occurs in some elderly patients but not others is unclear.

Mucociliary clearance of potentially pathogenic organisms caught in secreted mucous is an important host defense in the upper airways and conducting airways. Nasal mucociliary clearance, which correlates with that of the trachea, has been shown to be slower and less efficient in older nonsmokers and has been postulated to lead to pneumonia [11].

A variety of age-related effects on cell-mediated immunity, humoral immunity, and phagocytic function have been observed, although their significance in the development of pneumonia in the elderly remains undetermined (Box 1) [7–9,12].

Many of the studies documenting changes in immune function due to age have been performed in animals. Human studies have sometimes involved patients who have been chronically institutionalized or recently hospitalized. These factors have clouded the true role of aging on host defenses by introducing the effects of malnutrition, bacterial colonization associated with health care facilities, and comorbid conditions on the parameters studied.

Box 1. Age-related changes in pulmonary host defenses[a]

Upper airway host defenses
↓ Oropharyngeal clearance[b]
↑ Aspiration
↓ Mucociliary function

Conducting airways host defenses
↓ Mucociliary function

Lower respiratory tract (terminal airways, alveoli)

Cell-mediated immunity
↓ T-cell numbers
↓ Naive T cells; ↑% memory cells
↓ Helper T-cell activity
↓ T-cell response to antigens

Humoral immunity
↓ B-cell numbers
↓ Response to antigens
↓ Antibody production

Phagocytes
↓ Toll-like receptors
↓ Phagocytosis

---

[a] *Data* derived from animal and human studies; the former may or may not apply to elderly humans.
[b] Occurs in the elderly but may be due to factors other than age.

In addition to the effects of aging on specific areas of host defense, dysregulation of the immune response occurs in the elderly [13]. In nonsmoking adults in good health who underwent bronchoscopy with bronchoalveolar lavage, increases in neutrophil number, total cell numbers, and immunoglobulin content were noted in the greater than 65-year-old age group when compared with younger age groups. Interleukin-6 concentrations in bronchoalveolar lavage were increased, as was superoxide anion production by stimulated cells. The presence of what appears to be low-grade inflammation in the absence of clinically detectable disease suggests the loss of immune regulation in the elderly.

Although the effects of age on the host defense system may be an important predisposing factor in the development of pneumonia, a great deal of individual variation in these effects has been noted. Age effects may be determined in part genetically but may also be due to changes in gene expression that occur over the lifetime of the individual [14].

Underlying disease states and the therapy given for them may also influence host defenses and may have a role in the development of pneumonia in aging populations. Malnutrition manifested by hypoalbuminemia and the risk for large-volume aspiration have been identified as important factors in the development of pneumonia [15]. Changes in the flow of saliva and in pH, common in the elderly, have been associated with increased adherence of some strains of *Klebsiella* to oral epithelial cells [16]. These changes have been associated with xerostomia due to Sjögren's syndrome, radiotherapy, or drugs such as antidepressants, diuretics, antihistamines, and antihypertensives, drugs with anticholinergic effects, and drugs used to treat Parkinson's disease [8,9,17].

Although other comorbidities have been associated with pneumonia in the elderly, the exact mechanisms involved in the association have not been well established. These comorbidities include diabetes, cancer, chronic pulmonary disease, heart failure, renal failure, alcoholism, asthma, and immune suppression [8,18].

Clinical presentation

The clinical presentation of community-acquired pneumonia in older populations varies greatly and, at times, may be more subtle or atypical when compared with that in younger populations (Box 2) [18–22]. It has been postulated that the presence of dementia may be a major reason for differences in the clinical presentation of pneumonia in the elderly [23]. A limited number of studies have stratified the presence of the classic signs, symptoms, and physical findings of pneumonia with age. Hospitalized patients have made up the majority of patient populations studied, shifting observations toward the more seriously ill. Metlay and colleagues [19] examined four patient age groups including a 64- to 74-year-old group and a greater than 75-year-old group. Fernandez-Sabé and colleagues [20] stratified patients as either less than or greater than 80 years of age. Symptoms were present longer before presentation in the older age groups. Respiratory symptoms such as cough, dyspnea, and sputum production were present 1 to 2.5 days longer before presentation than in the younger groups. Nonrespiratory symptoms such as fatigue were present 2 days longer, whereas fever and chills were present 1 day less in a comparison with younger age groups [19].

Respiratory signs and symptoms such as cough and dyspnea were less frequent in older age groups, although the vast majority of subjects had these symptoms. Pleuritic chest pain and hemoptysis were seen in 31% and 12%

Box 2. Signs and symptoms of pneumonia in the elderly[a,b] (% in patients >65 years)

Respiratory symptoms
Cough (66%–84%)
Sputum production (53%–55%)
Pleuritic chest pain (17%–45%)
Hemoptysis (3%–13%)
Dyspnea (70%–82%)

Non-respiratory symptoms
Chills (23%–51%)
Sweats (45%–55%)
Fatigue (84%–88%)
Abdominal pain (18%)
Anorexia (57%–64%)
Altered mental status (11%–45%)
Myalagia (8%–23%)

Findings on physical examination
Fever (40%–78%)
Tachypnea (65%–68%)
Tachycardia (37%–40%)
Rales (77%–84%)

---

[a] *Adapted from* Refs. [14,17–20,22,23].
[b] Values of patients ≥65 years of age.

---

of older patients, respectively, compared with 60% and 19% of patients in the younger age groups [19]. The majority of non-respiratory symptoms were less common in the elderly, with fewer than half demonstrating findings such as headache, myalgia, or decreased appetite. Chills and sweats were present in approximately 40% to 50% of the older age groups compared with more than 80% of younger groups [19,20]. In the older age groups, physical findings consistent with the diagnosis of pneumonia were totally absent in 20% to 47% of patients. In contrast tachypnea and the presence of rales were noted more commonly in the elderly.

Although these studies show that the elderly may demonstrate fewer signs, symptoms, and physical findings of pneumonia, 60% of younger and older age groups manifested a "classical bacterial pneumonia syndrome" defined as three or more of the findings of acute onset, chills, chest pain, or purulent sputum in the setting of bacteremic pneumococcal pneumonia [20]. Changes in functional status, metabolic disarray, new or more frequent episodes of falling, or exacerbation of comorbid disease states may be the most prominent or only manifestations of community-acquired pneumonia in the elderly [21].

Given the variation and subtlety of presentation of pneumonia in the elderly, the role of chest radiography takes on added importance. Unfortunately, the radiographic manifestations of pneumonia in the elderly may be difficult to interpret. The presence of underlying disease such as chronic obstructive pulmonary disease, congestive heart failure, and malignancy may make diagnosing pneumonia difficult radiographically. Despite limited data to substantiate the finding, it has been observed by some clinicians that the chest radiograph may initially be normal in elderly patients with pneumonia and subsequently blossom with hydration [22]. Progression of radiographic abnormalities occurs more frequently in older populations [24]. Although the chest radiograph is a vital component of making the diagnosis of pneumonia, and, in fact, should be obtained in everyone in whom the diagnosis of pneumonia is being entertained, it is not definitive. In the setting of patients with clinical findings consistent with pneumonia but with a negative chest radiograph, 26% of patients in one study were shown to have abnormalities consistent with the diagnosis of pneumonia on high-resolution chest CT [25]. Although chest CT is not suggested for routine use in the work-up of patients with pneumonia, it may be useful in certain settings.

Etiology

The etiology of community-acquired pneumonia in the elderly is similar to that observed in younger populations [26]. A major limitation in discussions of this aspect of the disease is that only 5% to 50% of patients have a microbiologically proven diagnosis [19,20,24]. The absence of productive cough and the common use of antibiotics before any cultures are obtained help explain this observation. As is true for younger populations, *Streptococcus pneumoniae* is the predominant organism involved, accounting for 20% to 60% of cases [8,26,27]. Non-typeable strains of *Haemophilus influenzae* are commonly the second most frequently detected organisms, isolated in 7% to 11% of microbiologically defined cases. Other gram-negative bacilli including *Pseudomonas aeruginosa* have a variable but overall small role as etiologic agents. Although many studies fail to differentiate between colonization and true infection, it is estimated that approximately 1% to 3% of community-acquired pneumonias in the elderly involve gram-negative organisms. *Staphylococcus aureus* occurs in 0% to 7% of cases of community-acquired pneumonia, although it is thought to have a greater role in nursing home–associated pneumonias [8].

Older adults are at greater risk for the development of pneumonia caused by group B streptococci, *Moraxella catarrhalis*, and *Legionella* sp, but the overall incidence of disease caused by these organisms is small.

Pneumonia caused by mixed aerobe/anaerobe pathogens due to aspiration is estimated to occur in 5% of elderly populations. The incidence increases in the setting of dysphagia, cerebrovascular accidents, and dementia [28]. Atypical pathogens have a variable role in causing pneumonia in the elderly. *Mycoplasma pneumoniae* is a rare cause of pneumonia, whereas *Chlamydophila* sp infections occur in 16% to 28% of cases [8,27,29].

Clinical evaluation

Once the diagnosis of pneumonia is made, the next decision is whether the patient should be hospitalized or treated as an outpatient. A variety of models have been developed to address this issue. The PORT study developed the most widely used predictive model in the United States by analyzing over 14,000 hospitalized patients and applying the model to over 40,000 patients in the outpatient and inpatient setting [30]. This system uses 20 parameters including age, the presence of defined comorbid conditions, physical findings, and laboratory and radiographic findings to place patients into one of five risk groups with varying associated mortalities. Patients falling into the lowest two groups with the lowest potential mortalities are usually treated as outpatients, whereas those in the highest groups with the highest potential mortality risks are treated as inpatients. Similar prediction models have been developed that use only five parameters and may be more easily applied in a variety of clinical settings [31–34]. Although many of these prediction models have used patients of varying ages, others have been developed using only older populations [33,34]. Prediction models that have been based on mortality have limitations in that the mortality risk is not the only reason for hospitalization. Social circumstances, the ability to take oral medications, reliability, and the ability to recognize when help is needed should all be factors in the decision to treat a patient with pneumonia in the hospital [35,36]. In addition, the presence of hypoxia (oxygen tension <60 mm Hg or oxygen saturation <90%), tachypnea, or the suspicion of sepsis have all been causes for hospitalization, even when the prediction score would have suggested that outpatient therapy would have been appropriate. Prediction models should serve as guidelines and not mandates or standards of care; clinical judgment and commonsense must be used as well [35,37]. The fact that mortality has been higher in "low-risk" patients with pneumonia who have been hospitalized further substantiates this idea [38].

Diagnosis

Making a specific etiologic diagnosis of pneumonia in elderly populations remains a clinical challenge for a variety of reasons. The subtle and often nonspecific presentation of disease leads to delays in obtaining and examining appropriate diagnostic material such as sputum and blood. Even when the diagnosis of pneumonia is made early, obtaining the material to analyze may be difficult. Because empiric therapy guidelines are frequently successfully used, the need for aggressive diagnostic interventions in often frail and debilitated patients may be questioned.

A staged approach to diagnostic testing in patients with community-acquired pneumonia has recently been suggested [39]. For all patients with pneumonia, a specific etiologic diagnosis would help the clinician narrow, broaden, or change antibiotic coverage completely. Knowledge of the specific etiology allows the clinician to be aware of the natural course of disease as well as potential complications. In an era of ever-increasing antibiotic resistance patterns, susceptibility testing of isolated organisms may provide important information to care givers as well as those who track the epidemiology of disease regionally and nationally. The more ill the patient, the more important making a specific diagnosis becomes in impacting appropriate therapy, including the need for more aggressive diagnostic interventions.

The major diagnostic interventions used for community-acquired pneumonia have been reviewed [40]. Microscopic examination and culture of sputum samples representative of lower respiratory tract secretions represents a noninvasive, relatively inexpensive, and potentially useful diagnostic test. Unfortunately, 30% to 40% of patients fail to produce sputum. Furthermore, in many cases, antibiotics are received for varying periods of time before sputum is obtained, leading to a marked decrease in the yield for Gram's stain and culture [40]. When the culture of sputum is delayed, isolation of organisms such as *Streptococcus pneumoniae* is less likely owing to overgrowth of oropharyngeal flora. When adequate sputum samples are collected before antibiotics have been given, Gram's stain sensitivity of approximately 80% has been noted in patients with bacteremic pneumococcal pneumonia, with culture sensitivities ranging from 80% to 90% [41]. Yields of Gram's stain and culture are lower for organisms other than the pneumococcus, including *Haemophilus influenzae* [42]. Although adequate samples of sputum that are evaluated promptly may be extremely useful in establishing the etiologic diagnosis of community-acquired pneumonia, such samples are provided in as few as 14% of patients [43].

Blood cultures may be positive in 1% to 16% of patients hospitalized with community-acquired pneumonia [44,45]. As is true for sputum analysis, prior antibiotic therapy greatly diminishes the diagnostic yield. Blood cultures have no real role in the evaluation of outpatient pneumonia but should be acquired in patients who are hospitalized and more severely ill.

The incidence of pleural effusions in community-acquired pneumonia varies with the organism involved. Pleural effusions may be seen in 10% of patients with infection caused by *Streptococcus pneumoniae,* 50% to 70% of patients infected with aerobic gram-negative bacilli, and as many as 95% of patients infected with group A streptococci [40]. Obtaining pleural fluid for culture and chemical analysis may provide the clinician with a specific diagnosis, may rule in or out other components of the differential diagnosis including tuberculosis, malignancy, and collagen vascular disease, and may determine when drainage is necessary.

Although serologic assays have been used for decades to try to identify the etiology of pneumonia, their reliability and overall usefulness remain unclear. In contrast, urinary antigen tests for *S pneumoniae* and *Legionella pneumophila* serogroup 1 have been widely accepted [46–49]. An immuno-chromatographic membrane assay has been developed to detect the C-poly-saccharide cell wall antigen of *S pneumoniae* in urine. Sensitivities of 70% to 80% and specificities of 77% to 97% have been noted [46,47]. Unlike in the culture of sputum or blood, prior antibiotic use does not seem to affect the test [48]. The legionella antigen assay has a sensitivity of 80% to 97% and a specificity of 99%. The assay detects only serogroup 1, which accounts for approximately 80% of legionella infections [49].

Fiberoptic bronchoscopy and bronchoalveolar lavage are usually used in patients who have severe pneumonia, usually requiring mechanical ventilation, or in patients who have pneumonia that has not resolved or have clearly failed appropriate antibiotics.

Antibacterial selection

Once pneumonia has been documented, a determination is made as to where the patient will be treated and, once diagnostic tests are obtained, as to what antibiotics need to be given.

The guidelines for antibacterial selection for elderly patients with community-acquired pneumonia do not differ from those for immunocompetent adults [37]. Several professional societies have outlined recommendations for the empiric treatment of community-acquired pneumonia, all of which are organized according to the clinical setting in which treatment is provided [50–52]. The most recent guidelines published by the Infectious Diseases Society of America and the American Thoracic Society are summarized in Table 1 [39].

Outpatient treatment

Empiric therapy for ambulatory patients with community-acquired pneumonia should provide activity against *S pneumoniae* and atypical pathogens. Macrolide (erythromycin, clarithromycin, or azithromycin) monotherapy is recommended for previously healthy patients who have not received antibiotic therapy in the previous 3 months. Recent antibiotics or comorbidities (eg, chronic heart, lung, liver, or renal disease, alcoholism, malignancy) predispose the patient to an increased risk for infection with drug-resistant *S pneumoniae*. In these cases, a respiratory fluoroquinolone (gemifloxacin, levofloxacin, moxifloxacin) or combination therapy with a macrolide plus a beta-lactam is recommended. Preferred oral beta-lactams include high-dose amoxicillin or amoxicillin-clavulanate. Alternatively, cepodoxime or

Table 1
Empiric treatment of community-acquired pneumonia [39]

Patient category	Empiric therapy
Outpatient	
Previously healthy	
No risk factors for DRSP	Macrolide[a] or doxycycline
Comorbidities or recent antibiotic therapy	Advanced macrolide[b] plus a β-lactam[c] or respiratory fluoroquinolone[d] Amoxicillin-clavulanate or clindamycin
Aspiration with infection	
Influenza with bacterial superinfection	β-lactam[c] or respiratory fluoroquinolone[d]
Inpatient	
Medical ward	Advanced macrolide[b] plus a β-lactam[e] or respiratory fluoroquinolone[d]
ICU	
Pseudomonas not suspected	β-lactam[e] plus ozithromycin[b] or β-lactam[e] plus respiratory fluoroquinolone[d]
Pseudomonas suspected	Anti-pseudomonal β-lactam[f] plus ciprofloxacin or levofloxacin (750 mg) or anti-pseudomonal β-lactam[f] plus an aminoglycoside plus a respiratory fluoroquinolone[d] or a ezithromycin[a]
Pseudomonas suspected, β-lactam allergy	Aztreonam plus levofloxacin (750 mg) or aztreonam plus moxifloxacin or gemifloxacin, with or without an aminoglycoside

Abbreviation: DRSP, drug-resistant *Streptococcus pneumoniae.*
[a] Erythromycin, azithromycin, or clarithromycin.
[b] Azithromycin or clarithromycin.
[c] Amoxicillin, 1 g PO TID; amoxicillin-clavulanate, 2 g PO BID; cefpodoxime, cefprozil, or cefuroxime.
[d] Levofloxacin (750 mg), moxifloxacin, or gemifloxacin.
[e] Cefotaxime, ceftriaxone, ampicillin-sulbactam, or ertapenem.
[f] Piperacillin, piperacillin-tazobactam, cefepime, imipenem, or meropenem.
Adapted from Mandell LA, Wunderink RG, Anzueto A, et al. Infectious Disease Society of America/America Thoracic Society census guidelines on the management of community-acquired pneumonia in adults. Clin Infect Dis 2007;44(Suppl 2):S45; with permission.

cefuroxime may be used. For patients with allergy or intolerance to macrolides, doxycycline remains a less expensive option, albeit, one with limited in vivo data supporting its use as monotherapy [53]. Because recent therapy or repeated courses with the same antibiotic class are risk factors for subsequent pneumococcal resistance, patients requiring new or ongoing therapy should receive treatment with a different antibacterial class [39]. The British Thoracic Society guidelines do not recommend macrolides as first-line therapy, because high-level resistance in *S pneumoniae* infection is common [52].

Inpatient treatment, non–intensive care unit

Patients requiring hospital admission should receive an anti-pneumococcal fluoroquinolone or combination therapy with a beta-lactam plus a macrolide. Beta-lactam monotherapy is not recommended largely owing to observational evidence that the addition of a macrolide is associated with reduced mortality [54,55] and a shorter length of stay [56]. Among elderly patients hospitalized for pneumonia, empiric treatment with a second-generation cephalosporin plus a macrolide, a non-pseudomonal third-generation cephalosporin plus a macrolide, or fluoroquinolone monotherapy was associated with a lower 30-day mortality when compared with treatment with a non-pseudomonal cephalosporin alone [55]. The reason for this finding remains unclear. It may relate to a higher than suspected prevalence of pneumonia caused by atypical pathogens or to the immunomodulating effects of macrolides [54,57]. No well-designed, randomized studies have confirmed the superiority of combination therapy over beta-lactam monotherapy.

Inpatient treatment, intensive care unit

Therapy for ICU patients should include an anti-pneumococcal beta-lactam plus either a macrolide or respiratory fluoroquinolone, thereby providing adequate coverage for *S pneumoniae* and *Legionella*. The role of anti-pneumococcal fluoroquinolone monotherapy in severe community-acquired pneumonia has not been established. In addition, patients with risk factors for *pseudomonas* infection (eg, structural lung disease, corticosteroid therapy, and recent broad-spectrum antibacterial therapy [50]) should receive anti-pseudomonal combination therapy, because inadequate empiric treatment has been associated with increased mortality [58–60]. Once susceptibilities are available, antibacterial selection may be narrowed accordingly. Recommendations for the empiric treatment of community-acquired pneumonia in which *pseudomonas* is suspected are summarized in Table 1.

Although primarily described in the young and immunocompetent necrotizing pneumonias caused by community-acquired methicillin-resistant *Staphylococcus aureus* (CA-MRSA) have been reported [61–64]. Many of these patients had preceding influenza infection, and most strains were known to produce Panton-Valentine leukocidin, a virulence factor associated with tissue necrosis. Vancomycin is a therapeutic option for suspected CA-MRSA pneumonia; however, the addition of clindamycin or linezolid should be considered given the potential for toxin production [64,65]. Empiric clindamycin monotherapy is not recommended owing to the possibility of inducible resistance and subsequent clinical failure. Daptomycin, which is effective against CA-MRSA at other body sites, should not be used for pneumonia because the drug is inhibited by pulmonary surfactant [66].

Special considerations in the elderly

Choosing antibacterials in elderly patients requires careful consideration of age-related differences in pharmacokinetics and pharmacodynamics, comorbid conditions, and the consequences of polypharmacy. Decreased gastric acid secretion may enhance the absorption of acid-labile antimicrobials, and drug serum half-lives may be prolonged as a result of reduced hepatic metabolism or renal elimination. Prudent drug and dosage selection together with a thorough review of possible drug-disease and drug-drug interactions serve to maximize efficacy while minimizing the potential for adverse drug events. Table 2 summarizes common serious adverse effects, significant drug-drug interactions, and agents requiring dosage adjustment in renal insufficiency among therapeutic options for community-acquired pneumonia [67–71]. A comprehensive discussion of the principles related to antimicrobial use in older adults has been described elsewhere [71].

Although members of the beta-lactam class are typically well tolerated and exhibit few drug-drug interactions, almost all require dosage adjustment in renal insufficiency. Recent case reports of cefepime-related neurotoxicity have identified excessive dosage and reduced renal clearance among predisposing factors [72]. This observation highlights the importance of ensuring optimal estimates of creatinine clearance, the parameter upon which dosing recommendations for renally eliminated drugs are based. Avoiding overestimation in the elderly is of particular relevance, given that a serum creatinine within normal limits may represent low muscle mass rather than the absence of reduced renal drug clearance.

Within the macrolide class, erythromycin is not routinely used due to its lack of activity against *Haemophilus influenzae* (of particular concern in cigarette smokers) and a higher incidence of gastrointestinal intolerance [73]. In addition, as substrates and potent inhibitors of cytochrome P450 3A4, both erythromycin and clarithromycin demonstrate greater potential for drug-drug interactions when compared with azithromycin. Concurrent use may increase serum concentrations of CYP 3A4 substrates such as digoxin, cyclosporine, HMG-CoA reductase inhibitors, and warfarin. Clarithromycin inhibition of CYP3A4 and P-glycoprotein may have contributed to fatal colchicine toxicity in elderly patients with concomitant gout and renal insufficiency [74]. Telithromycin, a ketolide and semisynthetic macrolide derivative, was approved by the Food and Drug Administration in 2004 for the treatment of mild to moderately severe community-acquired pneumonia [75]. Despite activity against drug-resistant strains of *Streptococcus pneumoniae*, similar difficulty with drug-drug interactions in addition to strengthened warnings for loss of consciousness, visual disturbances, and life-threatening hepatotoxicity have limited significant use of this agent [75,76].

Fluoroquinolones have become increasingly popular in therapy for community- acquired pneumonia given that they are typically well tolerated, convenient, highly bioavailable, and provide excellent activity against common community-acquired pneumonia pathogens, including drug-resistant pneumococci. Nevertheless, gatifloxacin was voluntarily withdrawn from the market in 2006 because of its effect on glucose control [77]. When compared with macrolides, gatifloxacin was associated with an increased risk of hypoglycemia and hyperglycemia among patients with and without diabetes mellitus [78]. Apart from an increased risk of hypoglycemia in patients receiving levofloxacin, no significant associations were noted in patients receiving other fluoroquinolones. Although gatifloxacin appears to carry the highest risk of dysglycemia, elderly patients receiving fluoroquinolones may benefit from blood glucose monitoring and an instruction in the recognition of symptoms of hypo- and hyperglycemia.

Reports of fluoroquinolone-resistant pneumococci are well documented. Because clinical failure due to resistant isolates has only been reported with the less active anti-pneumococcal fluoroquinolones (ciprofloxacin and levofloxacin) [79], is it unclear whether moxifloxacin and gemifloxacin carry the same risk [39]. Widespread use of fluoroquinolones in the elderly evokes additional concern due to their apparent association with a hypervirulent strain of *Clostridium difficile* [80,81]. In a Québec outbreak for which age was an independent risk factor, fluoroquinolones emerged as the highest risk antimicrobial class [80]. Loo and colleagues [81] subsequently described 1719 episodes of *C difficile*–associated diarrhea in 12 Québec hospitals where a predominantly fluoroquinolone-resistant strain may have selected for its spread. An overall attributable 30-day mortality rate of 6.9% increased to 10.2% and 14% in patients aged greater than 80 years and 90 years, respectively.

Outcome of community-acquired pneumonia

The development of community-acquired pneumonia in elderly populations is associated with an in-hospital mortality and 30-day mortality rate of 11% to 20% [15,18,20,33,82–84]. Mortality may be increased for the next several years [85]. Predictors of mortality have varied among studies and have included advanced age (>85 years), abnormal vital signs (temperature >36.1–37°C, blood pressure <90 mm Hg, pulse >110 beats/min), failure to respond to stimuli, aggravation of comorbid disease, prior swallowing disorders, multi-lobar pneumonia, a bed-ridden status, and an elevated C-reactive protein [15,33,34].

Prevention

Vaccination remains the primary preventative strategy for community-acquired pneumonia in the elderly. Persons older than 50 years should receive inactivated influenza vaccine annually; pneumococcal vaccination should be given once to persons aged more than 65 years. A second pneumococcal vaccination is recommended after 5 years for those persons in whom the first dose was administered before age 65 years [39]. Vaccination may be provided before hospital discharge in patients hospitalized for any reason or as follow-up in the primary care setting.

Table 2
Considerations among antibacterial agents commonly prescribed for the treatment of community-acquired pneumonia

Antibacterial agent or class	Required dosage adjustment in renal insufficiency	Adverse effects (common/serious)	Significant drug-drug interactions
β-lactams	Yes Except ceftriaxone	Gastrointestinal intolerance, rash, blood dyscrasias, drug fever, interstitial nephritis, encephalopathy (cefepime)	↓ β-lactam excretion Uricosuric agents (eg, probenecid)
Doxycycline	No	Gastrointestinal intolerance, photosensitivity	↓ Doxycycline concentration Aluminum, calcium, or magnesium-containing antacids, bismuth subsalicylate, ferrous sulfate, sucralfate, CYP 3A4 inducers (eg, carbemazepine, phenytoin, rifampin) ↑ Concentration of interacting drug CYP 3A4 substrates (eg, cyclosporine, digoxin, HMG-CoA reductase inhibitors, sildenafil, verapamil, warfarin)
Fluoroquinolones	Yes Except moxifloxacin	Gastrointestinal intolerance, QT prolongation, CNS effects (dizziness, somnolence, confusion, delirium, hallucinations, ↓ seizure threshold), dysglycemias, photosensitivity	↓ Fluoroquinolone absorption Aluminum or magnesium-containing antacids, calcium-containing antacids (ciprofloxacin), bismuth subsalicylate, ferrous sulfate, sucralfate ↑ Risk of arrhythmia QT-prolonging agents (eg, class Ia/III antiarrhythmics) ↑ Concentration of interacting drug (concurrent ciprofloxacin) CYP 1A2 substrates (eg, duloxetine, mirtazapine, theophylline, tizanidine, warfarin)

Macrolides Ketolide	Yes Except azithromycin	Gastrointestinal intolerance, QT prolongation, ototoxicity	↓ Macrolide concentration CYP 3A4 inducers (eg, carbemazepine, phenytoin, rifampin)
		Telithromycin: hepatotoxicity, loss of consciousness, visual disturbances	↑ Concentration of interacting drug CYP 3A4 substrates (eg, cyclosporine, digoxin, HMG-CoA reductase inhibitors, sildenafil, tacrolimus, verapamil, warfarin) ↑ Risk of arrhythmia QT-prolonging agents (eg, class Ia/III antiarrhythmics)

Abbreviations: CYP, cytochrome P450; HMG-CoA, hydroxymethylglutaryl-coenzyme A.

The effectiveness of the influenza vaccine depends on host factors in addition to the degree of match with circulating strains. A meta-analysis evaluating influenza vaccine efficacy in primarily institutionalized elderly [86] and a subsequent cohort study of the benefits of influenza vaccination in elderly members of a large health maintenance organization [87] identified significant reductions in hospitalization, pneumonia, and death in vaccinated patients. In a more recent evaluation of 17,393 adults aged 18 years or older and hospitalized with community-acquired pneumonia during influenza season, vaccine recipients were significantly less likely to die during hospitalization than were nonrecipients [88]. When compared with vaccination in younger groups, influenza vaccination in subjects 65 years or older was not less effective in preventing in-hospital mortality.

Although a mortality benefit following pneumococcal vaccination has not been definitively established, administration of the pneumococcal polysaccharide vaccine to adults and the conjugate vaccine to children has been associated with a reduced risk of invasive disease in persons 65 years or older [89,90]. A survival benefit was observed for subjects with prior pneumococcal vaccination in a concurrent review of 62,918 adults hospitalized with community-acquired pneumonia between 1999 and 2003 [91]. All-cause in-hospital mortality was significantly lower for subjects with documented prior pneumococcal vaccination when compared with vaccine nonrecipients or those with unknown vaccination status. The survival advantage was maintained following an adjustment for the severity of illness, medical comorbidities, the receipt of influenza vaccine, and varied assumptions regarding subjects with unknown pneumococcal vaccination status. Furthermore, subgroup analyses among only vaccine recipients revealed no significant differences in mortality related to older age.

Other preventative strategies may reduce the incidence of pneumonia in the elderly. Jackson and colleagues estimated that nearly one third of pneumonia episodes in the elderly could be attributed to smoking [3]. Cigarette smoking was also an independent risk factor for invasive pneumococcal disease in a case-control study of nonelderly adults [92]. Smoking cessation should be attempted during hospitalization and encouraged upon discharge and in the outpatient setting. Additional measures may be useful in patients with comorbid conditions that predispose to aspiration of colonized oropharyngeal secretions (eg, stroke, degenerative central nervous system disease). Aggressive oral care, swallowing evaluation, and reducing the use of sedating and anticholinergic medications may lower the risk for aspiration pneumonia [28].

References

[1] Silvermanm ME, Murray TJ, Bryan CS. The quotable Osler. Am Coll Physicians Obs 1998;139.

[2] Minino A, Heron AP, Smith BL. Deaths, preliminary data for 2004. National Vital Statistics Report 2006;54(19):1–52.
[3] Jackson ML, Neuzil KM, Thompson WW, et al. The burden of community-acquired pneumonia in seniors: results of a population based study. Clin Infect Dis 2004;39:1651–3.
[4] May DS, Kelly JJ, Mendlein JM, et al. Surveillance of major causes of hospitalization among the elderly 1988. MMWR CDC Surveill Summ 1991;40:7–21.
[5] Strausbaugh LJ. Emerging health care associated infections in the geriatric population. Emerg Infect Dis 2001;7:268–71.
[6] Gyetko MR, Toews GB. Immunology of the aging lung. Clin Chest Med 1993;14:379–91.
[7] Meyer KC. Aging. Proc Am Thorac Soc 2005;2:433–9.
[8] Janssens P, Krause KH. Pneumonia in the very old. Lancet Infect Dis 2004;4:112–24.
[9] Palmer LB, Albulack K, Fields S, et al. Oral clearance and pathogenic oropharyngeal colonization of the elderly. Am J Respir Crit Care Med 2001;164:464–8.
[10] Kikuchi R, Watabe N, Konno T, et al. High incidence of silent aspiration in elderly patients with community acquired pneumonia. Am J Respir Crit Care Med 1994;150:251–3.
[11] Ho JC, Chan KN, Hu WH, et al. The effect of aging on nasal mucocilliary clearance, beat frequency, and ultrastructure of respiratory cilia. Am J Respir Crit Care Med 2001;163: 983–8.
[12] Meyer KC. The role of immunity in susceptibility to respiratory infection in the aging lung. Respir Physiol 2001;128:23–31.
[13] Meyer KC, Ershler W, Rosenthal NS, et al. Immune dysregulation in the aging human lung. Am J Respir Crit Care Med 1996;153:1072–9.
[14] Fraga MF, Ballestar E, Paz MF, et al. Epigenetic differences arise during the lifetime of monozygotic twins. Proc Natl Acad Sci U S A 2005;102:10604–9.
[15] Riquelme R, Torres A, El-Ebiary M, et al. Community-acquired pneumonia in the elderly: a multivariate analysis of risk factors and prognostic factors. Am J Respir Crit Care Med 1996;154:1450–5.
[16] Ayers GH, Altman LC, Fretwell MD. Effect of decreased salivation and pH on the adherence of Klebsiella species to human buccal epithelial cells. Infect Immun 1982;38: 179–82.
[17] Smaldone GC. Deposition and clearance: unique problems in the proximal airways and oral cavity in the young and elderly. Respir Physiol 2001;128:33–8.
[18] Loeb M. Pneumonia in older persons. Clin Infect Dis 2003;37:1335–9.
[19] Metlay JP, Schulz R, Li H, et al. Influence of age on symptoms at presentation in patients with community-acquired pneumonia. Arch Intern Med 1997;157:1453–9.
[20] Fernandez-Sabe N, Carratala J, Roson B, et al. Community-acquired pneumonia in very elderly patients: causative organism, clinical characteristics and outcomes. Medicine 2003; 82:159–69.
[21] Granton JT, Grossman RF. Community-acquired pneumonia in the elderly patient: clinical features, epidemiology, and treatment. Clin Chest Med 1993;14(3):537–53.
[22] Feldman C. Pneumonia in the elderly. Clin Chest Med 1999;20:563–73.
[23] Johnson JC, Jayadevappa R, Baccash PD, et al. Nonspecific presentation of pneumonia in hospitalized older people: age effect or dementia. J Am Geriatr Soc 2000;48:1316–20.
[24] Marrie TJ, Haldane EV, Faulkner RS, et al. Community-acquired pneumonia requiring hospitalization: is it different in the elderly? J Am Geriatr Soc 1985;33:671–80.
[25] Syrjala H, Broas M, Suramo I, et al. High resolution computed tomography for the diagnosis of community-acquired pneumonia. Clin Infect Dis 1998;27:358–63.
[26] Ruiz M, Ewig S, Marcos MA, et al. Etiology, community-acquired pneumonia: impaired of age, comorbidity and severity. Am J Respir Crit Care Med 1999;160:397–405.
[27] Lim WS, Macfarland JT. A prospective comparison of nursing home acquired pneumonia with community acquired pneumonia. Eur Respir J 2001;18:362–8.
[28] Marik PE, Kaplan D. Aspiration pneumonia and dysphagia in the elderly. Chest 2003;124: 328–36.

[29] Janssens JP. Pneumonia in the elderly (geriatric) population. Curr Opin Pulm Med 2005;11: 226–30.

[30] Fine MJ, Auble TE, Yearly DM, et al. A prediction rule to identify low risk patients with community-acquired pneumonia. N Eng J Med 1997;336:1248–50.

[31] Fein AM. Pneumonia in the elderly: overview of diagnostic and therapeutic approaches. Clin Infect Dis 1999;28:726–9.

[32] Lim WS, Van der Eerden MM, Laing R, et al. Defining community-acquired pneumonia severity on presentation to hospital: an international derivation and validation study. Thorax 2003;58:377–82.

[33] Conte HA, Chen YT, Mehal W, et al. A prognostic rule for elderly patients admitted with community-acquired pneumonia. Am J Med 1999;106:20–8.

[34] Seppa Y, Bloigu A, Honkanen PO, et al. Severity assessment of lower respiratory tract infection in elderly patients in primary care. Arch Intern Med 2001;161:2709–13.

[35] Arnold FW, Ramirez JA, McDonald LC, et al. Hospitalization for community-acquired pneumonia: the pneumonia severity index vs clinical judgment. Chest 2003;124:121–4.

[36] Marras TK, Gutierrez C, Chan CK. Applying a prediction rule to identify low-risk patients with community-acquired pneumonia. Chest 2000;118:1339–43.

[37] Mandell LA, Bartlett JG, Dowel SF, et al. Update of practice guidelines for the management of community-acquired pneumonia in immunocompetent adults. Clin Infect Dis 2003;37: 1405–33.

[38] Labarere J, Stone RA, Obrosky S, et al. Comparison of outcomes for low-risk outpatients and inpatients with pneumonia. Chest 2007;131:480–8.

[39] Mandell LA, Wunderink RG, Anzueto A, et al. Infectious Disease Society of America/ America Thoracic Society census guidelines on the management of community-acquired pneumonia in adults. Clin Infect Dis 2007;44(Suppl 2):S27–72.

[40] Donowitz GR, Mandell GL, et al. Acute pneumonia. In: Mandell GL, Bennett JE, Dolin R, editors. Principles and practice of infectious diseases. 6th edition. Philadelphia: Elsevier Science; 2005. p. 819–45.

[41] Musher DM, Montoya R, Wanahita A. Diagnostic value of microscopic examination of Gram-stained sputum and sputum culture in patients with bacteremic pneumococcal pneumonia. Clin Infect Dis 2004;39:165–9.

[42] Fine MJ, Orloff JJ, Rihs JD, et al. Evaluation of housestaff physicians' preparation and interpretation of sputum Gram stains for community-acquired pneumonia. J Gen Intern Med 1991;6:189–98.

[43] Garcia-Vasquez E, Marcos MA, Mensa J, et al. Assessment of the usefulness of sputum culture for diagnosis of community-acquired pneumonia using the PORT predictive scoring system. Arch Intern Med 2007;164:1807–11.

[44] Bohte R, Van Furth R, Van den Broek PJ. Aetiology of community-acquired pneumonia: a prospective study among adults requiring admission to hospital. Thorax 1995;50:543–7.

[45] Campbell SG, Marrie TJ, Anstey R, et al. The contribution of blood cultures to the clinical management of adult patients admitted to the hospital with community-acquired pneumonia: a prospective observational study. Chest 2003;123:1142–50.

[46] Dominguez J, Gali N, Blanco S, et al. Detection of *Streptococcus pneumoniae* antigen by a rapid immunochromatographic assay in urine samples. Chest 2001;119:243–9.

[47] Murdoch DR, Laing TR, Mills GD. Evaluation of a rapid immunochromatographics test for detection of *Streptococcus pneumoniae* antigen in urine samples from adults with community-acquired pneumonia. J Clin Microbiol 2001;39:3495–8.

[48] Smith MD, Derrington P, Evans R, et al. Rapid diagnosis of bacteremic pneumococcal infection in adults by using the Binax now *Streptococcus pneumoniae* urine antigen test: a prospective, controlled clinical evaluation. J Clin Microbiol 2003;41:2810–3.

[49] Ruf B, Schurmann D, Horbach I, et al. Frequency and diagnosis of *Legionella pneumophilia*: a 3 year prospective study with emphasis on application of urine detection. J of Infect Dis 1990;162:1341–7.

[50] Niederman MS, Mandell LA, Anzueto A, et al. Guidelines for the management of adults with community-acquired pneumonia: diagnosis, assessment of severity, antimicrobial therapy, and prevention. Am J Respir Crit Care Med 2001;163:1730–54.

[51] Mandell LA, Marrie TJ, Grossman RF, et al. Canadian guidelines for the initial management of community-acquired pneumonia: an evidence-based update by the Canadian Infectious Diseases Society and the Canadian Thoracic Society. Clin Infect Dis 2000;31: 383–421.

[52] British Thoracic Society. Guidelines for the management of community-acquired pneumonia in adults. Thorax 2001;56(Suppl 4):iv1–64.

[53] Jacobs MR, Bajaksouzian S, Windau A, et al. Susceptibility of Streptococcus pneumoniae, Haemophilus influenzae, and Moraxella catarrhalis to 17 oral antimicrobial agents based on pharmacodynamic parameters. Clin Lab Med 2004;24:503–30.

[54] Garcia Vazquez E, Mensa J, Martinez JA, et al. Lower mortality among patients with community-acquired pneumonia treated with a macrolide plus a beta-lactam agent versus a beta-lactam agent alone. Eur J Clin Microbiol Infect Dis 2005;24:190–5.

[55] Gleason PP, Meehan TP, Fine JM, et al. Associations between initial antimicrobial therapy and medical outcomes for hospitalized elderly patients with pneumonia. Arch Intern Med 1999;159:2562–72.

[56] Stahl JE, Barza M, DesJardin J, et al. Effect of macrolides as part of initial empiric therapy on length of stay in patients hospitalized with community-acquired pneumonia. Arch Intern Med 1999;159:2576–80.

[57] Tamaoki J. The effects of macrolides on inflammatory cells. Chest 2004;125:41S–50S.

[58] Alvarez-Lerma F. Modification of empiric antibiotic treatment in patients with pneumonia acquired in the intensive care unit. Intensive Care Med 1996;22:387–94.

[59] Luna CM, Vujacich P, Niederman MS, et al. Impact of BAL data on the therapy and outcome of ventilator-associated pneumonia. Chest 1997;111:676–85.

[60] Rello J, Gallego M, Mariscal D, et al. The value of routine microbial investigation in ventilator-associated pneumonia. Am J Respir Crit Care Med 1997;156:196–200.

[61] Francis JS, Doherty MC, Lopatin U, et al. Severe community-onset pneumonia in healthy adults caused by methicillin-resistant Staphylococcus aureus carrying the Panton-Valentine leukocidin genes. Clin Infect Dis 2005;40:100–7.

[62] Fridkin SK, Hageman JC, Morrison M, et al. Methicillin-resistant Staphylococcus aureus disease in three communities. N Engl J Med 2005;352:1436–44.

[63] Gillet Y, Issartel B, Vanhems P, et al. Association between Staphylococcus aureus strains carrying the gene for Panton-Valentine leukocidin and highly lethal necrotizing pneumonia in young immunocompetent patients. Lancet 2002;359:753–9.

[64] Micek ST, Dunne M, Kollef MH. Pleuropulmonary complications of Panton-Valentine leukocidin-positive community-acquired methicillin-resistant Staphylococcus aureus. Chest 2005;128:3732–8.

[65] Bernardo K, Pakulat N, Fleer S, et al. Subinhibitory concentrations of linezolid reduce Staphylococcus aureus virulence factor expression. Antimicrob Agents Chemother 2004; 48(2):546–55.

[66] Silverman JA, Mortin LI, VanPraagh ADG, et al. Inhibition of daptomycin by pulmonary surfactant: in vitro modeling and clinical impact. J Infect Dis 2005;191:2149–52.

[67] Shakeri-Nejad K, Stahlmann R. Drug interactions during therapy with three major groups of antimicrobial agents. Expert Opin Pharmacother 2006;7:639–51.

[68] Cunha BA. Antibiotic side effects. Med Clin North Am 2001;85:149–85.

[69] Lipsky BA, Baker CA. Fluoroquinolone toxicity profiles: a review focusing on newer agents. Clin Infect Dis 1999;28:352–64.

[70] Owens RC, Ambrose PG. Antimicrobial safety: focus on fluoroquinolones. Clin Infect Dis 2005;41:S144–57.

[71] Faulkner CM, Cox HL, Williamson JC. Unique aspects of antimicrobial use in older adults. Clin Infect Dis 2005;40:997–1004.

[72] Lam S, Gomolin IH. Cefepime neurotoxicity: case report, pharmacokinetic considerations, and literature review. Pharmacotherapy 2006;26(8):1169–74.

[73] Zuckerman JM. Macrolides and ketolides: azithromycin, clarithromycin, telithromycin. Infect Dis Clin North Am 2004;18:621–49.

[74] Hung IFN, Wu AKL, Cheng VCC, et al. Fatal interaction between clarithromycin and colchicines in patients with renal insufficiency: a retrospective study. Clin Infect Dis 2005;41: 291–300.

[75] Ketek (telithromycin) [package insert]. Bridgewater (NJ): Sanofi-Aventis US; 2007.

[76] Clay KD, Hanson JS, Pope SD, et al. Brief communication: severe hepatotoxicity of telithromycin. Three case reports and literature review. Ann Intern Med 2006;144:415–20.

[77] Information for health care professionals: gatifloxacin (marketed as Tequin), Food and Drug Administration. Available at: http://www.fda.gov/cder/drug/InfoSheets/HCP/gatifloxacinHCP.htm. Accessed March 7, 2006.

[78] Park-Wyllie LY, Juurlink DN, Kopp A, et al. Outpatient gatifloxacin therapy and dysglycemia in older adults. N Engl J Med 2006;354:1352–61.

[79] Fuller JD, Low DE. A review of *Streptococcus pneumoniae* infection treatment failures associated with fluoroquinolone resistance. Clin Infect Dis 2005;41:118–21.

[80] Pépin J, Saheb N, Coulombe MA, et al. Emergence of fluoroquinolones as the predominant risk factor for *Clostridium difficile*–associated diarrhea: a cohort study during an epidemic in Québec. Clin Infect Dis 2005;41:1254–60.

[81] Loo VG, Poirier L, Miller MA, et al. A predominantly clonal multi-institutional outbreak of *Clostridium difficile*–associated diarrhea with high morbidity and mortality. N Engl J Med 2005;353:2442–9.

[82] Kaplan V, Clermont G, Griffin MF, et al. Pneumonia, still the old man's friend. Arch Intern Med 2003;103:317–23.

[83] Metersky ML, Tate JP, Fine MJ, et al. Temporal trends in outcomes of older patients with pneumonia. Arch Intern Med 2006;160:3385–91.

[84] Kaplan V, Angus DC, Griffin MF. Hospitalized community acquired pneumonia in the elderly: age and sex-related pattern of care and outcome in the United States. Am J Respir Crit Care Med 2002;165:766–72.

[85] Korvula I, Sten M, Makela PH. Prognosis after community-acquired pneumonia in the elderly: a population-based 12 year follow-up study. Arch Intern Med 1995;157:1550–5.

[86] Gross PA, Hermogenes AW, Sacks HS, et al. The efficacy of influenza vaccine in elderly persons. Ann Intern Med 1995;123(7):518–27.

[87] Nichol KL, Wuorenma J, von Sternberg T. Benefits of influenza vaccination for low-, intermediate-, and high-risk senior citizens. Arch Intern Med 1998;158:1769–76.

[88] Spaude KA, Abrutyn E, Kirchner C, et al. Influenza vaccination and risk of mortality among adults hospitalized with community-acquired pneumonia. Arch Intern Med 2007;167:53–9.

[89] Jackson LA, Neuzil KM, Yu O, et al. Effectiveness of pneumococcal polysaccharide vaccine in older adults. N Engl J Med 2003;348:1747–55.

[90] Whitney CG, Farley MM, Hadler J, et al. Decline in invasive pneumococcal disease after the introduction of protein-polysaccharide conjugate vaccine. N Engl J Med 2003;348:1737–46.

[91] Fisman DN, Abrutyn E, Spaude KA, et al. Prior pneumococcal vaccination is associated with reduced death, complications, and length of stay among hospitalized adults with community-acquired pneumonia. Clin Infect Dis 2006;42:1093–101.

[92] Nuorti JP, Butler JC, Farley MM, et al. Cigarette smoking and invasive pneumococcal disease. N Engl J Med 2000;342:681–9.

CLINICS IN
GERIATRIC
MEDICINE

ELSEVIER
SAUNDERS

Clin Geriatr Med 23 (2007) 535–552

Community-Acquired Viral Pneumonia

Ann R. Falsey, MD[a,b,*]

[a]*Division of Infectious Diseases, Department of Medicine at Rochester General Hospital,
1425 Portland Avenue, Rochester, NY 14621, USA*
[b]*Department of Medicine, University of Rochester School of Medicine and Dentistry,
601 Elmwood Avenue, Rochester, NY 16424, USA*

Respiratory viruses are ubiquitous pathogens that cause acute respiratory illnesses in all age groups [1]. Viral pneumonia occurs most frequently at the extremes of age—in young children and elderly adults. When respiratory viruses first are encountered by children who do not have immunity, particularly during infancy when airways are small and immature, pneumonia may result. Although infection in older adults represents reinfection, viruses again become a more frequent cause of pneumonia because of immunosenescence and the presence of chronic medical conditions. Influenza virus is the viral pathogen that is most well recognized in older adults and is the cause of significant morbidity and mortality in this age group [2,3]. In addition, several common respiratory viruses are implicated in the etiology of pneumonia in older adults (Table 1). Because of the fastidious nature of several of these viruses and imperfect diagnostic tools, the burden of disease likely is underestimated. Newer investigations using reverse transcription polymerase chain reaction (RT-PCR) and sensitive serologic techniques define the frequency of these agents in adults more accurately. Several other systemic viruses (see Table 1) also can cause pneumonia. Most are uncommon in immunocompetent older adults because of pre-existing immunity. Although viral pneumonia cannot be distinguished reliably on clinical grounds alone, some features can help clinicians judge the likelihood of viral infection and the need for laboratory testing (Table 2). The focus of this review is on the role of the common respiratory viruses in immunocompetent older adults who have community-acquired pneumonia, with a brief mention of other viruses that cause pneumonia less frequently. Epidemiology, clinical features, methods of diagnosis, and treatments are discussed.

———————
* Infectious Diseases Unit, Rochester General Hospital, 1425 Portland Avenue, Rochester, NY 14621.
E-mail address: ann.falsey@viahealth.org

Table 1
Viral causes of pneumonia

Respiratory viruses	Other viruses
Influenza viruses A and B	Herpes simplex virus type 1
RSV	Cytomegalovirus
PIVs 1–4	Varicella-zoster virus
hMPV	Epstein-Barr virus
Coronaviruses (CO43, 229,	Hantavirus
SARS, HKU1, and NL63)	
Adenoviruses	
Rhinoviruses	
Human bocaviruses	
Coxsackie viruses	

Epidemiology

The viral contribution to community-acquired pneumonia in adults is difficult to define precisely, because diagnostic tools generally are insensitive. In published series of adults, specifically the elderly, rates of viral pneumonia vary tremendously depending on the type of tests used, populations, and season studied. Viruses are identified in 0.3% to 30% of patients who have community-acquired pneumonia in studies using viral culture and serology for diagnosis (Table 3) [4,5]. Recent studies using RT-PCR for diagnosis have improved the ability to detect viruses considerably [6,7]. In a study of 105 patients who had community-acquired pneumonia, 50% of whom were over age 60, respiratory viruses were detected in 14% of patients using conventional techniques compared with 56% by RT-PCR [7]. In all studies of the etiology of community-acquired pneumonia, regardless of the diagnostic techniques used, influenza A is the viral pathogen identified most commonly, accounting for 4% to 19% of cases [5–12].

Table 2
Common respiratory viruses

Virus	Season	Clinical clues	Incubation	Treatment
Influenza	Winter	Abrupt onset, fever, myalgias	1–2 days	Oseltamivir, aanamivir
RSV	Late fall to late winter	Rhinorrhea, wheezing	2–8 days	Aerosolized ribavirin[a]
hMPV	Late winter	Nonspecific	5–6 days	None available
PIV	Fall to spring	Hoarseness	2–8 days	None available
Coronaviruses	Winter	Nonspecific	1–3 days	None available
Rhinoviruses	All year, fall	Rhinorrhea	8 hours to 2 days	None available

[a] Not approved for use in adults.

Table 3
Studies of community-acquired pneumonia, including viral diagnostics

Year	Location	Methods	Age (years)	% Viral	Most common virus	Second most common virus
1993–1995	Spain [9]	Serology	54 ± 21	14	Influenza	RSV/PIV
1998–1999	England [12]	Serology	65 ± 20	23	Influenza	RSV
1998–2000	Japan [11]	Serology	>65	13	NA	NA
1996–2001	Spain [8]	Serology	68 ± 18	18	Influenza	PIV
200–2002	USA [36]	Serology	61	10	Influenza	RSV
2000–2002	Netherlands [7]	Culture, serology, PCR	>60	46	Coronavirus/ rhinovirus	Influenza
2002–2004	Netherlands [6]	Culture, RT-PCR	64 ± 16	29	Influenza	Coronavirus
2003	Belgium [5]	Culture, serology	82 ± 7	30	Influenza	RSV
2003–2004	Spain [10]	Antigen, culture, RT-PCR	NA	23	Influenza	Rhinovirus/ adenovirus

Specific viruses

Influenza virus

Influenza viruses are segmented RNA viruses that are classified as A, B, or C, based on stable internal proteins [13]. Influenza viruses A and B are the most significant human pathogens and are capable of causing serious lower respiratory tract disease, whereas influenza C generally causes mild upper respiratory tract disease. Influenza A viruses are classified further based on the two surface envelope proteins, hemagglutinin (H) and neuraminidase (N). These glycoproteins are the primary targets of neutralizing antibody. At least 16 antigenically distinct hemagglutinin (H1–H16) and nine neuraminidase (N1–N9) proteins are described. H1–H3 viruses currently are the primary pathogens in humans, whereas the others generally are found in other mammals and aquatic birds. As with most RNA viruses, influenza A viruses are prone to a high degree of genomic mutations during replication, which leads to minor changes in the H and N proteins. These changes are referred to as antigenic "drift" and account for seasonal influenza epidemics. Because influenza A has a segmented genome, two influenza viruses can exchange H or N genes, with resultant viruses containing a completely new H or N gene. This phenomenon is referred to as antigenic "shift" and may result in worldwide pandemics. During the past century, three pandemics occurred: 1918 (H1N1), 1957 (H2N2), and 1968 (H3N2). Currently, two type A viruses circulate (H1N1 and H3N2) and influenza B. H3N2 viruses tend to be most severe in the elderly. Partial immunity to H1N1 virus, resulting from exposure in the early part of the twentieth century, is postulated as a mechanism for milder H1N1 disease in this age group.

In 1997, influenza A (H5N1), previously seen only in birds, crossed the species barrier and human infection occurred in Southeast Asia [14]. This highly pathogenic avian influenza has spread in bird populations throughout Asia and into Europe. To date, human infection is rare and transmission has occurred primarily by direct contact with infected birds. Transmission between humans is limited but the possibility of mutation allowing efficient person-to-person spread makes avian influenza (H5N1) the greatest pandemic threat since 1918.

Seasonal influenza virus is a predictable cause of wintertime respiratory disease. Epidemics usually last 6 to 8 weeks and can occur anytime between November and April, with highly variable severity. The virus is transmitted most efficiently by small particle aerosols generated by coughing and sneezing; thus, explosive outbreaks can occur in closed settings, such as nursing homes [15]. Influenza results in approximately 36,000 deaths and more than 200,000 hospital admissions in the United States every year [16]. Age-specific hospitalization rates resulting from influenza form a J-shaped curve in which rates are high in ages below 5, decline in ages 5 to 49, and rise significantly for those age 50 or older [3]. Rates of hospitalization rise significantly with each decade over age 60, rising from 190 per 100,000 for ages 65 to 69 to 1195 per 100,000 for those over age 85. Increases in mortality are more dramatic, rising from 19 to 358 per 100,000 for the previously noted age groups.

The classic description of influenza pneumonia was by Louria and colleagues [17] after the 1957 to 1958 H2N2 pandemic. Lower tract disease was classified into four categories: (1) no radiographic pneumonia; (2) viral infection followed by bacterial pneumonia; (3) rapidly progressive viral pneumonia; and (4) concomitant viral-bacterial pneumonia. Diffuse infiltrates previously were seen in patients who had rheumatic heart disease–associated mitral stenosis (Fig. 1). Although age is a significant risk factor for the development of lower respiratory tract complications to influenza, pure viral pneumonia is uncommon outside pandemic settings in nonimmunocompromised hosts [18,19]. Most elderly persons have partial immunity resulting from previous vaccination or natural infections. In a recent study of highly vaccinated elderly in the community who subsequently were documented to have influenza, approximately 5% developed pneumonia [20]. In a survey of 193 patients hospitalized with influenza A, approximately half (101) had radiographic findings consistent with acute disease [21]. Of these, 33% had definitive infiltrates, 45% had atelectasis versus pneumonia, 15% had edema, and 7% had edema versus infiltrates. Most infiltrates were subtle and unilateral and involved the left lower lobe (Fig. 2). Documented bacterial infection was observed in 8% of cases. Pneumonia and progression to acute respiratory distress syndrome (ARDS) and death are common with influenza A (H5N1). Limited microbiologic data indicate that this syndrome is a primary viral pneumonia. Unlike epidemic influenza, avian influenza to date is most severe in children under age 15.

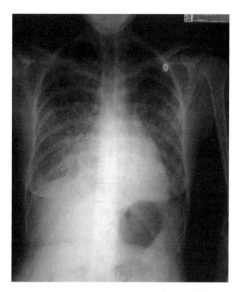

Fig. 1. Chest radiograph of a 63-year-old woman who had mitral stenosis admitted to the hospital with severe respiratory distress and culture positive influenza A infection. Diffuse pulmonary infiltrates are illustrated.

The typical manifestations of influenza (abrupt fever, cough, myalgias, and headache) may be altered in somewhat older persons [22,23]. Fever, although still common, may be lower and the presence of underlying cardiac and pulmonary conditions may obscure the diagnosis. In addition, patients who have cognitive impairment may be unable to articulate their symptoms.

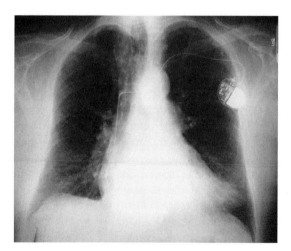

Fig. 2. Chest radiograph of a 75-year-old man admitted to the hospital with fever, cough, and dyspnea. Influenza A was diagnosed by RT-PCR and confirmed by serology. A patchy opacity is demonstrated in the left lung base.

Among elderly outpatients, cough, fever, and acute onset of symptoms had a positive predictive value for influenza of 30% in contrast to young adults, in whom this triad of symptoms had a value of 78% [23]. The presence of gastrointestinal complaints, fever, and myalgias, with a lack of significant rhinorrhea and wheezing, may help distinguish influenza from respiratory syncytial virus (RSV), another common winter virus [24,25]. Because of infection control issues and potential therapeutic interventions, clinicians should have a high index of suspicion for influenza during the winter months, particularly when viral activity is high.

The diagnosis of influenza frequently is made on the basis of clinical presentation when viral activity is high in the community. Because of cocirculation of several other respiratory viruses, however, laboratory confirmation generally is recommended. Viral diagnostics include culture, antigen detection, RT-PCR, and serology [26]. Nasal swabs are believed better specimens than throat swabs to detect influenza viruses [13]. Sputum, endotracheal secretions, and bronchoalveolar lavage specimens also can be used to detect virus. Viral culture is the time-honored technique for identifying influenza infection. Influenza virus is hardy and grows well in culture but generally 2 to 3 days is required for cytopathic effect to be evident. Thus, culture is of limited value for making therapeutic or isolation decisions. The use of shell viral culture can shorten time to detection to approximately 24 hours [27]. Rapid antigen testing is available for influenza A and B and offers immediate results. These tests offer a sensitivity of approximately 50% to 60% and sensitivity of 90% or greater in adults [28]. Because false-negative results are common, patients who have pneumonia and negative test in whom a high index of suspicion of influenza based on clinical grounds exists should be considered for empiric treatment. Molecular testing, such as RT-PCR, offers the best combination of sensitivity and specificity for diagnosis of acute influenza but is labor intensive, expensive, and currently not widely available. Most assays use primers complementary to the conserved matrix gene [26]. RT-PCR can be useful in patients who are immunocompromised. Because all adults have antibody, a single serologic test is not useful for the acute diagnosis of influenza. Serologic testing demonstrating a fourfold or greater rise in influenza-specific antibody can be used to make a diagnosis as long as vaccine effect does not complicate interpretation.

Four antivirals—amantadine, rimantadine, zanamivir, and oseltamavir—are approved for the treatment of influenza infection [13]. Amantadine and rimantadine are active against influenza A, whereas zanamivir and oseltamavir are active against influenza A and B. These agents are 70% to 90% effective for prophylaxis and reduce illness severity, duration of symptoms, and viral shedding when given within 48 hours of symptom onset in uncomplicated influenza. Data are limited regarding the effectiveness of antiviral treatment of influenza pneumonia. The duration of patients' symptoms before admission usually presents a dilemma, because the average number of days most are ill is 3 to 4 days, falling outside the recommended 48-hour window of symptom duration for drug treatment [29]. Although no official recommendation can be made because risks and benefits must be weighed in individual clinical situations, many authorities believe treatment of patients who are antigen positive is reasonable because a significant viral load in secretions is needed to generate a positive rapid test. If a decision is made to use antiviral therapy, it is important to consider the type of influenza being treated (A or B), issues of drug resistance, and the possible adverse reactions of specific medications. The Centers for Disease Control and Prevention recently reported that 92% of influenza A (H3N2) and 25% of influenza A (H1N1) were resistant to the adamantanes [13]. Although only a total of 217 isolates was tested, isolates were obtained from 26 states and for this reason, use of this class of drugs is not recommended at the present time. Zanamivir and oseltamivir are effective for influenza A and B and, currently, rates of resistance are low. Each antiviral agent has different side-effect profiles that must be considered in treatment selection (Table 4). Zanamivir is associated with bronchospasm and decline in forced expiratory volume in 1 second in some patients who have underlying lung disease and is not recommended for patients who have asthma or chronic obstructive pulmonary disease (COPD) [30]. Oseltamivir generally is well tolerated, although approximately 10% of recipients experience associated nausea and vomiting. The precise rate of bacterial complications of nonpandemic influenza is difficult to ascertain. Observational studies report ranges of 8% to 36% [31]. Physicians treating frail, elderly patients who have pneumonia and who have documented influenza face a challenge when deciding if antibiotics

Table 4
Influenza antivirals

Drug/use	Route	Treatment dose	Renal impairment (creatine clearance 10–30 mL/min)	Adverse effects
Zanamivir				
Treatment	Inhaled	10 mg (2 inhalations) twice daily for 5 days	No adjustment	Bronchospasm; inhaler system may be difficult for older adults to use
Chemoprophylaxis	Inhaled	10 mg (2 inhalations) twice daily for 5 days	No adjustment	
Oseltamivir				
Treatment	Oral	75 mg twice daily for 5 days	75 mg once daily	Nausea and vomiting
Chemoprophylaxis	Oral	75 mg twice daily for 5 days	75 mg every other day	

Adapted from Prevention and control of influenza: recommendations of the advisory committee of immunization practices (ACIP). MMWR Recomm Rep 2006;55:1–48.

are needed. Decisions must be individualized based on duration of symptoms, patient stability, white blood cell count, and results of blood and sputum cultures.

Respiratory syncytial virus

RSV is a common wintertime respiratory virus that affects persons of all ages and is the major cause of serious lower respiratory tract infections in young children [32]. For many years after its discovery in 1956, RSV was considered strictly a pediatric pathogen; however, it recently has been recognized increasingly as a serious adult pathogen [20]. Human RSV is an enveloped RNA virus and is a member of the family, Paramyxoviridae, classified within the genus, *Pneumovirus* [33]. RSV can be classified into two major groups, A and B, based primarily on antigenic differences found in one of the surface glycoproteins but, unlike in influenza, major antigenic shifts do not occur. RSV is a predictable cause of yearly epidemics of winter respiratory illnesses in temperate climates and activity typically begins in late fall and generally lasts 4 to 5 months, ending in late spring. Unlike influenza, which tends to produce a sharp peak in respiratory illness over 6 to 8 weeks, the epidemic curve of RSV generally is broader.

Estimates using national health care databases and viral surveillance data indicate that approximately 10,000 deaths in persons over age 65 in the United States each year are attributable to RSV. Several epidemiologic studies and mathematic models indicate that RSV is second to influenza as a cause of serious viral respiratory disease in adults [16,34]. Several studies have examined the frequency of RSV as a cause of community-acquired pneumonia and estimates vary widely (0–14%) depending on the diagnostic tools used and season of study [35]. In a large study of approximately 1200 adults admitted to the hospital with a diagnosis of pneumonia, investigators found that RSV was identified in 4.4% of cases and was the pathogen identified third most commonly after *Streptococcus pneumoniae* and influenza [36]. A recent study of community-acquired pneumonia from Spain using a combination of diagnostic techniques found RSV to be the cause of 5 of 198 (3%) of adult patients who had pneumonia [10]. In composite, using data from the past 30 years, RSV accounts for 2% to 5% of pneumonia throughout the year and 5% to 15% during the winter months.

Although the clinical manifestations are difficult to distinguish from influenza, there are a few helpful clinical clues that suggest RSV infection. In a recent study of 118 RSV- and 133 influenza A–infected hospitalized patients, several signs and symptoms were found significantly different. RSV-infected subjects were more likely to have nasal congestion, wheezing, and a productive cough compared with influenza-infected patients and less likely to have high-grade fever [37]. In addition, the duration of symptoms before admission was 1.3 days longer for patients who had RSV compared with those who had influenza. Thus, in elderly patients who present to the hospital with pneumonia and have a low-grade fever and wheezing, particularly if preceded by a "cold," the diagnosis of RSV infection should be entertained.

The radiographic findings associated with RSV vary from patchy subsegmental alveolar densities to lobar consolidation [36]. In a recent review of chest radiographs from 118 elderly adults hospitalized with RSV in whom known concomitant bacterial infections were excluded, opacities consistent with pneumonia were described in 20% of chest radiographs and an additional 13% had infiltrates believed to be atelectasis or pneumonia. Opacities generally were basilar, unilateral, and relatively subtle (Fig. 3). Few patients had diffuse interstitial infiltrates considered typical for viral pneumonia. Bacterial pathogens are demonstrated in up to 30% of adult RSV cases, although the adequacy of specimens commonly is not addressed [35]. In Walsh and colleagues' [37] recent study of 132 hospital patients who had RSV, 15% had a potential pathogen identified in an adequate sputum sample and 3% had positive blood cultures. Unlike those who had only virus identified, 5 of 14 of these individuals had large pulmonary infiltrates with consolidation.

Because RSV does not produce a distinctive clinical syndrome in adults, laboratory testing is required for specific viral diagnosis. The first diagnostic hurdle for RSV is consideration of the diagnosis. Because RSV is known best as a pediatric pathogen, it is not considered frequently in adults. In addition, the labile nature of the virus and low titers of virus in nasal secretions in the elderly make diagnosis of acute RSV infection problematic. Viral culture, rapid antigen tests, and RT-PCR can be used for diagnosis of acute infection and serology for retrospective diagnosis. A variety of specimens can be tested by the means described previously, including nasopharyngeal swabs, nasal washes, sputum, or bronchiolar lavages. Under ideal

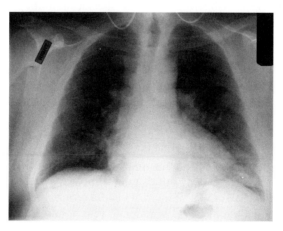

Fig. 3. Chest radiograph of a 68-year-old man who had a history of emphysema admitted to the hospital with a history of recent "cold," low-grade fever, wheezing, and dyspnea. RSV infection was documented by viral culture and serology. Patchy airspace disease is seen in the lung bases bilaterally.

circumstances, viral culture is only 20% to 50% sensitive compared with serology using enzyme immunoassay (EIA) [35]. Unlike for influenza, commercial rapid antigen tests for RSV have poor sensitivity in adults. In a study of 60 older persons who had RSV documented by serology or RT-PCR, rapid testing by indirect fluorescence assay was positive in only 23% and by EIA in only 10% [38]. RT-PCR is used more successfully to detect RSV in adult populations [39]. In a study of more than 1000 adult nasal samples, RT-PCR was 73% sensitive and 99% specific compared with viral culture, which was 39% sensitive and 100% specific [40]. Although RT-PCR is sensitive and specific, the test currently is limited by expense, labor intensity, and limited commercial availability. The NucliSens EasyQ RSV A+B assay is a commercial real-time nucleic acid sequence amplification system that uses molecular beacons [41]. This assay is simpler to perform than traditional RT-PCR and may represent a method that can be used by clinical laboratories for adult diagnosis. Recent data suggest that sputum may be a better sample than nasal specimens if RT-PCR is used for diagnosis [42]. Infection also can be demonstrated retrospectively by a fourfold or greater rise in RSV-specific IgG, either by complement fixation or EIA. Because RSV in adults always represents reinfection, a single elevated titer is not useful for acute diagnosis. RSV-specific IgM has been detected in 11% to 81% of older subjects who have acute RSV, but its clinical usefulness has yet to be defined [43].

The treatment of RSV pneumonia in elderly adults largely is supportive with antipyretics, intravenous fluids, and oxygen as needed. It may be reasonable to administer corticosteroids and bronchodilators to patients who are wheezing acutely, although no formal controlled trials to use such agents for treatment of RSV-related wheezing have been performed. Antiviral therapy with aerosolized ribavirin and RSV-specific immunoglobulin are approved for high-risk infants, but only anecdotal data are available in adults [32]. Although the general use of ribavirin cannot be recommended, its use may be considered in selected cases, such as for patients who are immunocompromised. Anecdotal experience suggests that high-dose, short-duration therapy (60 mg/mL for 2 hours given by mask 3 times a day) in nonintubated adults is tolerated better than tent treatment [44].

Parainfluenza viruses

Parainfluenza viruses (PIVs) are single-stranded RNA viruses belonging to the paramyxovirus family. Four distinct serotypes are recognized, termed 1, 2, 3, and 4A and 4B [45]. These viruses cause croup, bronchitis, and pneumonia in young children. PIV-3 is endemic year round, whereas PIV-1 and PIV-2 tend to peak during the fall months. PIV-3 is associated most often with pneumonia in children [1]. Infection recurs throughout adulthood, accounting for 1% to 15% of acute respiratory illnesses with occasional reports of pneumonia in young adults. The burden of disease resulting from

PIV in the elderly is not well studied, but pneumonia is reported [46]. Investigators in Sweden found that 11% of elderly persons who had community-acquired pneumonia had serologic evidence of recent PIV-1 or PIV-3 [47]. Prospective studies in nursing homes have documented PIV infection in 4% to 14% of respiratory illnesses and fatal cases of bronchopneumonia are described [48]. PIV also is implicated as a precursor to an outbreak of invasive pneumococcal disease in a long-term care facility [49]. Clinical syndromes, characterized by fever, rhinorrhea, hoarseness, cough, and sore throat, are not distinctive. Viral culture, RT-PCR, and serologic tests can be used to diagnose PIV infection. At the present time there are no commercially available rapid antigen tests. Ribavirin has activity in vitro against PIV but is not approved for treatment of PIV pneumonia [45].

Human metapneumovirus

Human metapneumovirus (hMPV) was identified by Dutch researchers, in 2001, in young children who had bronchiolitis [50]. hMPV also is an RNA virus in the paramyxovirus family. The virus is shown to have worldwide distribution; by age 5, all children are infected. In temperate climates, the virus circulates predominantly in the winter months overlapping with activity of influenza virus and RSV. Several studies suggest there may be significant year-to-year variation in incidence rates [51]. Infection with hMPV in young children causes a syndrome similar to RSV, with bronchiolitis and pneumonia the most common manifestations. Asymptomatic infection, colds, asthma exacerbations, and flu-like illnesses are documented in older children and healthy young adults [52]. Pneumonia and exacerbation of COPD are documented in elderly adults; however, comprehensive studies have not yet been published [53]. In a 2-year study of elderly and high-risk adults, hMPV infection was identified in 4.1%, using RT-PCR and serology for diagnosis [51]. Twenty-five percent of patients hospitalized with hMPV had infiltrates on chest radiographs. Illness may be more severe in frail elderly, as evidenced by a Canadian study in which pneumonia was documented in 40% of hMPV-infected nursing home residents [54]. The clinical characteristics of hMPV pneumonia in older adults do not appear distinctive from the other wintertime respiratory viruses, although rates of fever seem higher than with RSV and are similar to influenza. Diagnosis of hMPV outside research settings is difficult. The virus has special growth requirements and cytopathic effect can take up to 3 weeks to be detectable [50]. RT-PCR and serology are used successfully in research settings and transplant units, but these assays are not widely available commercially. Similar to PIV, ribavirin has activity in vitro but is not approved for treatment of hMPV infection.

Coronaviruses

Coronaviruses are RNA viruses, discovered in 1965, and are the second most frequent cause of the common cold after rhinoviruses [55]. Similar to hMPV, studies of human illness are limited by the inability to grow the virus under routine conditions. Two groups of coronaviruses are identified and four strains identified as causes of acute respiratory illnesses, ranging from colds to pneumonia, and include group 1 (229E and NL63) and group 2 (OC43 and HKU1) [56]. A novel coronavirus, SARS-CoV, which represents an early split from group 2, was identified in 2002 as the cause of the severe acute respiratory syndrome (SARS) epidemic, which originated in China and spread quickly to distant locations around the world [57].

OC43 and 229E occur most often in late winter and early spring demonstrating 2- to 3-year periodicity. Infection in healthy adults is characterized by low-grade fever, malaise, and nasal symptoms. Pneumonia is described in young children, patients who are immunocompromised, and the elderly [58,59]. Using RT-PCR, coronaviruses were identified in 17% of community elderly who had acute respiratory illnesses in a recent Dutch study and 50% had lower respiratory tract symptoms [59]. Coronavirus lower respiratory tract disease is described in frail elderly attending senior daycare, where 66% of infected persons complained of a productive cough and 34% were short of breath [60]. In a study from China, investigators examined the frequency and clinical features of the newly described coronavirus HKU1 [61]. Of 418 patients admitted to the hospital with community-acquired pneumonia, 2.4% had evidence of coronavirus HKU1 by RT-PCR. All cases occurred between January and May. Of the 10 patients identified, eight were over age 65. Preceding upper respiratory tract symptoms were noted in only two patients. Clinically, illnesses were not distinguishable from other causes of community-acquired pneumonia. Two patients who had multiple chronic medical problems died. Another new strain of coronavirus discovered recently, HCOV-NL63, is found to circulate in summer and autumn and is associated with upper respiratory infection, bronchiolitis, and asthma exacerbations in children [62]. Little data on H COV-NL63 in the elderly exist. Nineteen of 525 respiratory specimens collected from patients who had winter respiratory illnesses in Canada were positive by RT-PCR for this pathogen [63]. Nine of 19 (47%) were elderly persons. Symptoms primarily were fever, sore throat, and cough. Most coronavirus studies to date do not describe radiographic findings; thus, the frequency of coronavirus pneumonia remains unknown.

Although SARS-CoV currently is quiescent, the clinical syndrome is worth describing, because older age is a significant risk factor for death [57]. Infected persons present initially with fever, myalgias, cough, and chills. Unlike other respiratory viruses, rhinorrhea and sore throat are uncommon symptoms. Approximately two thirds of patients develop persistent fever, tachypnea, hypoxia, and diarrhea. Serial chest radiographs reveal progressive multifocal airspace disease. Age and coexisting medical conditions are independent risk factors for risk for death, and in patients older than 65, the mortality rate exceeds 50%. Although therapies, such as ribavirin, corticosteroids, and intravenous gamma globulin, are used for treatment of SARS, there are no randomized placebo controlled trials by which to assess benefit.

Rhinoviruses

Rhinoviruses, the most frequent cause of the common cold, circulate throughout the year but have peaks in the fall and spring [64]. Infections are common at all ages, including the elderly, and account for approximately 25% to 50% of respiratory illnesses in community-dwelling elderly [65]. Outbreaks also are documented in long-term care facilities and senior daycare centers [60,66]. Prominent nasal congestion, cough, and constitutional symptoms characterize illnesses. The role of rhinoviruses in pneumonia remains somewhat controversial. Replication of rhinoviruses is restricted at core body temperature and for this reason rhinoviruses once were dismissed as a cause of pneumonia. Recently, rhinoviruses have been recovered from lower airways after experimental challenge and cases of pneumonia described in very young children and patients who are severely immunocompromised [67]. The role of rhinoviruses as a cause of community-acquired pneumonia in older adults remains to be determined.

Herpes simplex virus

Herpes simplex virus (HSV) rarely causes lower respiratory tract disease in adults despite the fact the mucocutaneous reactivation of HSV during periods of stress is common [68]. Patients at risk for HSV pneumonia include those who have immunosuppression, severe burns, AIDS, or trauma. Age per se is not a specific risk factor, but older adults may reactivate HSV because of any of these factors. Because the isolation of HSV is possible as a result of asymptomatic reactivation, interpretation of cultures may be difficult. For example, HSV was isolated in 74% and 65% of upper and lower respiratory tract samples in one series of patients who had ARDS; however, pathogenicity was unclear [69].

Herpetic pneumonia can present either as localized or a disseminated pneumonia. Focal pneumonia is attributed to direct spread or a virus from the upper tract with tracheitis or esophagitis to the lower tract from aspiration of infected secretion [70]. The disseminated form results from viremia and occurs in patients who are severely immunocompromised. Fever is common as are cough and dyspnea. Chest pain and hemoptysis also may occur and mucocutaneous lesions are present in all patients. Because oral lesions in the majority of patients are not associated with lung involvement and contamination of bronchoalveolar lavage, specimens from upper airway secretions are a problem, definitive diagnosis requires the finding of histologic or cytologic examination of lower tract specimen showing necrotizing or hemorrhagic pneumonia with viral inclusion bodies [70]. Infection is localized mainly to the trachea and large bronchi, and a thick inflammatory membrane and mucosal ulcerations may be seen. Endobronchial biopsy is preferred for diagnosis compared with open lung biopsy. Acyclovir is active against HSV and has decreased mortality in disseminated HSV and pneumonia in children; however, in adults who have ARDS, the benefit is less clear [69]. No controlled trials of acyclovir for pneumonia have been done, and risks and benefits must be weighed in individual cases.

Other viruses

Several other viruses are implicated as causes of pneumonia in children or young adults; however, data in the elderly are lacking. Adenoviruses, in particular types 4 and 7, are linked to large outbreaks of respiratory disease and severe pneumonia in young adults living in congregate settings [71]. In the author's experience, adenovirus is not a frequent pathogen in elderly adults. Human bocavirus is a newly discovered parvovirus [72]. The virus has been identified by RT-PCR in respiratory samples from children who have lower respiratory tract illnesses; however, no data are available in adults. Several systemic viruses, such as varicella zoster and measles, not uncommonly cause pneumonia when acquired in adulthood, yet are uncommon in the elderly because of pre-existing immunity. Hantaviruses primarily are pathogens of rodents but may be transmitted to humans by contact with rodent excrement or bites [73]. Cases are reported in the southwestern United States. Human infection results in a febrile prodrome followed by pulmonary edema and shock. Progression may be rapid, and laboratory findings include elevated hematocrit and white blood cell count with thrombocytopenia. Treatment is supportive. Although primary Epstein-Barr virus is uncommon in the elderly, when it occurs, clinical syndromes can be atypical and pneumonia is described [74].

Summary

Aging can be associated with functional and immunologic decline and chronic cardiopulmonary diseases that predispose to pneumonia when viral infection occurs. Influenza virus remains the primary viral pathogen in the elderly, although the true impact of the other respiratory viruses remains to be defined as more sensitive diagnostic tools are developed. Unfortunately, the clinical syndromes associated with respiratory viruses frequently are indistinguishable from one another and bacterial pathogens. Because healthy elderly persons may visit exotic locations, which place them at risk for emerging pathogens, a travel history is important in the workup of pneumonia of older adults. Antiviral therapy is available for influenza A and B; thus, specific viral diagnosis may be useful for clinical management. Rapid antigen tests, although not as sensitive as viral culture or new molecular techniques, are widely available and offer quick turnaround times. RSV, PIV, hMPV, and coronaviruses in composite contribute to a substantial proportion of the community-acquired pneumonia cases in the elderly but at the present time treatment primarily is supportive.

References

[1] Treanor JJ. Viral infections of the respiratory tract: prevention and treatment. Int J Antimicrob Agents 1994;4:1–22.

[2] Barker WH, Mullooly JP. Impact of epidemic a influenza in a defined adult population. Am J Epidemiol 1980;112:798–811.

[3] Thompson WW, Shay DK, Weintraub E, et al. Influenza-associated hospitalizations in the united states. JAMA 2004;292:1333–40.

[4] Fang G, Fine M, Orloff J, et al. New and emerging etiologies for community-acquired pneumonia with implications for therapy. A prospective multicenter study of 359 cases. Medicine 1990;69:307–15.

[5] Flamaing J, Engelmann I, Joosten E, et al. Viral lower respiratory tract infection in the elderly: a prospective in-hospital study. Eur J Clin Microbiol Infect Dis 2003;22:720–5.

[6] Oosterheert JJ, van Loon AM, Schuurman R, et al. Impact of rapid detection of viral and atypical bacterial pathogens by real-time polymerase chain reaction for patients with lower respiratory tract infection. Clin Infect Dis 2005;41:1438–44.

[7] Templeton KE, Scheltinga SA, van den Eeden WC, et al. Improved diagnosis of the etiology of community-acquired pneumonia with real-time polymerase chain reaction. Clin Infect Dis 2005;41:345–51.

[8] de Roux A, Marcos MA, Garcia E, et al. Viral community-acquired pneumonia in nonimmunocompromised adults. Chest 2004;125:1343–51.

[9] Almirall J, Bolibar I, Vidal J, et al. Epidemiology of community-acquired pneumonia in adults: a population-based study. Eur Respir J 2000;15:757–63.

[10] Angeles Marcos M, Camps M, Pumarola T, et al. The role of viruses in the aetiology of community-acquired pneumonia in adults. Antivir Ther 2006;11:351–9.

[11] Kobashi Y, Okimoto N, Matsushima T, et al. Clinical analysis of community-acquired pneumonia in the elderly. Intern Med 2001;40:703–7.

[12] Lim WS, Macfarlane JT, Boswell TC, et al. Study of community acquired pneumonia aetiology (SCAPA) in adults admitted to hospital: implications for management guidelines. Thorax 2001;56:296–301.

[13] Prevention and control of influenza: recommendations of the advisory committee of immunization practices (ACIP). MMWR Recomm Rep 2006;55:1–48.

[14] World health organization. Current concepts: avian influenza A (H5N1) infection in humans. N Engl J Med 2005;353:1374–85.

[15] Gravenstein S, Miller BA, Drinka P. Prevention and control of influenza a outbreaks in long term care facilities. Infect Control Hosp Epidemiol 1992;13:49–54.

[16] Thompson WW, Shay DK, Weintraub E, et al. Mortality associated with influenza and respiratory syncytial virus in the united states. J Am Med Assoc 2003;289:179–86.

[17] Louria DE, Blumenfeld HL, Ellis JT, et al. Studies on influenza in the pandemic of 1957–1958. II. Pulmonary complications of influenza. J Clin Invest 1959;38:213–65.

[18] Fry J. Influenza, 1959: the story of an epidemic. Br Med J 1959;2:135–8.

[19] Foy HH, Cooney MK, Allan I, et al. Rates of pneumonia during influenza epidemics in seattle 1964–1975. JAMA 1979;241:253–8.

[20] Falsey AR, Hennessey PA, Formica MA, et al. Respiratory syncytial virus infection in elderly and high-risk adults. N Engl J Med 2005;352:1749–59.

[21] Murata Y, Walsh EE, Falsey AR. Pulmonary complication of influenza a infections in the inter-pandemic era. J Infect Dis, in press.

[22] Cate TR. Clinical manifestations and consequences of influenza. Am J Med 1987;82:15–9.

[23] Govaert TME, Dinant GJ, Aretz K, et al. The predictive value of influenza symptomatology in elderly peole. Fam Pract 1998;15:16–22.

[24] Mathur U, Bentley DW, Hall CB. Concurrent respiratory syncytial virus and influenza a infections in the institutionalized elderly and chronically ill. Ann Intern Med 1980; 93:49–52.

[25] Wald TG, Miller BA, Shult P, et al. Can respiratory syncytial virus and influenza a be distinguished clinically in institutionalized older persons? J Am Geriatr Soc 1995;43: 170–4.

[26] Petric M, Comanor L, Petti CA. Role of the laboratory in diagnosis of influenza during seasonal epidemics and potential pandemics. J Infect Dis 2006;194(Suppl 2):S98–110.

[27] Schirm J, Luijt DS, Pastoor GW, et al. Rapid detection of respiratory viruses using mixtures of monoclonal antibodies on shell viral cultures. J Med Virol 1992;38:147–51.

[28] Storch GA. Rapid tests for influenza. Curr Opin Pediatr 2003;15:77–84.

[29] Walsh EE, Cox C, Falsey AR. Clinical features of influenza a virus infection in elderly hospitalized persons. J Am Geriatr Soc 2002;50:1498–503.

[30] Williamson JC, Pegram PS. Respiratory distress associated with zanamivir. N Engl J Med 2000;342:661–2.

[31] Falsey AR, Murata Y, Walsh EE. Impact of rapid diagnosis on management of adults hospitalized with influenza. Arch Intern Med 2007;167:354–60.

[32] Hall CB. Respiratory syncytial virus and parainfluenza virus. N Engl J Med 2001;334: 1917–28.

[33] Collins P. The molecular biology of human respiratory syncytial viruses (RSV) of the genus pneumovirus. In: Kingsbury DW, editor. The paramyxoviruses. New York: Plenum Publishing; 1991. p. 103–62.

[34] Nicholson KG. Impact of influenza and respiratory syncytial virus on mortality in England and Wales from january 1975 to december 1990. Epidemiol Infect 1996;116:51–63.

[35] Falsey AR, Walsh EE. Respiratory syncytial virus infection in adults. Clin Microbiol Rev 2000;13:371–84.

[36] Dowell SF, Anderson LJ, Gary HEJ, et al. Respiratory syncytial virus is an important cause of community-acquired lower respiratory infection among hospitalized adults. J Infect Dis 1996;174:456–62.

[37] EE Walsh, DR Peterson, AR Falsey. Clinical recognition of respiratory syncytial virus infection in hospitalized elderly and high-risk adults possible? J Infect Dis 2007;195:1046–51.

[38] Casiano-Colon AE, Hulbert BB, Mayer TK, et al. Lack of sensitivity of rapid antigen tests for the diagnosis of respiratory syncytial infection in adults. J Clin Virol 2003;28:169–74.

[39] Zambon MC, Stockton JD, Clewley JP, et al. Contribution of influenza and respiratory syncytial virus to community cases of influenza-like illness: an observational study. Lancet 2001; 358:1410–6.

[40] Falsey AR, Formica MA, Walsh EE. Diagnosis of respiratory syncytial virus infection: comparison of reverse transcription-PCR to viral culture and serology in adults with respiratory illness. J Clin Microbiol 2002;40:817–20.

[41] Moore C, Valappil M, Corden S, et al. Enhanced clinical utility of the NucliSens EasyQ RSV A+B assay for tapid detection of respiratory syncytial virus in clinical samples. Eur J Clin Microbiol Infect Dis 2006;25:167–74.

[42] Falsey AR, Formica MA, Hennessey PA, et al. Detection of respiratory syncytial virus in adults with chronic obstructive pulmonary disease. Am J Respir Crit Care Med 2005;173: 639–43.

[43] Vikerfors T, Grandien M, Johansson M, et al. Detection of an immunoglobulin M response in the elderly for early diagnosis of respiratory syncytial virus infection. J Clin Microbiol 1988;26:808–11.

[44] Englund JA, Piedra P, Jefferson LS, et al. High-dose, short duration ribavirin aerosol therapy in children with suspected respiratory syncytial virus infection. J Pediatr 1990;117: 313–20.

[45] Henrickson KJ. Parainfluenza viruses. Clin Micro Rev 2003;16:242–64.

[46] Marx A, Gary HE, Martston BJ, et al. Parainfluenza virus infection among adults hospitalized for lower respiratory tract infection. Clin Infect Dis 1999;29:134–40.

[47] Fransen H, Heigl Z, Wolontis S, et al. Infections with viruses in patients hospitalized with acute respiratory illness, stockholm 1963–1967. Scand J Infect Dis 1969;1:127–36.

[48] Public Health Laboratory Service Communicable Disease Surveillance Centre. Parainfluenza infections in the elderly 1976–82. Br Med J 1983;287:1619.

[49] Fiore AE, Iverson C, Messmer T, et al. Outbreak of pneumonia in a long-term care facility: antecedent human parainfluenza virus 1 infection may predispose to bacterial pneumonia. J Am Geriatr Soc 1998;46:1112–7.

[50] van den Hoogen BG, DeJong JC, Groen J, et al. A newly discovered human pneumovirus isolated from young children with respiratory tract disease. Nat Med 2001;7:719–24.

[51] Falsey AR, Erdman D, Anderson LJ, et al. Human metapneumovirus infections in young and elderly adults. J Infect Dis 2003;187:785–90.

[52] Hamelin ME, Abed Y, Boivin G. Human metapneumovirus: a new player among respiratory viruses. Clin Infect Dis 2004;38:983–90.

[53] Hamelin ME, Cote S, Laforge J, et al. Human metapneumovirus infection in adults with community-acquired pneumonia and exacerbation of chronic obstructive pulmonary disease. Clin Infect Dis 2005;41:498–502.

[54] Boivin G, Abed Y, Pelletier G, et al. Virological features and clinical manifestations associated with human metapneumovirus: a new paramyxovirus responsible for acute respiratory-tract infections in all age groups. J Infect Dis 2002;186:1330–4.

[55] Larson HE, Reed SE, Tyrrell DAJ. Isolation of rhinoviruses and coronaviruses from 38 colds in adults. J Med Virol 1980;5:221–9.

[56] Lau SK, Woo PC, Yip CC, et al. Coronavirus HKU1 and other coronavirus infections in Hong Kong. J Clin Microbiol 2006;44:2063–71.

[57] Peiris JSM, Yuen KY, Osterhaus AD, et al. The severe acute respiratory syndrome. N Engl J Med 2003;349:2431–41.

[58] El-Sahly HM, Atmar RL, Glezen WP, et al. Spectrum of clinical illness in hospitalized patients with "common cold" virus infections. Clin Infect Dis 2000;31:96–100.

[59] Graat JM, Schouten EG, Heijnen MA, et al. A prospective, community-based study on virologic assessment among elderly people with and without symptoms of acute respiratory infection. J Clin Epidemiol 2003;56:1218–23.

[60] Falsey AR, McCann RM, Hall WJ, et al. The "common cold" in frail older persons: impact of rhinovirus and coronavirus in a senior daycare center. J Am Geriatr Soc 1997;45:706–11.

[61] Woo PC, Lau SK, Tsoi HW, et al. Clinical and molecular epidemiological features of coronavirus HKU1-associated community-acquired pneumonia. J Infect Dis 2005;192:1898–907.

[62] Chiu SS, Chan KH, Chu KW, et al. Human coronavirus NL63 infection and other coronavirus infections in children hospitalized with acute respiratory disease in Hong Kong, China. Clin Infect Dis 2005;40:1721–9.

[63] Bastien N, Anderson K, Hart L, et al. Human coronavirus NL63 infection in canada. J Infect Dis 2005;191:503–6.

[64] Gwaltney JM, Hendley JO, Simon G, et al. Rhinovirus infections in an industrial population–I. The occurrence of illness. N Engl J Med 1966;275:1261–8.

[65] Nicholson KG, Kent J, Hammersley V, et al. Acute viral infections of upper respiratory tract in elderly people living in the community: comparative, prospective, population based study of disease burden. Br Med J 1997;315:1060–4.

[66] Wald TG, Shult P, Krause P, et al. A rhinovirus outbreak among residents of a long-term care facility. Ann Intern Med 1995;123:588–93.

[67] Papadopoulos NG, Bates PJ, Bardin PG, et al. Rhinoviruses infect the lower airways. J Infect Dis 2000;181:1875–84.

[68] Cherr GS, Meredith JW, Chang M. Herpes simplex virus pneumonia in trauma patients. J Trauma 2000;49:547–9.

[69] Tuxen DV, Wilson JW, Cade JF. Prevention of lower respiratory herpes simplex virus infection with acyclovir in patients with the adult respiratory distress syndrome. Am Rev Respir Dis 1987;136:402–5.

[70] Ruben FL, Nguyen M. Viral pneumonitis. Clin Chest Med 1991;12:223–35.

[71] Dudding BA, Wagner SC, Zeller JA, et al. Fatal pneumonia associated with adenovirus type 7 in three military trainees. N Engl J Med 1972;286:1289–92.

[72] Manning A, Russell V, Eastick K, et al. Epidemiological profile and clinical associations of human bocavirus and other human parvoviruses. J Infect Dis 2006;194:1283–90.

[73] Miedzinski L. Community-acquired pneumonia: new facets of an old disease—hantavirus pulmonary syndrome. Respir Care Clin N Am 2005;11:45–58.

[74] Schmader K, van der Horst, Charles M, et al. Epstein-Barr virus and the elderly host. Rev Infect Dis 1989;11:64–73.

ELSEVIER
SAUNDERS

CLINICS IN
GERIATRIC
MEDICINE

Clin Geriatr Med 23 (2007) 553–565

Nursing Home–Associated Pneumonia

Joseph M. Mylotte, MD

Departments of Medicine and Microbiology, School of Medicine and Biomedical Sciences,
State University of New York, Buffalo, NY 14215, USA

Nursing home–associated pneumonia (NHAP) affects the most fragile and debilitated residents in long-term care settings and is associated with considerable morbidity and mortality [1]. Despite increasing research into various aspects of NHAP, there are many important unanswered questions related to this infection, some of which are listed in Box 1. The goal of this review is to address some of these questions based on recently published studies.

Classification of nursing home–associated pneumonia

Since the early 1990s, NHAP has been included in published studies of CAP. It is suggested, however, that NHAP should be considered a distinct clinical entity separate from CAP because of the unique population involved and the higher case-fatality rate [2]. Most recently, NHAP has been classified as a HCAP [3]. The rationale for categorizing NHAP as a health care–associated infection is the notion that, compared with people who have CAP, nursing home residents are at greater risk for developing pneumonia as a result of antibiotic-resistant organisms, including gram-negative bacilli and methicillin-resistant *Staphylococcus aureus* (MRSA) [3]. The variation in classification of NHAP is related, in part, to the debate regarding the etiology of this infection; this is discussed in more detail later, in the etiology section.

Epidemiology

Muder [4] reviewed studies published before 1998 and found that the reported incidence of NHAP varied between 0.3 and 2.5 episodes per 1000 resident care days. Factors that may explain this variation include a change in

E-mail address: mylotte@buffalo.edu

doi:10.1016/j.cger.2007.02.003
geriatric.theclinics.com

Box 1. Important unanswered questions regarding nursing home–associated pneumonia

1. Should NHAP be considered a health care–associated pneumonia (HCAP) or a unique entity to be distinguished from community-acquired pneumonia (CAP) and HCAP?
2. What bedside criteria are most accurate in identifying residents who have pneumonia in nursing home settings?
3. What laboratory tests should be done in residents suspected of having pneumonia in nursing home settings?
4. What are the causes of NHAP?
5. Can severity of NHAP be assessed adequately in nursing home settings in the absence of laboratory testing?
6. What factors should be considered in making a hospitalization decision?
7. What is the most appropriate antibiotic treatment regimen for NHAP in nursing homes? In hospitals?
8. Are recently published recommendations for treating NHAP in CAP or HCAP guidelines appropriate?
9. Should antibiotic treatment be withheld in residents who have severe dementia and pneumonia?
10. Does influenza or pneumococcal vaccination significantly reduce the risk for pneumonia in nursing home residents?

---

incidence over time, differences in study design, number of facilities studied, intensity of surveillance, and facility affiliation (Veterans Affairs versus community). Prospective studies indicate that the incidence of NHAP is 0.7 to 1.0 episodes per 1000 resident care days [5,6].

Independent predictors of NHAP include poor functional status; presence of a nasogastric tube; difficulty swallowing; occurrence of an unusual event, defined as confusion, agitation, falls, or wandering; chronic lung disease; tracheostomy; increasing age; male gender; and inadequate oral care [1,4,7]. Together the findings indicate that the most debilitated nursing home residents, especially those at risk for aspiration, are most likely to develop pneumonia.

The reported case-fatality rate for NHAP treated in nursing homes is 8.8% to 28% and in hospitals 17.6% to 53% [1,4]. The variation in reported case-fatality rate is related to differences in study design and definitions. Overall, the trend is for higher mortality in those treated in hospitals compared with nursing homes. Risk factors for death in nursing home residents who have pneumonia include prepneumonia functional status, dementia, increased respiratory rate, increased pulse, change in mental status, witnessed aspiration, use of sedatives, and comorbidity score [1,4]. Three models have been derived to predict mortality in residents who have pneumonia [8–10]. None of these models, however, has been validated extensively and one model [9] requires specific laboratory testing. The role of these models in the management of NHAP remains to be determined.

Pathogenesis

Microaspiration of oropharyngeal secretions into the lung and failure of host defense mechanisms to eradicate aspirated bacteria is the pathogenesis for pneumonia in most adults, including those residing in nursing homes [11]. There is a subset of nursing home residents, however, who have impaired swallowing or decreased cough reflex resulting from dementia, stroke, Parkinson's disease, or other neurologic deficits at risk for macroaspiration of oropharyngeal secretions and development of aspiration pneumonia [12,13]. Aspiration pneumonia should be distinguished from "aspiration pneumonitis" that is the result of aspiration of gastric contents into the lung that produces an acute inflammatory response that is noninfectious [13].

Etiology

Earlier studies of NHAP relied on sputum cultures to make an etiologic diagnosis [4]. Using sputum cultures to identify the causative agent of NHAP, however, is problematic. First, sputum specimens for culture in residents who have suspected pneumonia are obtained infrequently in clinical practice because of the difficulty in obtaining samples [14]. Second, when sputum specimens are obtained for culture, interpretation is confounded by the high rate of oropharyngeal colonization by aerobic enteric gram-negative bacilli, *Pseudomonas aeruginosa*, and *S aureus* in nursing home residents [15]. To minimize contamination of sputum by oropharyngeal bacteria, the reliability of specimens needs to be evaluated [16].

Muder [4] reviewed 18 studies of NHAP published between 1978 and 1994 in which causes were sought specifically using sputum cultures. In studies that used strict criteria [16] for evaluating reliability of sputum specimens, the organisms isolated most commonly were *Streptococcus pneumoniae* and *Haemophilus influenzae*. In contrast, in studies that used no criteria or modified criteria for assessing sputum adequacy, gram-negative bacilli and *S aureus* were isolated more commonly. Loeb and colleagues [5] performed one of the most extensive studies of causes of lower respiratory tract infection in nursing home residents, and viruses were the organisms isolated most commonly (60 of 272 episodes). Severe pneumonia is defined as infection associated with acute respiratory failure requiring intubation and mechanical ventilation and represents less than 2% of all episodes of NHAP. Two studies of nursing home residents who had severe pneumonia found a predominance of resistant gram-negative bacilli and *S aureus* as causative agents [17,18]. The importance of these studies [17,18] is that they formed the basis for the American Thoracic Society/Infectious Diseases Society of America (ATS/IDSA) recommendation for the management of NHAP in residents admitted to hospitals for treatment [3].

Clinical presentation

Summarizing the findings from multiple studies, the frequency of respiratory signs and symptoms related to NHAP was cough in approximately 60% and dyspnea in 40%, whereas nonspecific symptoms, such as fever, occurred in 65% and altered mental status in 50% to 70%. Johnson and colleagues [19] found that nonspecific symptoms (eg, weakness, anorexia, falls, delirium, and incontinence) were more common in the presentation of pneumonia in elderly people compared with those less than 65 years old, and this was because of the confounding effect of dementia. Mehr and colleagues [20] found that in residents who had pneumonia, 80% had three or fewer respiratory or nonspecific symptoms or signs, suggesting this diagnosis, but 92% had at least one respiratory symptom or sign.

Diagnosis

An expert panel recommends the following diagnostic testing when pneumonia is suspected: white blood cell count with differential, pulse oximetry if the respiratory rate is greater than 25 breaths per minute, chest radiograph, and Gram's stain and culture of sputum [21]. Pulse oximetry may be useful particularly in identifying residents who have pneumonia; an oxygen saturation of less than 94% breathing room air has a sensitivity of 80% and specificity of 91% for pneumonia with a positive predictive value of 95% [22]. Mehr and colleagues [20] developed a prediction model for pneumonia that consisted of the following predictors: increased pulse, respiratory rate greater than or equal to 30 breaths per minute, temperature greater than or equal to 38°C, decreased alertness, acute confusion, lung crackles on examination, absence of wheezes, and increased white blood cell count.

Other factors should be considered when trying to identify NHAP. First, agreement among radiologists regarding the interpretation of chest radiographs in residents who have suspected pneumonia is found fair at best [23]. This suggests that treatment decisions should not be based on chest radiographic interpretation alone. Second, gastric content aspiration into the lung and development of an acute inflammatory response (pneumonitis) results in signs and symptoms identical to pneumonia [13]. Recent studies suggest that there may be a substantial number of nursing home residents who have a diagnosis of pneumonia who actually have pneumonitis and do not need antibacterial therapy [24,25].

Treatment

Hospitalization decision

Rates of hospitalization for initial treatment of NHAP vary from 22% to 37% [1,4]. How physicians make a decision to hospitalize residents who have pneumonia remains undetermined. Predictors of hospital transfer have included deterioration after regular working hours or a respiratory rate greater than 40 breaths per minute [26]. There is evidence, however, that there is no significant difference in case-fatality rate when NHAP is treated in nursing homes versus hospitals [27]. Hutt and Kramer [28] recommend hospitalization if two or more of the following are present: oxygen saturation less than 90% on room air, systolic blood pressure less than 90 mm Hg, respiratory rate greater than 30 breaths per minute, necessity for 3 L of oxygen per minute, unstable chronic lung disease, heart failure, diabetes, patient unarousable if previously conscious, and new or increased agitation.

Other factors may influence a decision to hospitalize residents who have pneumonia. Because nursing homes are not responsible for the cost of hospital care and may not be reimbursed fully for caring for residents who have pneumonia in a facility, the facility has a financial incentive to transfer residents to hospitals for treatment [29]. Lack of bedside assessment by a physician also may be a factor influencing a hospitalization decision [30]. Family or resident preferences or pressure from facility staff may have a greater influence in the decision-making process than clinical factors [31]. Payer source for a resident and facility ownership also may influence a decision to hospitalize [32]. In a randomized trial of a clinical pathway to reduce hospitalizations in nursing home residents who had lower respiratory tract infection, nursing homes randomized to the pathway had a significantly lower proportion of hospitalizations (10%) compared with homes randomized to usual care (22%; $P = .001$), and there was no significant difference in mortality between management strategies [33].

In summary, the evidence suggests that treatment of NHAP in nursing homes is safe and inexpensive compared with treatment in hospitals. There are, however, barriers to the management of NHAP in nursing homes, including obtaining laboratory testing in a timely fashion, adequate documentation of resident or surrogate wishes for site of treatment, and logistic issues related to treating sick residents in nursing homes (oxygen, fluid replacement, and need for isolation) [34].

Initial route of antibiotic administration for those treated in nursing homes

Parenterally administered antibiotics (usually via intramuscular injection) are prescribed for the initial treatment of NHAP in 16% to 44% of episodes treated in nursing homes [1,4]. No significant difference in case-fatality rate between those treated with an oral versus a parenteral agent initially for NHAP in nursing homes is identified [35]. The process whereby physicians decide to initiate parenteral treatment of NHAP in nursing homes, however, remains unclear.

Timing of switch to an oral regimen in nursing homes or hospitals

In a study of treatment of NHAP, 75% of residents prescribed a parenteral antibiotic initially for pneumonia in a nursing home received this therapy for less than or equal to 3 days, whereas those treated in a hospital received intravenous antibiotic therapy for a median of 5 days [26]. Based on these findings, it is suggested that residents should be assessed for switch to an oral agent beginning on day 2 of parenteral therapy, if treated in a nursing home, and on day 3 if treated in a hospital [26].

Duration of treatment

In one study, the seventy-fifth percentile for duration of therapy was 10 days for residents treated in a nursing home, whereas if treatment was initiated in a hospital the seventy-fifth percentile for duration of treatment was 14 days [35]. In a subset analysis of a larger trial, patients 65 years of age or older who had CAP (nursing home residents were excluded) treated with levofloxacin (750 mg daily for 5 days) had a clinical success rate equivalent to levofloxacin (500 mg daily for 10 days) [36]. Whether or not such recommendations apply to NHAP remains to be determined but it is likely that it will apply to many episodes, especially those treated with an oral agent in a nursing home setting.

Choosing an antibiotic regimen for nursing home–associated pneumonia

There are no clinical trials of treatment of NHAP available on which to base recommendations for this infection. There are several factors to consider in making empiric antibiotic treatment decisions. First, recent antibiotic therapy increases the risk for antibiotic resistance of organisms causing pneumonia [37]. Second, recent (within 3 months) hospitalization also increases the risk for colonization with a resistant organism.

Two guidelines provide specific recommendations for the treatment of NHAP in nursing home settings (Table 1) [38,39]. These guidelines have similar recommendations and are based on the assumption that *S pneumoniae* and *H influenzae* are the most common etiologic agents of NHAP. A fluoroquinolone (gatifloxacin, levofloxacin, or moxifloxacin) may be the preferred regimen because it also has activity against all of the important typical and atypical pathogens and Enterobacteriaceae that may cause NHAP; it only requires one dose daily; and it is tolerated reasonably well.

The Canadian [38] and American [39] CAP guidelines provide similar recommendations for treatment of NHAP in hospital settings (see Table 1).

Table 1
Empiric antibiotic treatment of nursing home–acquired pneumonia: guideline recommendations

Treatment location	IDSA[a]	Canadian[b]	ATS/IDSA[c]
Nursing home	Oral fluoroquinolone (levofloxacin, gatifloxacin, or moxifloxacin) or amoxicillin/clavulanate + macrolide (axithromycin or clarithromycin)	First choice: oral fluoroquinolone (levofloxacin, gatifloxacin, or moxifloxacin) or amoxicillin/ clavulanate + macrolide Second choice: second-generation oral cephalosporin + macrolide	Not applicable
Hospital ward	Parenteral third-generation cephalosporin or ampicillin/ sulbactam + macrolide (azithromycin or clarithromycin) or parenteral fluoroquinolone alone (levofloxacin, gatifloxacin, or moxifloxacin)	First choice: parenteral fluoroquinolone (levofloxacin, gatifloxacin, or moxifloxacin) Second choice: parenteral second-, third-, or fourth-generation cephalosporin + macrolide (oral or parenteral)	Cefepime or ceftazidime or Imipenem or meropenem or piperacillin/tazobactam + ciprofloxacin + vancomycin or linezolid

Abbreviation: Canadian, Canadian Infectious Diseases Society and Canadian Thoracic Society.

[a] *From* Mandell LA, Bartlett JG, Dowell SF, et al. Update of practice guidelines for the management of community-acquired pneumonia in immunocompetent adults. Clin Infect Dis 2003;37:1405–33.

[b] *From* Mandell LA, Marrie TJ, Grosman RF, et al. Canadian guidelines for the initial management of community-acquired pneumonia: an evidence-based update by the Canadian Infectious Diseases Society and the Canadian Thoracic Society. Clin Infect Dis 2000;31:383–421.

[c] *From* American Thoracic Society and Infectious Diseases Society of America. Guidelines for the management of adults with hospital-acquired, ventilator-associated, and healthcare-associated pneumonia. Am J Respir Crit Care Med 2005;171:388–416.

These two guidelines do not consider resistant organisms (*P aeruginosa* and MRSA) to be major etiologic agents of NHAP. In contrast, the ATS/IDSA guideline [3] assumes that nursing home residence is a major risk factor for infection because of these resistant organisms; this guideline is based exclusively on the findings of intubated residents in an ICU setting [17,18] and, therefore, the empiric treatment recommendation focuses specifically on these pathogens (see Table 1). There is no evidence, however, that the broad-spectrum regimen recommended by the ATS/IDSA guideline is more efficacious compared with the regimens recommended by the Canadian [38] and American [39] CAP guidelines for residents who have NHAP requiring hospitalization and who are not intubated or ventilated.

Hutt and Kramer [28] developed a guideline for the management of NHAP based on the consensus opinion of a multispecialty panel, but some recommendations have little or no literature support. This guideline is an attempt to develop standards of care for nursing home residents who have pneumonia in the United States that can be used to assess quality of care. It will have to be demonstrated, however, that the guideline recommendations are true measures of quality of care and have an impact on outcome before they can be recommended for general use.

Withholding antibiotic treatment for pneumonia in residents who have advanced dementia

Pneumonia is a common terminal event in nursing home residents who have advanced dementia [40]. Severity of dementia is an independent predictor of short-term (1 week; 28% mortality) and long-term (3 month; 50% mortality) mortality in NHAP after adjusting for multiple confounding factors, including with or without antibiotic therapy [41]. These findings raise questions about the benefit of aggressive therapy (with antibiotics, intravenous hydration, and so forth) in residents who have advanced dementia and pneumonia [42]. It is suggested that prolonging the life of those who have advanced dementia and pneumonia by administering antibiotic therapy only serves to expose them to the continuing deterioration of their dementia [43]. van der Steen and colleagues [44] found that care for nursing home residents who had lower respiratory tract infection and dementia was more aggressive in the United States than in the Netherlands, regardless of the severity of dementia. These differences in management reflect differences in attitudes by physicians and families about the use of aggressive interventions in this group of people and the fact that in the Netherlands, unlike in the United States, physicians ultimately are responsible for decision making in consultation with families [43,45]. van der Steen and colleagues [46] found that there was no difference in level of discomfort in those dying who had pneumonia with or without antibiotic therapy.

In summary, when pneumonia occurs in nursing home residents who have advanced dementia, consideration needs to be given to whether or not curative (antibiotic) therapy is appropriate. Curative treatment may lead to resolution of the pneumonia but usually there is no impact on the mental or physical status of residents.

Prevention

The burden of pneumococcal disease in terms of morbidity and mortality is substantial for nursing home populations [47]. This is the rationale for recommending pneumococcal vaccination for nursing home residents. There is, however, considerable debate regarding the efficacy of pneumococcal vaccine in the elderly because of the lack of clinical trials [48]. The immunogenicity of pneumococcal vaccine decreases with age and efficacy diminishes rapidly after vaccination, especially in individuals vaccinated for the first time at an advanced age [49]. Despite these limitations, experts recommend vaccination of all elderly people because the vaccine is safe, inexpensive, and cost effective [50]. The rapid decline in efficacy of pneumococcal vaccine, especially in the very aged, and evidence of safety of revaccination [51] argue for periodic revaccination of nursing home residents (eg, every 5 years). The latest recommendation from the Advisory Committee on Immunization Practice is for a one-time revaccination in individuals age 65 or older if vaccination had first occurred before age 65 and it was 5 or more years since the first vaccination [50].

Influenza also has its greatest impact on the elderly in terms of morbidity and mortality. Influenza vaccine is recommended strongly for all residents of nursing homes despite the fact that its efficacy in preventing acute influenza is no better than 40% [52]. There are additional benefits, however, to influenza vaccination in the elderly, including reduction in the risk for hospitalization for cardiac problems, stroke, and pneumonia and a reduction of 50% in all-cause mortality [53]. On the basis of these findings, therefore, annual influenza vaccination is recommended strongly for all nursing home residents.

Previously it was postulated that oral hygiene and periodontal status of nursing home residents had an impact on the burden and quality of the bacterial flora in the mouth [54]. Subsequent studies verify that poor oral hygiene in nursing home residents is associated with preferential colonization of teeth and dentures by potential respiratory pathogens rather than mucosal surfaces [55]. Thus, improving oral hygiene in nursing home residents should reduce plaque load, thereby reducing oropharyngeal colonization with potential respiratory pathogens that can be aspirated into the lung, with a resulting decrease in the risk for bacterial pneumonia in this vulnerable population.

In a clinical trial, nursing home residents randomized to an intensive oral care regimen (caregivers brushed teeth after each meal and dentists or hygienists provided care weekly) had a significantly lower rate of pneumonia compared with standard oral care [56]. This level of intensity of oral care, however, may not be practical for most nursing homes. There also are several barriers to oral care for nursing home residents, including lack of designated personnel motivated to perform oral care on a regular basis, resident noncompliance, and the lack of a standard method to provide oral care (tooth brushing, mouthwash, and disinfectants) [57]. Although feasible methods to improve oral hygiene in nursing home residents need to be identified, this approach has the potential to reduce the risk for bacterial pneumonia significantly and further study is warranted.

Several studies published as letters to the editor suggest that angiotensin-converting enzyme inhibitors (ACEIs) reduce the risk for pneumonia in selected populations prone to aspiration related to dysphagia by increasing the cough reflex [12,58]. Retrospective cohort and case-control studies find a decreased rate of pneumonia in patients treated with an ACEI [59–61]. There are no clinical trials published to date, however, to support using ACEI therapy to prevent NHAP when there is no other indication for prescribing these agents. Other pharmacologic approaches, such as treatment with capsaicin or amantadine to stimulate the cough reflex, are not studied adequately to date [62].

In a systematic review of various interventions to prevent aspiration pneumonia in the elderly who have dysphagia, no evidence was found that changes in diet consistency or use of thickened liquids or positioning strategies reduces the risk for aspiration pneumonia [62]. Feeding tubes are inserted in the elderly most often because of severe dysphagia with recurrent aspiration events. There is evidence, however, that feeding tubes do not prevent aspiration in nursing home residents who have dysphagia and investigators suggest that their use be discouraged [63]. Loeb and colleagues [62] found no published studies demonstrating that tube feeding prevents aspiration in the elderly who have dysphagia.

In summary, at the present time influenza and pneumococcal vaccination seems to be the most appropriate approach to preventing NHAP. Whether or not pharmacologic approaches or improvement in oral hygiene will be used in the future to prevent NHAP depends on well-designed, randomized, controlled trials proving the efficacy of one or more of these approaches.

References

[1] Mylotte JM. Nursing home-acquired pneumonia. Clin Infect Dis 2002;35:1205–11.

[2] Zimmer JG, Hall WJ. Nursing home-acquired pneumonia: avoiding the hospital. J Am Geriatr Soc 1997;45:380–1.

[3] American Thoracic Society and Infectious Diseases Society of America. Guidelines for the management of adults with hospital-acquired, ventilator-associated, and healthcare-associated pneumonia. Am J Respir Crit Care Med 2005;171:388–416.

[4] Muder RR. Pneumonia in residents of long-term care facilities: epidemiology, etiology, management, and prevention. Am J Med 1998;105:319–30.

[5] Loeb M, McGeer A, McArthur M, et al. Risk factors for pneumonia and other lower respiratory tract infections in elderly residents of long-term care facilities. Arch Intern Med 1999; 159:2058–64.

[6] Jackson MM, Fierer J, Barrett-Connor E, et al. Intensive surveillance for infections in a three-year study of nursing home patients. Am J Epidemiol 1992;135:685–96.

[7] Quagliarello V, Ginter S, Han L, et al. Modifiable risk factors for nursing home-acquired pneumonia. Clin Infect Dis 2005;40:1–6.

[8] Naughton BJ, Mylotte JM, Tayara A. Outcome of nursing home-acquired pneumonia: derivation and application of a practical model to predict 30 day mortality. J Am Geriatr Soc 2000;48:1292–9.

[9] Mehr DR, Binder EF, Kruse RL, et al. Predicting mortality in nursing home residents with lower respiratory tract infectin: the Missouri LRI study. JAMA 2001;286:2427–36.

[10] van der Steen JT, Mehr DR, Kruse RL, et al. Predictors of mortality for lower respiratory infections in nursing home residents with dementia were validated internationally. J Clin Epidemiol 2006;59:970–9.

[11] Verghese A, Berk SL. Bacterial pneumonia in the elderly. Medicine 1983;62:271–85.

[12] Kaikawada M, Iwamoto T, Takasaki M. Aspiration and infection in the elderly: epidemiology, diagnosis, and management. Drugs Aging 2005;22(2):115–30.

[13] Marik PE. Aspiration pneumonitis and aspiration pneumonia. N Engl J Med 2001;344: 665–71.

[14] Mylotte JM, Naughton B, Saludades C, et al. Validation and application of the pneumonia prognosis index to nursing home residents with pneumonia. J Am Geriatr Soc 1998;46: 1538–44.

[15] Nicolle LE, McLeod J, McIntyre M, et al. Significance of pharyngeal colonization with aerobic gram-negative bacilli in elderly institutionalized men. Age Aging 1986;15:47–52.

[16] Murray PR, Washington JA. Microscopic and bacteriologic analysis of expectorated sputum. Mayo Clin Proc 1975;50:339–44.

[17] El-Solh AA, Sikka P, Ramadan F, et al. Etiology of severe pneumonia in the very elderly. Am J Respir Crit Care Med 2001;163:635–51.

[18] El-Solh AA, Pietrantoni C, Bhat A, et al. Microbiology of severe aspiration pneumonia in institutionalized elderly. Am J Respir Crit Care Med 2003;167:1650–4.

[19] Johnson JC, Jaydevappa R, Baccash PD, et al. Nonspecific presentation of pneumonia in hositalizated older people: age effect or dementia? J Am Geriatr Soc 2000;48:1316–20.

[20] Mehr DR, Binder EF, Kruse RL, et al. Clinical findings associated with radiographic pneumonia in nursing home residents. J Fam Pract 2001;50:931–7.

[21] Bentley DW, Bradley S, High K, et al. Practice guideline for evaluation of fever and infection in long-term care facilities. Clin Infect Dis 2000;31:640–53.

[22] Kaye KS, Stalam M, Shersen WE, et al. Utility of pulse oximetry in diagnosing pneumonia in nursing home residents. Am J Med Sci 2002;324:237–42.

[23] Loeb MB, Carusone SBC, Marrie TJ, et al. Interobserver reliability of radiologists' interpretations of mobile chest radiographs for nursing home-acquired pneumonia. J Am Med Dir Assoc 2006;7:416–9.

[24] Mylotte JM, Goodnugh S, Naughton BJ. Pneumonia versus pneumonitis in nursing home residents: diagnosis and management. J Am Geriatr Soc 2003;51:1–7.

[25] Mylotte JM, Gould M. Pneumonia versus aspiration pneumonitis in nursing home residents: prospective application of a clinical algorithm. J Am Geriatr Soc 2005;53:755–61.

[26] Fried TR, Gillick MR, Lipsitz LA. Whether to transfer? Factors associated with hospitalization and outcome of elderly long-term care patients with pneumonia. J Gen Intern Med 1995;10:246–50.

[27] Kruse RL, Mehr DR, Boles KE, et al. Does hospitalization impact survival after lower respiratory infection in nursing home residents? Med Care 2004;42:860–70.

[28] Hutt E, Kramer AM. Evidence-based guidelines for management of nursing home-acquired pneumonia. J Fam Pract 2002;51:709–16.

[29] Kruse RL, Boles KE, Mehr DR, et al. The cost of treating pneumonia in the nursing home setting. J Am Med Dir Assoc 2003;4:81–9.

[30] Brooks S, Harshaw G, Hasse L, et al. The physician decision-making process in transferring nursing home patients to the hospital. Arch Intern Med 1994;154:902–8.

[31] Cohen-Mansfield J, Lipson S. Medical staff's decision-making process in the nursing home. J Gerontol A Biol Sci Med Sci 2003;58:271–8.

[32] Konetzka T, Spector W, Shaffer T. Effects of nursing home ownership type and resident payor source on hospitalization for suspected pneumonia. Med Care 2004;42:1001–8.

[33] Loeb M, Carusone SC, Goeree R, et al. Effect of a clinical pathway to reduce hospitalizations in nursing home residents with pneumonia. A randomized controlled trial. JAMA 2006;295: 2503–10.

[34] Dosa D. Should I hospitalized my resident with nursing home-acquired pneumonia? J Am Med Dir Assoc 2005;6:327–33.

[35] Naughton BJ, Mylotte JM. Treatment guideline for nursing home-acquired pneumonia based on community practice. J Am Geriatr Soc 2000;48:82–8.

[36] Shorr AF, Zadeikis N, Xiang JX, et al. A multicenter, randomized, double-blind, retrospective comparison of 6- and 10-day regimens of levofloxacin in a subgroup of patients aged >65 years with community-acquired pneumonia. Clin Ther 2005;22:1251–9.

[37] Vanderkooi OG, Low DE, Green K, et al. Predicting antimicrobial resistance in invasive pneumococcal disease. Clin Infect Dis 2005;40:1288–97.

[38] Mandell LA, Marrie TJ, Grosman RF, et al. Canadian guidelines for the initial management of community-acquired pneumonia: an evidence-based update by the Canadian Infectious Diseases Society and the Canadian Thoracic Society. Clin Infect Dis 2000;31:383–421.

[39] Mandell LA, Bartlett JG, Dowell SF, et al. Update of practice guidelines for the management of community-acquired pneumonia in immunocompetent adults. Clin Infect Dis 2003;37: 1405–33.

[40] Brandt HE, Deliens L, Ooms ME, et al. Symptoms, signs, problems, and diseases of terminally ill nursing home patients. Arch Intern Med 2005;165:314–20.

[41] van der Steen JT, Ooms ME, Mehr DR, et al. Severe dementia and adverse outcomes of nursing home-acquired pneumonia: evidence for medication by functional and pathophysiological decline. J Am Geriatr Soc 2002;50:439–48.

[42] Morrison RS, Siu AL. Survival in end-stage dementia following acute illness. JAMA 2000; 284:47–52.

[43] Hertogh CMPM, Ribbe MW. Ethical aspects of medical decision-making in demented patients: a report from the Netherlands. Alzheimer Dis Associ Dis 1996;10:11–9.

[44] van der Steen JT, Kruse RL, Ooms ME, et al. Treatment of nursing home residents with dementia and lower respiratory tract infection in the United States and the Netherlands: an ocean apart. J Am Geriatr Soc 2004;52:691–9.

[45] Helton MR, van der Steen JT, Daaleman TP, et al. A cross-cultural study of physician treatment decisions for demented nursing home patients who develop pneumonia. Ann Fam Med 2006;4:221–7.

[46] van der Steen JT, Ooms ME, van der Wal G, et al. Pneumonia: the demented patient's best friend? Discomfort after starting or withholding antibiotic treatment. J Am Geriatr Soc 2002;50:1681–8.

[47] Centers for Disease Control and Prevention. Active Bacterial Core Surveillance Report, Emerging Infections Program Network, Streptococcus pneumoniae, 2005—Provisional. Available at: http://www.cdc.gov/ncidod/dbmd/abcs/survreports/spneu05prelim.pdf. Accessed December 18, 2006.

[48] Watson L, Wilson BJ, Waugh N. Pneumococcal polysaccharide vaccine: a systematic review of clinical effectiveness in adults. Vaccine 2002;20:2166–73.

[49] Shapiro ED, Berg AT, Austrian R, et al. The protective efficacy of polyvalent pneumococcal polysaccharide vaccine. N Engl J Med 1991;325:1453–60.

[50] Centers for Disease Control and Prevention. Prevention of pneumococcal disease: recommendations of the Advisory Committee on Immunization Practice (ACIP). MMWR Recomm Rep 1997;46(RR-8):1–24.

[51] Artz AS, Ershler WB, Longo DL. Pneumococcal vaccination and revaccination of older adults. Clin Microbiol Rev 2003;16:308–18.

[52] Bradley SF. Prevention of influenza in long-term care facilities. Infect Control Hosp Epidemiol 1999;20:629–37.

[53] Nichol KL, Nordin J, Mullooly J, et al. Influenza vaccination and reduction in hospitalizations for cardiac disease and stroke among the elderly. N Engl J Med 2003;348:1322–32.

[54] Scannapieco FA, Mylotte JM. Relationships between periodontal disease and bacterial pneumonia. J Periodontol 1996;67:1114–22.

[55] Sumi Y, Kagami H, Ohtsuka Y, et al. High correlation between the bacterial species in denture plaque and pharyngeal microflora. Gerodontology 2003;20:84–7.

[56] Yoneyama T, Mitsuyoshi Y, ohrui T, et al. Oral care reduces pneumonia in older patients in nursing homes. J Am Geriatr Soc 2002;50:430–3.

[57] Terpenning M. Geriatric oral health and pneumonia risk. Clin Infect Dis 2005;40:1807–10.

[58] Yamaya M, Yanai M, Ohrui T, et al. Interventions to prevent pneumonia among older adults. J Am Geriatr Soc 2001;49:85–90.

[59] Ohkubo T, Chapman N, Neal B, et al. Effects of an antigiotensin converting enzyme inhibitor-based regimen on pneumonia risk. Am J Respir Crit Care Med 2004;169:1041–5.

[60] van de Garde EM, Souverein PC, van den Bosch JM, et al. Angiotensin-converting enzyme inhibitor use and pneumonia risk in a general population. Eur Respir J 2006;27:1217–22.

[61] Mortensen EM, Restrepo MI, Anzueto A, et al. The impact of prior outpatient ACE inhibitor use on 30-day mortality for patients hospitalized with community-acquired pneumonia. BMC Pulm Med 2005;5:12.

[62] Loeb MB, Becker M, Eady A, et al. Interventions to prevent aspiration pneumonia in older adults: a systemic review. J Am Geriatr Soc 2003;51:1018–22.

[63] Gillick M. Rethinking the role of tube feeding in patients with advanced dementia. N Engl J Med 2000;342:206–10.

ELSEVIER
SAUNDERS

Clin Geriatr Med 23 (2007) 567–583

CLINICS IN
GERIATRIC
MEDICINE

HIV Infection in Older Adults

Vera P. Luther, MD*,
Aimee M. Wilkin, MD, MPH

*Section on Infectious Diseases, Department of Internal Medicine, Wake Forest University
Health Sciences, Medical Center Boulevard, Winston-Salem, NC 27157-1042, USA*

Epidemiology

There is variability in the definition of "older adult" in previous studies of persons who have HIV infection or AIDS, although the term, "older adult," in those who have HIV traditionally has been reserved for individuals age 50 or older. The decision to use age 50 or older as the definition of an "older adult" is based on an early bell-shaped demographic distribution of United States HIV/AIDS cases reported to the Centers for Disease Control and Prevention (CDC) [1–3]. Currently, it is estimated that more than 116,000 persons age 50 or older are living with HIV/AIDS in the United States [4], and the number of older adults who are infected with HIV continues to rise (Fig. 1) [3–5]. As of December 2005, the CDC estimated that adults age 50 or older comprise 29% of the individuals living with AIDS in the United States, compared with 20% in the year 2001 [4]. The growing number of older adults living with HIV/AIDS is the result of the dramatically improved survival of people living with HIV due to highly active antiretroviral therapy (HAART) and an increase in new diagnoses of HIV/AIDS in this age group [2]. Both trends likely will continue in the future. The United States Senate Special Committee on Aging predicts that by the year 2015, 50% of persons living with HIV/AIDS will be age 50 and older [6].

Similar to that in younger persons, the route of exposure to HIV reported most commonly in persons ages 50 and over who are newly diagnosed with AIDS in the United States is sexual contact among men who have sex with men, followed by injection drug use, then heterosexual sex (Table 1). Although men account for the majority of HIV-infected older adults, older women are acquiring HIV at a higher rate than older men [7,8]. The number of new AIDS diagnoses in women age 50 and over more than doubled from

---

* Corresponding author.
E-mail address: vluther@wfubmc.edu (V.P. Luther).

0749-0690/07/$ - see front matter © 2007 Published by Elsevier Inc.
doi:10.1016/j.cger.2007.02.004

geriatric.theclinics.com

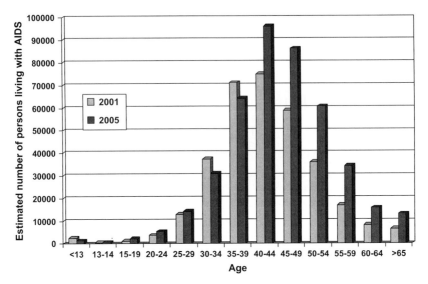

Fig. 1. Estimated number of persons in the United States living with AIDS, by age, in 2005 compared with 2001. (*Adapted from* HIV/AIDS Surveillance Report, 2005. Available at: http://www.cdc.gov/hiv/topics/surveillance/resources/reports/. Accessed January 11, 2007.)

1990 to 1999. Among these women, heterosexual sex is the route of exposure reported most commonly (see Table 1) [9]. In recent years, from 1999 to 2004, women over age 50 made up 12.4% of new HIV diagnoses in women in the United States [10]. Early in the HIV epidemic, blood and blood product transfusion was a significant source of infection in older age groups. After the introduction of blood and blood product screening in 1986, this route of exposure to HIV decreased significantly [9].

Similar to the HIV-positive population at large, the racial and ethnic makeup of new diagnoses of AIDS cases in persons ages 50 and older also has changed over time. In 1990, the majority of persons age 50 or older who were newly diagnosed with AIDS were white men. In 1999, the majority of persons age 50 or older were black men. In men and women ages 50 and older, the number of new diagnoses of AIDS has decreased in whites but increased in blacks and Hispanics (Table 2) [9]. Although rates decreased significantly for women in all age groups, it was not as prominent for women ages 50 and older [10]. This disparity in rates of HIV infection is stark, particularly for black women, who have up to 21 times the risk for being diagnosed with HIV compared with white women [10].

Clinical characteristics and natural history

In general, the clinical characteristics of HIV-infected older adults are similar to that of younger adults [11]. Symptom expression, however, may vary between older and younger people who have HIV/AIDS. For example,

Table 1

Estimated number of new AIDS cases in the United States in older adults compared with younger adults and adolescents by exposure category

Exposure category	1990		1999	
	Age at diagnosis		Age at diagnosis	
	13–49	50+	13–49	50+
Men				
MSM*	23,619 (61.7%)	2676 (63.0%)	12,046 (44.7%)	1589 (34.2%)
Injection drug use	8497 (22.2%)	648 (15.3%)	5517 (20.5%)	960 (20.6%)
MSM* and injection drug use	3585 (9.4%)	127 (3.0%)	1515 (5.6%)	123 (2.6%)
Hemophilia	388 (1.0%)	51 (1.2%)	75 (0.3%)	9 (0.2%)
Heterosexual contact	824 (2.1%)	199 (4.7%)	2,303 (8.6%)	593 (12.8%)
Blood transfusion	192 (0.5%)	230 (5.4%)	83 (0.3%)	40 (0.9%)
Exposure not reported	1152 (3.0%)	314 (7.4%)	5400 (20.1%)	1335 (28.7%)
Total	38,257 (100%)	4245 (100%)	26,939 (100%)	4649 (100%)
Women				
Injection drug use	3135 (55.7%)	118 (20.9%)	2,455 (27.7%)	221 (17.8%)
Hemophilia	13 (0.2%)	5 (0.9%)	3 (0.0%)	0 (0.0%)
Heterosexual contact	1973 (35.0%)	233 (41.2%)	3639 (41.4%)	526 (42.4)
Blood transfusion	164 (2.9%)	128 (22.7%)	73 (0.8%)	33 (2.7%)
Exposure not reported	345 (6.1%)	81 (14.3%)	2680 (30.3%)	462 (37.2%)
Total	5630 (100%)	565 (100%)	8850 (100%)	1242 (100%)

* Men who have sex with Men.

Adapted from AIDS public use data set through year-end 2000. Available at: http://www.cdc.gov/hiv/software/apids.htm. Accessed January 11, 2007.

cross-sectional data from the HIV Cost and Service Utilization Study (HCSUS) and Veterans Aging Cohort 3-Site Study indicate that HIV-infected older adults report a fewer number of symptoms to their health care providers than their younger counterparts. Specifically, these data indicate that older HIV-infected adults are less likely to report headache, fever, chills, sweats, nausea, vomiting, or feeling down or blue compared with their younger counterparts. Furthermore, older adults in the HCSUS were less likely to report diarrhea, white oral patches, or sinus trouble compared with younger adults. Older adults, however, in the HCSUS were more likely to report neuropathic symptoms or weight loss [12].

Older HIV-infected adults experience a similar number and array of AIDS-defining illnesses as younger adults, with *Pneumocystis jiroveci* (previously *Pneumocystis carinii*) pneumonia (PCP) the most common [12–17]. Additionally, some studies note an increased incidence of HIV encephalopathy or HIV dementia [15,18–20] and HIV wasting syndrome [18,19] in older adults. Although the overall prevalence of AIDS-defining illnesses seems similar, older HIV-infected individuals often experience worse outcomes in association with opportunistic infections compared with younger patients, particularly for PCP and tuberculosis. This increased morbidity may be related to more rapid disease progression and a higher risk for systemic dissemination [21].

Table 2
Estimated number of new AIDS cases in the United States in older adults compared with younger adults and adolescents by race/ethnicity

| | 1990 | | 1999 | |
| | Age at diagnosis | | Age at diagnosis | |
Race/ethnicity	13–49	50+	13–49	50+
Men				
White	20,428 (53.4%)	2485 (58.5%)	9142 (33.9%)	1585 (34.1%)
Black	10,905 (28.5%)	1124 (26.5%)	11,611 (43.1%)	2132 (46.0%)
Hispanic	6516 (17.0%)	597 (14.0%)	5730 (21.3%)	863 (18.6%)
Asian or Pacific Islander	257 (0.7%)	30 (0.7%)	273 (1.0%)	41 (0.9%)
American Indian/Alaska native	107 (0.3%)	6 (0.1%)	103 (0.4%)	14 (0.3%)
Unknown race	44 (0.1%)	3 (0.0%)	80 (0.3%)	14 (0.3%)
Total	38,257 (100%)	4245 (100%)	26,939 (100%)	4649 (100%)
Women				
White	1288 (22.9%)	216 (38.2%)	1507 (17.0%)	239 (19.2%)
Black	3077 (54.7%)	239 (42.3%)	5683 (64.2%)	730 (58.8%)
Hispanic	1225 (21.8%)	104 (18.4%)	1544 (17.4%)	254 (20.5%)
Asian or Pacific Islander	20 (0.4%)	5 (0.9%)	65 (0.7%)	6 (0.5%)
American Indian/Alaska native	11 (0.2%)	1 (0.2%)	36 (0.4%)	12 (1.0%)
Unknown race	9 (0.2%)	0 (0.0%)	15 (0.2%)	1 (0.0%)
Total	5630 (100%)	565 (100%)	8850 (100%)	1242 (100%)

Data from AIDS public use data set through year-end 2000. Available at: http://www.cdc.gov/hiv/software/apids.htm. Accessed January 11, 2007.

Plasma HIV viral load also may differ in older HIV-infected adults compared with those who are younger. Although a high HIV viral load after seroconversion is reported in older patients [22,23], Goodkin and colleagues [24] found that adults ages 50 and older had significantly lower levels of HIV-1 replication. This reduction in viral replication was independent of antiretroviral therapy usage, regimen adherence, and disease stage compared with adults ages 18 to 39. The reason for this difference in viral replication is not clear, but the investigators speculate that changes in viral evolution or immunologic monitoring in older adults may be responsible for this phenomenon.

Advanced age is associated with increased morbidity in HIV-infected individuals. This may be the result, in part, of the delay in diagnosis of HIV infection that often occurs in older adults [12,14,16,18,25–29]. There are many explanations for delays in diagnosis of HIV/AIDS in older people. As discussed previously, there are some differences in symptom expression in older adults [12]. Also, older adults may have more comorbid illnesses that confuse or confound the diagnosis. Multiple descriptions of elderly persons who have AIDS presenting "atypically" with malignancies, dermatologic manifestations, or new-onset dementia are reported [30]. Additionally, older patients often are hesitant to discuss or ask about HIV or

AIDS and providers do not ask about HIV risk factors in patients ages 50 and older compared with their younger patients [31].

Mortality and prognosis

Several investigations and observational data indicate that advanced age is associated with increased mortality in HIV-positive persons [13,14,16,18,19,29,32,33]. CDC surveillance statistics suggest that adults ages 50 and older are more likely to die within a month of the diagnosis of AIDS compared with younger adults [18,29]. Data from the 6656 participants in the multicenter AIDS in Europe Study Group show that higher age was associated with a shortened survival after an AIDS diagnosis [19]. Butt and colleagues [13] found that persons age 60 or older had an increased risk for death after adjusting for their stage of HIV infection, CD4 lymphocyte count, or history of opportunistic infection. Others have confirmed these findings by noting that an older age at the time of HIV seroconversion increases the risk for death in patients who acquire HIV from blood transfusions [17,34].

It is unclear, however, if this increase in mortality, and its assumed associated decline in immune function, is related solely to being elderly or if it is a function of age across the continuum. In fact, some investigators have found that an accelerated decline in immune status occurs at much younger ages than what is traditionally considered elderly. For instance, Operskalski and colleagues [35] studied 743 HIV-positive persons for nearly a decade and found that persons ages 40 and older experienced a more rapid decline in CD4 cell count. Phillips and colleagues [28] observed an increased risk for progression to AIDS in hemophiliacs ages 30 and over compared with younger adults, and Soriano and colleagues [23] showed that the duration of HIV infection and the age at seroconversion were associated independently with a reduction in CD4 cell counts. Moreover, CDC surveillance data from 1996 to 2001 show that people who are older at the time of HIV diagnosis are more likely to develop AIDS within in 1 to 3 years than those in younger age groups. Although 75% of 20 to 29 year olds who had HIV did not progress to AIDS within 1 year, only 45% of the 50-to-59-year-old age group and 38% of those 60 and older avoided progression to AIDS in 1 year [36].

To explain the increased rate of disease progression seen in older HIV-infected individuals, Adler and colleagues [37] studied T-cell dynamics in older and younger HIV-positive adults. They found that although the rate of T-cell death was similar in both groups, T-cell replacement was attenuated in older HIV-positive persons. They concluded that the mechanism of accelerated progression to AIDS seen in older persons is related to an impaired ability to replace functional T cells after T-cell death has occurred.

The majority of studies reporting an accelerated rate of HIV disease progression in older individuals were published based on data from the pre-HAART era. Prognosis of older adults since the advent of HAART is discussed later.

Antiretroviral therapy

The indications for initiation of antiretroviral therapy, choices of antiretroviral medication, and goals of treatment of older adults are the same as those for younger adults. Guidelines that include these treatment considerations of older patients are published by the Department of Health and Human Services and the International AIDS Society-USA panel and are updated regularly [38,39]. Nonetheless, the care of older HIV-positive patients should be individualized, taking into consideration each patient's comorbid conditions and the potential for adverse drug events, toxicities, and drug-drug interactions. Table 3 [40] lists selected adverse events and drug-drug interactions that may be important particularly in older patients.

Data regarding the immunologic and virologic response to HAART in older HIV-infected individuals are conflicting [41]. Some studies show that the immunologic response to HAART, as measured by CD4 cell count increases, of older HIV-positive adults is no different from the response seen in younger adults [42–46]. Other studies indicate, however, that the CD4 count response to HAART is not as robust in older persons as that seen in younger HIV-infected adults [47,48]. For instance, the EuroSIDA cohort noted that age was related inversely to maximal CD4 cell response and CD4 cell count increase [49]. The blunted immunologic response to HAART in older age groups does not seem related to impaired virologic responses. Data from a large cohort study in France show that older adults starting HAART had less immune reconstitution and more risk for disease progression despite higher rates of viral load suppression below 500 copies/mL [50]. Although many investigations have shown that the virologic response to HAART is similar in older adults and younger adults who have HIV [42–45,47,48], one study found that a higher percentage of older adults were able to achieve an undetectable viral load compared with younger adults [46]. This observation likely was a result of the improved adherence with HAART seen in the older group. Supporting this observation, others also have found a positive association between increasing age and HAART adherence [51,52]. Hinkin and colleagues [51] found that older patients were 3 times more likely to be adherent with greater than or equal to 95% of their HAART regimen compared with younger patients.

Regarding mortality in older adults infected with HIV who were treated with HAART, Perez and Moore [53] reported that HIV-infected adults ages 50 and older who were on HAART had similar survival death rates compared with younger adults who were on HAART. They did note, however, that older persons who did not receive HAART had double the risk for death compared with younger untreated adults. The ART Cohort Collaboration study, combining information from 13 different cohort studies, found

Table 3
Selected adverse reactions and drug-drug interactions

Selected antiretroviral medications	Selected adverse reaction	Selected drug-drug interactions
Nucleoside/Nucleotide reverse transcriptase inhibitors		
Abacavir	Nausea	Methadone
	Vomiting	
	Diarrhea	
	Hypertriglyceridemia	
Didanosine	Nausea	Itraconazole
	Vomiting	Hydroxyurea
	Diarrhea	Methadone
	Abdominal pain	Ciprofloxacin
	Peripheral neuropathy	
	Pancreatitis	
	Lactic acidosis	
Lamivudine	Headache	Cimetidine
	Fatigue	
	Nausea	Ethambutol
	Vomiting	
	Diarrhea	
	Skin rash	
	Peripheral neuropathy	
Stavudine	Headache	Antineoplastics
	Skin rash	Disulfiram
	Nausea	Zidovudine
	Peripheral neuropathy	Ribavirin
	Pancreatitis	
	Lactic acidosis	
Zidovudine	Anemia	Antineoplastics
	Granulocytopenia	Fluconazole
	Headache	Methadone
	Myopathy	Probenecid
	Liver toxicity	Phenytoin
		Valproic acid
		Rifampin
Tenofovir	Headache	Didanosine
	Diarrhea	Atazanavir
	Myalgias	Cidofovir
	Renal failure	Ganciclovir
	Hepatotoxicity	Valganciclovir
Non-nucleoside reverse transcriptase inhibitors		
Delavirdine	Headache	Simvastatin
	Fatigue	Lovastatin
	Abdominal discomfort	Rifampin
	Rash	Rifapentine
		Rifabutin
		Astemizole
		Terfenadine
		Cisapride
		H_2-blockers

(*continued on next page*)

Table 3 (*continued*)

Selected antiretroviral medications	Selected adverse reaction	Selected drug-drug interactions
		Proton pump inhibitors
		Alprazolam
		Midazolam
		Triazolam
		St. John's wort
		Amprenavir
		Fosamprenavir
		Carbamazepine
		Phenobarbital
		Phenytoin
Efavirenz	Rash	Rifapentine
	Neurologic symptoms	Astemizole
	Fatigue	Terfenadine
	Diarrhea	Cisapride
	Hyperlipidemia	Midazolam
		Triazolam
		St. John's wort
		Voriconazole
Nevirapine	Rash	Rifampin
	Headache	Rifapentine
	Diarrhea	St. John's wort
	Nausea	
	Liver toxicity	
Protease inhibitors		
Fosamprenavir	Rash	Bepridil
	Nausea	Simvastatin
	Vomiting	Lovastatin
	Abdominal pain	Rifampin
	Perioral tingling	Rifapentine
	Hypertriglyceridemia	Astemizole
		Terfenadine
		Cisapride
		Pimozide
		Midazolam
		Triazolam
		St. John's wort
		Delavirdine
		Fluticasone
Atazanavir	Rash	Bepridil
	Abdominal pain	Simvastatin
	Nausea	Lovastatin
	Diarrhea	Rifampin
	Unconjugated hyperbilirubinemia	Rifapentine
	Headache	Astemizole
	Prolonged P–R interval	Terfenadine
	First degree atrioventricular block	Cisapride
		Proton pump inhibitors

(*continued on next page*)

Table 3 (*continued*)

Selected antiretroviral medications	Selected adverse reaction	Selected drug-drug interactions
	Lactic acidosis	Pimozide
		Midazolam
		Triazolam
		St. John's wort
		Fluticasone
		Indinavir
		Irinotecan
Darunavir	Hypertriglyceridemia	Simvastatin
	Hyperamylasemia	Lovastatin
	Diarrhea	Rifampin
	Nausea	Rifapentine
	Headache	Astemizole
	Nasopharyngitis	Terfenadine
	Rash	Cisapride
		Pimozide
		Midazolam
		Triazolam
		St. John's wort
		Carbamazepine
		Phenobarbital
		Phenytoin
		Fluticasone
Indinavir	Headache	Amiodarone
	Nausea	Simvastatin
	Metallic taste	Lovastatin
	Hypertriglyceridemia	Rifampin
	Glucose intolerance	Rifapentine
		Astemizole
		Terfenadine
		Cisapride
		Pimozide
		Midazolam
		Triazolam
		St. John's wort
		Atazanavir
Lopinavir/ritonavir	Diarrhea	Flecainide
	Hypercholesterolemia	Propafenone
	Hypertriglyceridemia	Simvastatin
		Lovastatin
		Rifampin
		Rifapentine
		Astemizole
		Terfenadine
		Cisapride
		Pimozide
		Midazolam

(*continued on next page*)

Table 3 (*continued*)

Selected antiretroviral medications	Selected adverse reaction	Selected drug-drug interactions
		Triazolam
		St. John's wort
		Fluticasone
Nelfinavir	Glucose intolerance	Simvastatin
	Rash	Lovastatin
	Abdominal pain	Rifampin
	Diarrhea	Rifapentine
	Hypertriglyceridemia	Astemizole
		Terfenadine
		Cisapride
		Pimozide
		Midazolam
		Triazolam
		St. John's wort
Ritonavir	Nausea	Bepridil
	Vomiting	Amiodarone
	Diarrhea	Flecainide
	Headache	Propafenone
	Hypertriglyceridemia	Quinidine
	Hypercholesterolemia	Simvastatin
	Glucose intolerance	Lovastatin
		Rifapentine
		Astemizole
		Terfenadine
		Cisapride
		Pimozide
		Midazolam
		Triazolam
		St. John's wort
		Fluticasone
		Voriconazole
Saquinavir	Nausea	Simvastatin
	Vomiting	Lovastatin
	Diarrhea	Rifampin
	Headache	Rifabutin
	Abdominal discomfort	Rifapentine
	Hypertriglyceridemia	Astemizole
	Glucose intolerance	Terfenadine
		Cisapride
		Pimozide
		Midazolam
		Triazolam
		St. John's wort
		Garlic supplements
		Fluticasone
Tipranavir	Rash	Bepridil
	Hypercholesterolemia	Amiodarone
	Diarrhea	Flecainide

(*continued on next page*)

Table 3 (*continued*)

Selected antiretroviral medications	Selected adverse reaction	Selected drug-drug interactions
	Nausea	Propafenone
	Vomiting	Quinidine
	Elevated liver function tests	Simvastatin
	Fatigue	Lovastatin
	Headache	Rifampin
		Rifapentine
		Astemizole
		Terfenadine
		Cisapride
		Pimozide
		Midazolam
		Triazolam
		St. John's wort
		Fluticasone
		Ritonavir

Note: This is not a comprehensive list.

Data from Guidelines for the use of antiretroviral agents in HIV-1-infected adults and adolescents. Available at: http://aidsinfo.nih.gov/ContentFiles/AdultandAdolescentGL.pdf. Accessed January 11, 2007; Dealing with antiretroviral side effects. Available at: http://www.projectinform.org/fs/sideeffects.html. Accessed January 11, 2007; Gebo KA. HIV in patients over 50: an increasing problem. Hopkins HIV Rep 2004;16:7–11; and manufacturers' product inserts.

that age remained a significant predictor of mortality, although CD4 count at the initiation of HAART was the most significant factor. The effect of age was most evident in the over-50 age group, with 3 times the risk for death compared with those ages 17 to 29 [54].

Comorbid conditions

Comorbid conditions are more common in older HIV-infected adults than their younger counterparts. It is reasonable to expect that the presence of additional comorbidities might affect the natural history, morbidity, and mortality of HIV infection in older adults. A higher rate of HIV-related and non–HIV-related comorbidity is observed in older adults [16,44]. Tumbarello and colleagues [44] found that HIV-positive individuals ages 50 and older experienced a significantly higher percentage of comorbid conditions than persons ages 20 to 35 as measured by the Charlson comorbidity index (44.8% versus 15.5%). In addition, a lower comorbidity index was associated with a higher baseline CD4 cell count and an improved immunologic response to HAART. Shah and colleagues [55] studied 165 people who had HIV ages 55 and older and found that 89% had comorbid conditions (mean number of conditions, 2.4). The comorbid conditions identified most frequently were hypertension, chronic airway disease, diabetes mellitus, arthritis, hepatitic C virus infection, coronary artery disease, depression, renal disease, visual abnormalities, and lipid disorders. Additionally, 81% were on chronic medications that were not related to their HIV infection.

Cognitive dysfunction is an important comorbidity associated with advanced age in HIV-positive individuals [56–59]. HIV-associated dementia (HAD) is a "subcortical" dementia defined as an abnormality in at least two cognitive domains plus an abnormality either in motor function or in motivation or emotional control that reduces the ability to complete daily activities or work [3]. Based on data reported to the CDC, there seems to be a linear increase in the incidence of HAD with increasing age (Fig. 2) [60]. Additionally, data from the Multicenter AIDS Cohort Study corroborate this association and show a 1.6-times higher risk for developing dementia for each decade of age [61]. Data from the Hawaii Aging with HIV-1 Cohort show that older patients are 3 times more likely to have HAD after controlling for duration of infection, use of HAART, and CD4 cell count. The investigators note that although the reason for this increased risk is not entirely clear, it does not seem related to duration of HIV infection [20]. Data from a large registry of patients who had HIV and neurologic diseases in Italy suggest that the age-related increase in HAD may be ameliorated by the use of HAART. Although the prevalence of HAD increased with age in this cohort, the prevalence in treatment-naïve, HIV-infected patients over age 50 was 27.3% compared with 11.7% in treatment-experienced patients [62]. Although this observation should be confirmed in

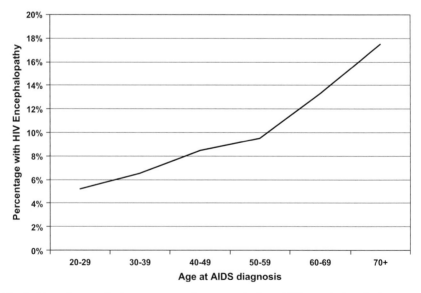

Fig. 2. Linear increase in the percentage of persons who have HIV encephalopathy by age at diagnosis of AIDS. (*Data from* Janssen RS, Nwanyanwu OC, Selik RM, et al. Epidemiology of human immunodeficiency virus encephalopathy in the United States. Neurology 1992;42: 1472–6.)

other settings, consideration of an increased risk for dementia in untreated older patients may have an impact on decisions regarding when to initiate antiretroviral therapy in this age group.

In addition to cognitive dysfunction, advanced age may be associated with other neuropsychiatric disorders. For example, besides experiencing an increase in memory problems, older HIV-positive individuals in the Veterans Aging Cohort Five-Site Study demonstrate a greater prevalence of depressive symptoms, alcohol use, and drug use [63]. Also, the risk for distal sensory polyneuropathy, a common neurologic complication of HIV, increases with age [64].

There is emerging evidence that other diseases associated with aging and not typically classified as HIV related may have a higher incidence in HIV-infected people compared with HIV-negative counterparts. Cancers of the skin (all types), prostate, colorectum, and anorectum and Hodgkin's disease are reported at higher rates than in age- and race-matched HIV-negative populations [65]. Although the risk for cardiovascular disease increases with age, and likely with exposure to antiretroviral therapy, it is not clear whether or not it is increased in HIV-positive compared with HIV-negative populations [66].

Prevention

Increased education and prevention efforts should target older adults and their younger counterparts, because older adults continue to participate in high-risk sexual behavior and likely are not tested for HIV. In a national sample of the National AIDS Behavioral Surveys, 92.4% of sexually active participants ages 50 to 75 reported never using condoms. Additionally, 96.5% never had been tested for HIV [67]. Similar data from the 1996 Behavioral Risk Factor Surveillance System reveal that 73.4% of older adults never had been tested for HIV [68]. The idea that the elderly are not at risk for HIV infection is a misconception and should be addressed as a part of preventive effort programs.

Preventive efforts should target older women and men. Such efforts should be tailored specifically for older women, because several factors put them uniquely at increased risk for HIV transmission. For example, physiologic changes, such as decrease in vaginal lubrication and a thinning of the vaginal mucosa, can predispose women to microscopic tears during intercourse, which increase the risk for HIV acquisition. Additionally, older women may change previous safer sex behaviors, such as condom use, because they no longer fear pregnancy [69].

Few HIV prevention and intervention efforts target older adults specifically. In a best-evidence review of HIV-prevention behavioral interventions performed by the CDC, none of the 18 interventions targeted older adults and only a few included participants over age 50 [70]. There are, however, examples of specific HIV prevention programs for older adults. One, the Senior HIV Intervention Project, was started in Florida in 1997. This project was designed to increase HIV awareness among senior citizens using peer educator and social marketing strategies and to provide counseling, testing, and referral [71]. Additionally, organizations, such as the National Association of HIV Over Fifty [72], function as resources for HIV education and prevention and provide service and health care programs and advocacy for older adults who are affected by HIV. Another organization, HIV Wisdom for Older Women [73], was created specifically to prevent HIV in this demographic group and to enrich the lives of those women infected with the virus [74]. Continued efforts to provide older adults with education about HIV and AIDS, HIV testing, and high-risk behaviors and risk-factor modification should be undertaken [71]. Furthermore, education and prevention campaigns also should include efforts geared toward health care providers, because health care providers often miss opportunities to discuss HIV/AIDS and risk-factor reduction with their older adult patients [31].

References

[1] Centers for Disease Control and Prevention. 1993 revised classification system for HIV infection and expanded surveillance case definition for AIDS among adolescents and adults. MMWR Recomm Rep 1992;41:1–19.

[2] Manfredi R. HIV infection and advanced age emerging epidemiological, clinical, and management issues. Ageing Res Rev 2004;3:31–54.

[3] Valcour V, Paul R. HIV infection and dementia in older adults. Clin Infect Dis 2006;42: 1449–54.

[4] Centers for Disease Control and Prevention. HIV/AIDS Surveillance Report, 2005. Available at: http://www.cdc.gov/hiv/topics/surveillance/resources/reports/. Accessed January 11, 2007.

[5] Levy JA, Ory MG, Crystal S. HIV/AIDS interventions for midlife and older adults: current status and challenges. J Acquir Immune Defic Syndr 2003;33(Suppl 2):S59–67.

[6] Statement of Senator Gordon H. Smith. Aging hearing: HIV over fifty, exploring the new threat. Available at: http://aging.senate.gov/hearing_detail.cfm?id=270655&. Accessed January 11, 2007.

[7] Phillips P. No plateau for HIV/AIDS epidemic in US women. JAMA 1997;277:1747.

[8] Waysdorf SL. The aging of the AIDS epidemic: emerging legal and public health issues for elderly persons living with HIV/AIDS. Elder Law J 2002;10:47–89.

[9] Centers for Disease Control and Prevention. AIDS public use data set through year-end 2000. Available at: http://www.cdc.gov/hiv/software/apids.htm. Accessed January 11, 2007.

[10] McDavid K, Li J, Lee LM. Racial and ethnic disparities in HIV diagnoses for women in the United States. J Acquir Immune Defic Syndr 2006;42:101–7.

[11] Manfredi R. HIV disease and advanced age: an increasing therapeutic challenge. Drugs Aging 2002;19:647–69.

[12] Zingmond DS, Kilbourne AM, Justice AC, et al. Differences in symptom expression in older HIV-positive patients: the Veterans Aging Cohort 3 Site Study and HIV Cost and Service Utilization Study experience. J Acquir Immune Defic Syndr 2003;33(Suppl 2): S84–92.

[13] Butt AA, Dascomb KK, DeSalvo KB, et al. Human immunodeficiency virus infection in elderly patients. South Med J 2001;94:397–400.

[14] Ferro S, Salit IE. HIV infection in patients over 55 years of age. J Acquir Immune Defic Syndr 1992;5:348–53.

[15] Inungu JN, Mokotoff ED, Kent JB. Characteristics of HIV infection in patients fifty years or older in Michigan. AIDS Patient Care STDS 2001;15:567–73.

[16] Skiest DJ, Rubinstien E, Carley N, et al. The importance of comorbidity in HIV-infected patients over 55: a retrospective case-control study. Am J Med 1996;101:605–11.

[17] Sutin DG, Rose DN, Mulvihill M, et al. Survival of elderly patients with transfusion-related acquired immunodeficiency syndrome. J Am Geriatr Soc 1993;41:214–6.

[18] Centers for Disease Control and Prevention. AIDS among persons aged > or = 50 years– United States, 1991–1996. MMWR Morb Mortal Wkly Rep 1998;47:21–7.

[19] Balslev U, Monforte AD, Stergiou G, et al. Influence of age on rates of new AIDS-defining diseases and survival in 6546 AIDS patients. Scand J Infect Dis 1997;29:337–43.

[20] Valcour V, Shikuma C, Shiramizu B, et al. Higher frequency of dementia in older HIV-1 individuals: the Hawaii aging with HIV-1 Cohort. Neurology 2004;63:822–7.

[21] Wallace JI, Paauw DS, Spach DH. HIV infection in older patients: when to suspect the unexpected. Geriatrics 1993;48:61–70.

[22] O'Brien TR, Blattner WA, Waters D, et al. Serum HIV-1 RNA levels and time to development of AIDS in the Multicenter Hemophilia Cohort Study. JAMA 1996;276: 105–10.

[23] Soriano V, Castilla J, Gomez-Cano M, et al. The decline in CD4+ T lymphocytes as a function of the duration of HIV infection, age at seroconversion, and viral load. J Infect 1998;36:307–11.

[24] Goodkin K, Shapshak P, Asthana D, et al. Older age and plasma viral load in HIV-1 infection. AIDS 2004;18(Suppl 1):S87–98.

[25] el Sadr W, Gettler J. Unrecognized human immunodeficiency virus infection in the elderly. Arch Intern Med 1995;155:184–6.

[26] Ena J, Valls V, Lopez AJ, et al. Clinical presentation of HIV infection in patients aged 50 years or older. J Infect 1998;37:213–6.

[27] Gordon SM, Thompson S. The changing epidemiology of human immunodeficiency virus infection in older persons. J Am Geriatr Soc 1995;43:7–9.

[28] Phillips AN, Lee CA, Elford J, et al. More rapid progression to AIDS in older HIV-infected people: the role of CD4+ T-cell counts. J Acquir Immune Defic Syndr 1991;4: 970–5.

[29] Ship JA, Wolff A, Selik RM. Epidemiology of acquired immune deficiency syndrome in persons aged 50 years or older. J Acquir Immune Defic Syndr 1991;4:84–8.

[30] Chiao EY, Ries KM, Sande MA. AIDS and the elderly. Clin Infect Dis 1999;28:740–5.

[31] Skiest DJ, Keiser P. Human immunodeficiency virus infection in patients older than 50 years. A survey of primary care physicians' beliefs, practices, and knowledge. Arch Fam Med 1997; 6:289–94.

[32] Adler WH, Nagel JE. Acquired immunodeficiency syndrome in the elderly. Drugs Aging 1994;4:410–6.

[33] Belanger F, Meyer L, Carre N, et al. Influence of age at infection on human immunodeficiency virus disease progression to different clinical endpoints: the SEROCO cohort (1988–1994). The Seroco Study Group. Int J Epidemiol 1997;26:1340–5.

[34] Blaxhult A, Granath F, Lidman K, et al. The influence of age on the latency period to AIDS in people infected by HIV through blood transfusion. AIDS 1990;4:125–9.

[35] Operskalski EA, Stram DO, Lee H, et al. Human immunodeficiency virus type 1 infection: relationship of risk group and age to rate of progression to AIDS. Transfusion Safety Study Group. J Infect Dis 1995;172:648–55.

[36] Hall HI, McDavid K, Ling Q, et al. Determinants of progression to AIDS or death after HIV diagnosis, United States, 1996 to 2001. Ann Epidemiol 2006;16:824–33.

[37] Adler WH, Baskar PV, Chrest FJ, et al. HIV infection and aging: mechanisms to explain the accelerated rate of progression in the older patient. Mech Ageing Dev 1997;96:137–55.

[38] Guidelines for the use of antiretroviral agents in HIV-1-Infected adults and adolescents. Available at: http://aidsinfo.nih.gov/ContentFiles/AdultandAdolescentGL.pdf. Accessed January 11, 2007.

[39] Hammer SM, Saag MS, Schechter M, et al. Treatment for adult HIV infection: 2006 recommendations of the International AIDS Society-USA panel. JAMA 2006;296:827–43.

[40] Dealing with antiretroviral side effects. Available at: http://www.projectinform.org/fs/sideeffects.html. Accessed January 11, 2007.

[41] Gebo KA. HIV in patients over 50: an increasing problem. Hopkins HIV Rep 2004;16:7–11.

[42] Grimes RM, Otiniano ME, Rodriguez-Barradas MC, et al. Clinical experience with human immunodeficiency virus-infected older patients in the era of effective antiretroviral therapy. Clin Infect Dis 2002;34:1530–3.

[43] Knobel H, Guelar A, Valldecillo G, et al. Response to highly active antiretroviral therapy in HIV-infected patients aged 60 years or older after 24 months follow-up. AIDS 2001;15:1591–3.

[44] Tumbarello M, Rabagliati R, De Gaetano DK, et al. Older HIV-positive patients in the era of highly active antiretroviral therapy: changing of a scenario. AIDS 2003;17:128–31.

[45] Tumbarello M, Rabagliati R, De Gaetano DK, et al. Older age does not influence CD4 cell recovery in HIV-1 infected patients receiving highly active antiretroviral therapy. BMC Infect Dis 2004;4:46.

[46] Wellons MF, Sanders L, Edwards LJ, et al. HIV infection: treatment outcomes in older and younger adults. J Am Geriatr Soc 2002;50:603–7.

[47] Lederman MM, McKinnis R, Kelleher D, et al. Cellular restoration in HIV infected persons treated with abacavir and a protease inhibitor: age inversely predicts naive CD4 cell count increase. AIDS 2000;14:2635–42.

[48] Manfredi R, Calza L, Cocchi D, et al. Antiretroviral treatment and advanced age: epidemiologic, laboratory, and clinical features in the elderly. J Acquir Immune Defic Syndr 2003;33: 112–4.

[49] Viard JP, Mocroft A, Chiesi A, et al. Influence of age on CD4 cell recovery in human immunodeficiency virus-infected patients receiving highly active antiretroviral therapy: evidence from the EuroSIDA study. J Infect Dis 2001;183:1290–4.

[50] Grabar S, Kousignian I, Sobel A, et al. Immunologic and clinical responses to highly active antiretroviral therapy over 50 years of age. Results from the French Hospital Database on HIV. AIDS 2004;18:2029–38.

[51] Hinkin CH, Hardy DJ, Mason KI, et al. Medication adherence in HIV-infected adults: effect of patient age, cognitive status, and substance abuse. AIDS 2004;18(Suppl 1): S19–25.

[52] Murphy DA, Marelich WD, Hoffman D, et al. Predictors of antiretroviral adherence. AIDS Care 2004;16:471–84.

[53] Perez JL, Moore RD. Greater effect of highly active antiretroviral therapy on survival in people aged > or = 50 years compared with younger people in an urban observational cohort. Clin Infect Dis 2003;36:212–8.

[54] Egger M, May M, Chene G, et al. Prognosis of HIV-1-infected patients starting highly active antiretroviral therapy: a collaborative analysis of prospective studies. Lancet 2002;360: 119–29.

[55] Shah SS, McGowan JP, Smith C, et al. Comorbid conditions, treatment, and health maintenance in older persons with human immunodeficiency virus infection in New York City. Clin Infect Dis 2002;35:1238–43.

[56] Becker JT, Lopez OL, Dew MA, et al. Prevalence of cognitive disorders differs as a function of age in HIV virus infection. AIDS 2004;18(Suppl 1):S11–8.

[57] Cherner M, Ellis RJ, Lazzaretto D, et al. Effects of HIV-1 infection and aging on neurobehavioral functioning: preliminary findings. AIDS 2004;18(Suppl 1):S27–34.

[58] Chiesi A, Vella S, Dally LG, et al. Epidemiology of AIDS dementia complex in Europe. AIDS in Europe Study Group. J Acquir Immune Defic Syndr Hum Retrovirol 1996;11: 39–44.

[59] Wilkie FL, Goodkin K, Khamis I, et al. Cognitive functioning in younger and older HIV-1-infected adults. J Acquir Immune Defic Syndr 2003;33(Suppl 2):S93–105.

[60] Janssen RS, Nwanyanwu OC, Selik RM, et al. Epidemiology of human immunodeficiency virus encephalopathy in the United States. Neurology 1992;42:1472–6.

[61] McArthur JC, Hoover DR, Bacellar H, et al. Dementia in AIDS patients: incidence and risk factors. Multicenter AIDS Cohort Study. Neurology 1993;43:2245–52.

[62] Larussa D, Lorenzini P, Cingolani A, et al. Highly active antiretroviral therapy reduces the age-associated risk of dementia in a cohort of older HIV-1-infected patients. AIDS Res Hum Retroviruses 2006;22:386–92.

[63] Justice AC, McGinnis KA, Atkinson JH, et al. Psychiatric and neurocognitive disorders among HIV-positive and negative veterans in care: Veterans Aging Cohort Five-Site Study. AIDS 2004;18(Suppl 1):S49–59.

[64] Watters MR, Poff PW, Shiramizu BT, et al. Symptomatic distal sensory polyneuropathy in HIV after age 50. Neurology 2004;62:1378–83.

[65] Burgi A, Brodine S, Wegner S, et al. Incidence and risk factors for the occurrence of non-AIDS-defining cancers among human immunodeficiency virus-infected individuals. Cancer 2005;104:1505–11.

[66] Friis-Moller N, Sabin CA, Weber R, et al. Combination antiretroviral therapy and the risk of myocardial infarction. N Engl J Med 2003;349:1993–2003.

[67] Stall R, Catania J. AIDS risk behaviors among late middle-aged and elderly Americans. The National AIDS Behavioral Surveys. Arch Intern Med 1994;154:57–63.

[68] Mack KA, Bland SD. HIV testing behaviors and attitudes regarding HIV/AIDS of adults aged 50-64. Gerontologist 1999;39:687–94.

[69] Lieberman R. HIV in older Americans: an epidemiologic perspective. J Midwifery Womens Health 2000;45:176–82.

[70] Lyles CM, Kay LS, Crepaz N, et al. Best-evidence interventions: findings from a systematic review of HIV behavioral interventions for US populations at high risk, 2000-2004. Am J Public Health 2007;97:133–43.

[71] Agate LL, Mullins JM, Prudent ES, et al. Strategies for reaching retirement communities and aging social networks: HIV/AIDS prevention activities among seniors in South Florida. J Acquir Immune Defic Syndr 2003;33(Suppl 2):S238–42.

[72] National Association of HIV Over Fifty. Available at: www.hivoverfifty.org. Accessed February 17, 2007.

[73] HIV Wisdom for Older Women. Available at: www.hivwisdom.org. Accessed February 17, 2007.

[74] Larkin M. HIV and older people: a growing concern. Lancet Infect Dis 2006;6:475.

CLINICS IN
GERIATRIC
MEDICINE

Clin Geriatr Med 23 (2007) 585–594

Asymptomatic Bacteriuria and Urinary Tract Infection in Older Adults

Manisha Juthani-Mehta, MD

Yale University School of Medicine, Department of Internal Medicine, Section of Infectious Disease, LMP 5040A, P.O. Box 208022, New Haven, CT 06520, USA

Asymptomatic bacteriuria

Asymptomatic bacteriuria (ASB) is a common occurrence in older adults. The major predisposing factors are physiologic changes related to aging (eg, decreased estrogen or changes in bactericidal activity of prostate secretions in men) and comorbid illnesses (eg, benign prostatic hypertrophy in men or cystocele in women). To date, short-term or long-term adverse outcomes attributable to the high incidence and prevalence of ASB are not demonstrated, and there is no evidence of impact on survival. The following sections review the diagnosis, prevalence, microbiology, management, and prevention of ASB in older adults.

Diagnosis of asymptomatic bacteriuria

The diagnosis of ASB is based on the result of a urine culture from a urine specimen that minimizes contamination from a person who does not have symptoms or signs referable to urinary infection [1]. For asymptomatic women, bacteriuria is defined as two consecutive voided urine specimens with isolation of the same bacterial strain in quantitative counts greater than or equal to 10^5 colony-forming units (cfu) per mL. For asymptomatic men, bacteriuria is defined as a single, clean-catch voided urine specimen with one bacterial species isolated in a quantitative count greater than or equal to 10^5 cfu/mL. For women and men, a single catheterized urine specimen with one bacterial species isolated in a quantitative count greater than or equal to 10^5 cfu/mL defines bacteriuria [2].

E-mail address: manisha.juthanimehta@yale.edu

doi:10.1016/j.cger.2007.03.001   *geriatric.theclinics.com*

Prevalence of asymptomatic bacteriuria

Studies of community populations throughout the world show a consistent increase in the prevalence of ASB with age. Young women have a prevalence of ASB of 1% to 2%. For women ages 65 to 90, the prevalence of ASB ranges from 6% to 16%. The prevalence is highest for women over the age of 90, with a prevalence of 22% to 43%. ASB is uncommon in young men, but for men over age 65, the prevalence ranges from 5% to 21%, highest in men over age 90 [3]. Among the institutionalized elderly, 25% to 50% of women and 15% to 35% of men have ASB. The prevalence increases with the severity of disability of nursing home residents. Up to 90% of institutionalized adults also have pyuria [4]. For those residents who have long-term indwelling catheters, 100% have ASB [5]. Elderly persons who have condom catheters, versus indwelling catheters, have a lower incidence of ASB or urinary tract infection (UTI) [6].

Microbiology of asymptomatic bacteriuria

The genitourinary tract usually is sterile except for the distal urethra. ASB occurs by ascension of bacteria up the urethra into the bladder with possible ascension to the kidneys. Bacteria causing ASB usually originate as colonizing flora of the gut, vagina, or periurethral area. *Escherichia coli* is the single most common organism isolated in women and men who have ASB 75% to 80% of the time [7,8]. Other organisms commonly identified include other Enterobacteriaceae (eg, *Klebsiella pneumoniae,* coagulase-negative staphylococci, *Enterococcus* species, group B streptococci, and *Gardnerella vaginalis*) [2]. Among community dwellers, *E coli* and coagulase-negative staphylococci are most common. *Proteus mirabilis, Providencia stuarti,* and *K pneumoniae* are more common in nursing home residents. Long-term indwelling catheters become coated with biofilm, and organisms, such as *P mirabilis, P stuarti,* and *Pseudomonas aeruginosa,* often are present in biofilm [9].

Management of asymptomatic bacteriuria

For elderly persons, routine screening for and treatment of ASB are not recommended. Based on recommendations of the Infectious Diseases Society of America, screening for or treatment of ASB are not recommended for the following persons: (1) diabetic women; (2) older persons living in the community or who are institutionalized; (3) persons who have spinal cord injury; and (4) catheterized patients while a catheter remains in situ [2]. Although a 3-day course of antibiotic therapy is shown to decrease the prevalence of bacteriuria at 6 months [10], no benefits in morbidity, mortality, and chronic urinary incontinence are demonstrated to date. The randomized trials leading to these recommendations are summarized in Table 1 [11–14]. Screening for and treatment of ASB in older persons is recommended only

Table 1
Prospective randomized studies of treatment of asymptomatic bacteriuria

Author	Subjects	Intervention	Outcome
Nicolle, et al [11]	Men, nursing home residents; median age 80 years	Treated: 16 Not treated: 20 Duration of study: 2 years	No differences in mortality or infectious morbidity between the two groups.
Nicolle, et al [12]	Women, nursing home residents; median age 83 years	Treated: 26 Not treated: 24 Duration of study: 1 year	No differences in mortality and genitourinary morbidity between the two groups. Increased adverse drug reactions and antimicrobial resistance in the treatment group.
Abrutyn, et al [13]	Women, ambulatory apartment and nursing home residents; mean age 82 years	Treated: 192 Not treated: 166 Duration of study: 8 years	No survival benefit from antimicrobial therapy in the treatment group compared with the control group.
Ouslander, et al [14]	Women and men, nursing home residents; mean age 85 years	Treatment: 33 No treatment: 38 Duration of study: 4 weeks	No differences in chronic urinary incontinence between the two groups.

in the following two circumstances: (1) before transurethral resection of the prostate and (2) before urologic procedures in which mucosal bleeding is anticipated [2]. Although it is shown that nonurinary symptoms and signs are an important factor in the prescription of antibiotics for ASB [15], there is no evidence to date to support this practice.

Prevention of asymptomatic bacteriuria

Few studies have been performed examining prevention strategies for ASB. In a randomized, double-blind, placebo-controlled trial in older, female, community-dwelling and nursing home residents, cranberry juice reduced the frequency of bacteriuria with pyuria in this population [16]. Because of several study design issues in this trial, however, the use of cranberry juice has not been advocated fully for the prevention of ASB. In a controlled trial of intravaginal estriol therapy in postmenopausal women who had recurrent UTI, the estriol group had fewer episodes of ASB than the placebo group [17]. This study was conducted, however, specifically in women who had a history of recurrent UTI. Intravaginal estriol therapy is not recommended for all postmenopausal women. Lastly, avoiding long-term indwelling catheter usage is optimal. If possible, using a condom catheter provides more comfort to patients and fewer adverse outcomes [6].

Urinary tract infection

UTI is the second most common cause of infectious disease hospitalization in adults 65 years or older after lower respiratory tract infections [18]. In 1998, UTI was the most costly and resource-intensive condition, causing more than 1.8 million physician office visits among Medicare beneficiaries. Total Medicare expenditures for UTI in all venues of care amounted to more than $1.4 billion, exclusive of medication costs [19].

Diagnosis of urinary tract infection

The diagnosis of UTI in community-dwelling older adults follows a similar paradigm to the diagnosis of UTI in younger adults, requiring significant bacteriuria ($\geq 10^5$ cfu/mL) associated with genitourinary symptoms. In older adults who are intact cognitively and can report symptoms, the diagnosis of UTI is made easily. Among institutionalized older adults, however, who often are impaired cognitively, distinguishing ASB from UTI often is problematic.

In older institutionalized adults, multiple comorbid illnesses may present with symptoms similar to UTI, and older adults who have cognitive impairment may not be able to report their symptoms [20]. Laboratory confirmation of UTI with significant bacteriuria ($\geq 10^5$ cfu/mL on urine culture) and pyuria (> 10 white blood cells on urinalysis) is an agreed-on minimum necessary but not sufficient criterion for diagnosis of UTI in this population [21]. Identifying symptoms that are present in older adults who have UTI is unclear, however. In a study of older adults who did not have dysuria, urinary symptoms (ie, incontinence, frequency, urgency, suprapubic pain, flank pain, or fever) and symptoms indicating a lack of well-being (anorexia, difficulty falling asleep, difficulty staying asleep, fatigue, malaise, or weakness) were present in equal frequency when these adults were bacteriuric or non-bacteriuric [22]. To date, no constellation of symptoms is identified in older adults who have bacteriuria that can distinguish symptomatic from asymptomatic patients reliably in all situations.

Although symptomatic UTI is defined by the presence of clinical symptoms attributed to the genitourinary tract in association with significant bacteriuria even in older institutionalized adults [4], experts recognize that elderly nursing home residents may present with biologically plausible, non-urinary-tract specific symptoms. With lack of empiric data, criteria for UTI surveillance, diagnosis, and treatment in nursing home residents have been developed by infectious diseases consensus group recommendations. Consensus-based criteria developed by McGeer and colleagues [23] were recommendations for surveillance and outcome assessment purposes in nursing homes. As per these criteria, for nursing home residents who do not have an indwelling catheter, three of the following criteria must be met to identify UTI: (1) fever greater than or equal to 100.4°F; (2) new or increased burning on urination, frequency, or urgency; (3) new flank or suprapubic pain or tenderness; (4) change in character of urine; and (5) worsening of mental or functional status. For residents who have a long-term indwelling catheter, two of the following criteria must be met: (1) fever greater than or equal to 100.4°F; (2) new flank or suprapubic pain or tenderness; (3) change in character of urine; and (4) worsening of mental or functional status [23]. These criteria are accepted as a standard for nursing homes by two national infection control organizations (the Association for Professionals in Infection Control and the Society for Healthcare Epidemiology of America) [24]. The Department of Health and Human Services and the Centers for Medicare and Medicaid Services issue yearly guidelines for nursing homes that state that only residents meeting the McGeer criteria should be treated for UTI [25]. Urine culture results are not required by these criteria because of the high prevalence of ASB; if an appropriately collected specimen is sent, the specimen must be reported as positive or contaminated [23]. Although these criteria are validated as a surveillance tool to compare rates of UTI in nursing homes [26], they could not be validated when used as "standard clinical criteria" [27]. Nevertheless, with no other diagnostic guidelines and with the endorsement of federal regulating agencies, most nursing homes use these criteria for diagnostic and treatment purposes [28].

Microbiology of urinary tract infection

Among community-dwelling older adults who have UTI associated with bacteremia, 80% of episodes are the result of gram-negative organisms (most commonly *E coli*) and 20% gram-positive organisms (eg, *Enterococcus* or methicillin-resistant *Staphylococcus aureus*) [29]. Among institutionalized older adults, *E coli* still is the pathogen identified most commonly, but nosocomial pathogens, such as *P aeruginosa,* vancomycin-resistant enterococci, *Candida* spp, and non–*E coli* Enterobacteriaceae, often are identified [9].

Management of urinary tract infection

For community-dwelling older adults presenting to an acute care hospital with presumed urosepsis, empiric therapy with a third-generation cephalosporin is appropriate single-agent therapy until culture and susceptibility reports are available. Unless specific risk factors for a gram-positive infection are identified (eg, pressure sores or concomitant pneumonia), vancomycin therapy is not required empirically [29]. For outpatient oral therapy, fluoroquinolones are appropriate first-line drugs for older adults who have UTI.

An appropriate first step in the evaluation of UTI in institutionalized older adults is performing a urinary dipstick. In nursing home residents who have suspected UTI, the negative predictive value of the urinary dipstick is 100% [30]. Performing this test in a nursing home setting obviates outsourcing urine cultures and urinalyses. Clinical criteria for empiric treatment of UTI in institutionalized adults also are consensus based. In 2001, Loeb and colleagues [31] recommended a minimum set of clinical criteria necessary to initiate antibiotic therapy for UTI. According to these criteria, for residents who do not have an indwelling catheter, minimum criteria for initiating antibiotics include acute dysuria alone *or* fever ($>37.9°C$ [100°F] or $1.5°C$ [2.4°F] increase above baseline temperature) *and* at least one of the following: new or worsening urgency, frequency, suprapubic pain, gross hematuria, costovertebral angle tenderness, or urinary incontinence. For residents who have a chronic indwelling catheter, minimum criteria for initiating antibiotics include the presence of at least one of the following: fever ($>37.9°C$ [100°F] or $1.5°C$ [2.4°F] increase above baseline temperature), new costovertebral angle tenderness, rigors (shaking chills) with or without an identified cause, or new onset of delirium. These criteria were the basis for a multifaceted intervention designed to reduce the number of antimicrobial prescriptions for suspected UTI in nursing home residents. The algorithm used in this trial is the best available approach to nursing home residents who have suspected UTI (Figs. 1 and 2).

In this clustered randomized controlled trial, fewer courses of antimicrobials were prescribed for suspected UTI. However, total antimicrobial use in the intervention and control groups did not differ. No significant difference was found in admissions to the hospital or mortality between the study arms [32]. Based on these results, it seems that nursing home practitioners suspected another infection instead of UTI in order to prescribe antibiotic therapy. Because these criteria currently are not evidence based, nursing home practitioners may not support using them and continue established antibiotic prescription patterns. Research that validates specific elements of these criteria is needed and will provide evidence to support their use in clinical practice.

Prevention of urinary tract infection

Although cranberry tablet or juice administration is an appealing prevention modality for UTI because of its low side-effect profile and ease of administration, it has not been investigated for the purposes of preventing UTI in older adults. As such, no data exist to date to demonstrate a benefit of long-term cranberry ingestion for the prevention of UTI. Intravaginal estriol therapy in postmenopausal women who have recurrent UTI is shown to decrease the number of episodes of UTI [17]. Antibiotic prophylaxis is highly effective at reducing the risk for recurrent UTI in older women. Continuous prophylaxis is recommended for women who experience two or

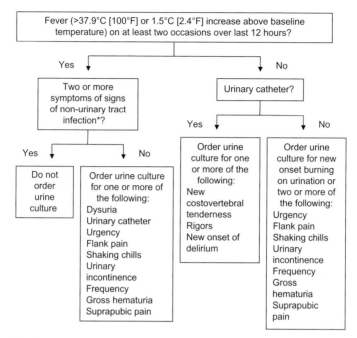

Fig. 1. Diagnostic algorithm for ordering urine cultures in nursing home residents. (*From* Loeb M, Brazil K, Lohfeld L, et al. Effect of a multifaceted intervention on number of antimicrobial prescriptions for suspected urinary tract infections in residents of nursing homes: cluster rand-omised controlled trial. BMJ 2005;331:669; with permission.)

more symptomatic UTIs over a 6-month period or three or more over a 12-month period, after an existing infection is eradicated. Most experts recommend a 6-month trial of a once-nightly prophylactic agent, after which the regimen is discontinued and patients observed for further infection. Some experts advocate prophylaxis for up to 2 years. Antimicrobial agents used for prophylaxis include trimethoprim-sulfamethoxazole, nitrofurantoin, and cefalexin [33].

Other risk factors for recurrent UTI are identified in older postmenopausal women; however, these risk factors are not shown to be modifiable to date. In postmenopausal women, a history of UTI in the premenopausal period, incontinence, presence of a cystocele, and postvoid residual urine predispose to UTI. In institutionalized older adults, catheterization, incontinence, antimicrobial exposure, and functional status are related most strongly to risk for recurrent UTI [34].

In older men, risk factors for UTI include dementia, incontinence of bladder and bowel, and use of condom or indwelling catheters [35,36].

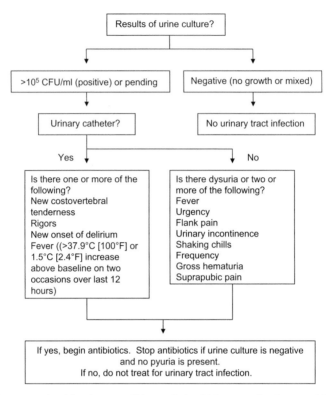

Fig. 2. Treatment algorithm for prescribing antimicrobials to nursing home residents. (*From* Loeb M, Brazil K, Lohfeld L, et al. Effect of a multifaceted intervention on number of antimicrobial prescriptions for suspected urinary tract infections in residents of nursing homes: cluster randomised controlled trial. BMJ 2005;331:669; with permission.)

Condom catheters are preferable to indwelling catheters; however, if an indwelling catheter is essential, staff should maintain a closed, dependent system to avoid introducing new organisms, be vigilant for the development of obstruction, and avoid trauma [37]. Severe benign prostatic hypertrophy often is implicated as a risk for recurrent UTI. When possible, resection of the prostate can assist in reducing recurrent episodes.

Summary

ASB is highly prevalent in older adults; however, with no short- or long-term adverse outcomes, screening and treatment are not recommended. UTI also is prevalent in older adults and is a source of considerable morbidity and mortality in this population, but the relation of ASB to UTI is uncertain. Those older adults who can report genitourinary symptoms associated with UTI can be identified easily. Distinguishing ASB from UTI in older adults, however, particularly in those who have cognitive impairment, remains a diagnostic challenge. Future studies should be focused on identifying mechanisms to distinguish older adults who have ASB from those who have UTI.

References

[1] Nicolle LE. Asymptomatic bacteriuria: when to screen and when to treat. Infect Dis Clin North Am 2003;17:367–94.

[2] Nicolle LE, Bradley S, Colgan R, et al. Infectious diseases society of America guidelines for the diagnosis and treatment of asymptomatic bacteriuria in adults. Clin Infect Dis 2005;40: 643–54.

[3] Nicolle LE. Asymptomatic bacteriuria in the elderly. Infect Dis Clin North Am 1997;11: 647–62.

[4] Nicolle LE. Urinary tract infections in long-term-care facilities. Infect Control Hosp Epidemiol 2001;22:167–75.

[5] Warren JW, Tenney JH, Hoopes JM, et al. A prospective microbiologic study of bacteriuria in patients with chronic indwelling urethral catheters. J Infect Dis 1982;146:719–23.

[6] Saint S, Kaufman SR, Rogers MA, et al. Condom versus indwelling urinary catheters: a randomized trial. J Am Geriatr Soc 2006;54:1055–61.

[7] Boscia JA, Kobasa WD, Knight RA, et al. Epidemiology of bacteriuria in an elderly ambulatory population. Am J Med 1986;80:208–14.

[8] Monane M, Gurwitz JH, Lipsitz LA, et al. Epidemiologic and diagnostic aspects of bacteriuria: a longitudinal study in older women. J Am Geriatr Soc 1995;43:618–22.

[9] Nicolle LE. Resistant pathogens in urinary tract infections. J Am Geriatr Soc 2002;50: S230–5.

[10] Boscia JA, Kobasa WD, Knight RA, et al. Therapy vs no therapy for bacteriuria in elderly ambulatory nonhospitalized women. JAMA 1987;257:1067–71.

[11] Nicolle LE, Bjornson J, Harding GK, et al. Bacteriuria in elderly institutionalized men. N Engl J Med 1983;309:1420–5.

[12] Nicolle LE, Mayhew WJ, Bryan L. Prospective randomized comparison of therapy and no therapy for asymptomatic bacteriuria in institutionalized elderly women. Am J Med 1987;83: 27–33.

[13] Abrutyn E, Mossey J, Berlin JA, et al. Does asymptomatic bacteriuria predict mortality and does antimicrobial treatment reduce mortality in elderly ambulatory women? Ann Intern Med 1994;120:827–33.

[14] Ouslander JG, Schapira M, Schnelle JF, et al. Does eradicating bacteriuria affect the severity of chronic urinary incontinence in nursing home residents? Ann Intern Med 1995;122: 749–54.

[15] Walker S, McGeer A, Simor AE, et al. Why are antibiotics prescribed for asymptomatic bacteriuria in institutionalized elderly people? A qualitative study of physicians' and nurses' perceptions. CMAJ 2000;163:273–7.

[16] Avorn J, Monane M, Gurwitz JH, et al. Reduction of bacteriuria and pyuria after ingestion of cranberry juice. JAMA 1994;271:751–4.

[17] Raz R, Stamm WE. A controlled trial of intravaginal estriol in postmenopausal women with recurrent urinary tract infections. N Engl J Med 1993;329:753–6.

[18] Curns AT, Holman RC, Sejvar JJ, et al. Infectious disease hospitalizations among older adults in the United States from 1990 through 2002. Arch Intern Med 2005;165:2514–20.

[19] Litwin MS, Saigal CS, Beerbohm EM. The burden of urologic diseases in America. J Urol 2005;173:1065–6.

[20] Yoshikawa TT, Nicolle LE, Norman DC. Management of complicated urinary tract infection in older patients. J Am Geriatr Soc 1996;44:1235–41.

[21] Garner JS, Jarvis WR, Emori TG, et al. CDC definitions for nosocomial infections, 1988. Am J Infect Control 1988;16:128–40.

[22] Boscia JA, Kobasa WD, Abrutyn E, et al. Lack of association between bacteriuria and symptoms in the elderly. Am J Med 1986;81:979–82.

[23] McGeer A, Campbell B, Emori TG, et al. Definitions of infection for surveillance in long-term care facilities. Am J Infect Control 1991;19:1–7.

[24] Smith PW, Rusnak PG. Infection prevention and control in the long-term-care facility. SHEA Long-Term-Care Committee and APIC Guidelines Committee. Infect Control Hosp Epidemiol 1997;18:831–49.

[25] Centers for Medicare and Medicaid (CMS) Manual System, State Operations Manual. Appendix PP. Section 483.25(d) vol; 2005:183–4.

[26] Stevenson KB, Moore J, Colwell H, et al. Standardized infection surveillance in long-term care: interfacility comparisons from a regional cohort of facilities. Infect Control Hosp Epidemiol 2005;26:231–8.

[27] Orr PH, Nicolle LE, Duckworth H, et al. Febrile urinary infection in the institutionalized elderly. Am J Med 1996;100:71–7.

[28] Juthani-Mehta M, Drickamer MA, Towle V, et al. Nursing home practitioner survey of diagnostic criteria for urinary tract infections. J Am Geriatr Soc 2005;53:1986–90.

[29] Ackermann RJ, Monroe PW. Bacteremic urinary tract infection in older people. J Am Geriatr Soc 1996;44:927–33.

[30] Juthani-Mehta M, Tinetti M, Perrelli E, et al. The role of dipstick testing in the evaluation of UTI in nursing home residents. Infect Control Hosp Epidemiol, in press.

[31] Loeb M, Bentley DW, Bradley S, et al. Development of minimum criteria for the initiation of antibiotics in residents of long-term-care facilities: results of a consensus conference. Infect Control Hosp Epidemiol 2001;22:120–4.

[32] Loeb M, Brazil K, Lohfeld L, et al. Effect of a multifaceted intervention on number of antimicrobial prescriptions for suspected urinary tract infections in residents of nursing homes: cluster randomised controlled trial. BMJ 2005;331:669.

[33] Hooton TM. Recurrent urinary tract infection in women. Int J Antimicrob Agents 2001;17: 259–68.

[34] Stamm WE, Raz R. Factors contributing to susceptibility of postmenopausal women to recurrent urinary tract infections. Clin Infect Dis 1999;28:723–5.

[35] Nicolle LE, Henderson E, Bjornson J, et al. The association of bacteriuria with resident characteristics and survival in elderly institutionalized men. Ann Intern Med 1987;106:682–6.

[36] Ouslander JG, Greengold B, Chen S. External catheter use and urinary tract infections among incontinent male nursing home patients. J Am Geriatr Soc 1987;35:1063–70.

[37] Drinka PJ. Complications of chronic indwelling urinary catheters. J Am Med Dir Assoc 2006;7:388–92.

CLINICS IN
GERIATRIC
MEDICINE

ELSEVIER
SAUNDERS

Clin Geriatr Med 23 (2007) 595–613

Skin and Soft Tissue Infections in Older Adults

Deverick J. Anderson, MD[a],*, Keith S. Kaye, MD, MPH[b]

[a]Division of Infectious Diseases, Duke University Medical Center, Box 3605, Durham, NC 27710, USA
[b]Division of Infectious Diseases, Duke University Medical Center, Box 3152, Durham, NC 27710, USA

Skin and soft tissue infections (SSTIs) are common in the general population and in older persons. Because of changes in skin consistency, immunosenescence, and the presence of underlying skin conditions and comorbid conditions, elderly persons are at high risk for SSTIs. This article discusses SSTIs acquired frequently in the community, such as cellulitis, necrotizing fasciitis, and carbunculosis, and infections that frequently are health care associated, such as pressure ulcers and surgical site infections (SSIs).

Infections in the community

Cellulitis and erysipelas

Overview, pathophysiology, and microbiology

Cellulitis is a common bacterial infectious disease of the skin and is managed by health care providers in various diverse fields. Cellulitis occurs frequently in long-term care facilities, affecting 1% to 9% of residents [1]. Cellulitis is caused by bacteria that breach the skin and sometimes involve the subcutaneous tissue. Thus, peripheral lymphedema, venous stasis, and the presence of tinea pedis are important in the pathogenesis of some cases.

Without the presence of underlying abscess or deeper infectious foci, the bacterial burden in the skin is low. Bacterial exotoxins play a prominent role in the inflammation and infectious symptoms associated with cellulites [2].

Dr. Anderson is the recipient of the Pfizer Fellowship in Infectious Disease.
* Corresponding author.
E-mail address: dja@duke.edu (D.J. Anderson).

The majority of cellulitis cases are caused by gram-positive organisms, most commonly *Streptococci* (group A most commonly and also groups B, C, and G). *Staphylococcus aureus* is another notable cause of cellulitis. Other pathogens do not cause cellulitis routinely but can in specific circumstances: *Pseudomonas aeruginosa* after puncture wounds through a sneaker, *Haemophilus influenzae* type b in children, *Pasteurella* spp after a cat bite or scratch, *Capnocytophaga canimorsus* after dog bite, *Eikenella corrodens* after a human bite, and *Aeromonas hydrophila* and *Vibrio* spp after trauma and water exposure.

Erysipelas is an infection involving the upper dermis that often is characterized by a raised rash with clearly demarcated borders. Erysipelas is caused most commonly by *Streptococcus pyogenes* (group A streptococcus) and *S aureus*. The presentation, diagnosis, and management for erysipelas are similar to those for other types of cellulitis.

Risk factors, presentation, and diagnosis

Knowledge of the clinical epidemiology of cellulitis almost exclusively comes from studies in the general population; the elderly have not been studied extensively as a group. Risk factors for cellulitis include conditions that compromise the integrity of the skin and associated host defenses, such as obesity, venous or lymph stasis, tinea pedis, recent trauma, and underlying skin conditions, such as eczema. Elderly patients have a high frequency of conditions that are associated with skin fragility, such as edema and trauma, that predispose them to cellulitis. For example, by age 70, approximately 70% of persons have at least one underlying skin problem [3]. Patients often present with rapidly spreading erythema, warmth, and edema. Occasionally, tenderness, lymphangitic streaking, and regional lymphadenopathy are present. Systemic symptoms occur less frequently and often are mild, including fever, tachycardia, hypotension, leukocytosis, and change in mental status. Cellulitis in the elderly, however, may present with atypical symptoms; fever often is low grade or absent and patients might present solely with changes in mental status or declining functional status [3].

The diagnosis of cellulitis usually is a clinical one. Blood cultures are positive in less than 5% of cases and cultures of soft tissue aspirate and punch biopsies generally are negative. Serologic tests sometimes are useful in culture-negative cases. Generally, cultures and serologies are not necessary to confirm a diagnosis of cellulitis, but these modalities might be considered if patients do not respond to standard antimicrobial therapy. The differential diagnosis for cellulitis includes deep venous thrombosis, herpes zoster, gout, and acute venous stasis dermatitis.

Treatment and outcomes

If patients are toxic, are septic, or have severe or rapidly spreading cellulitis, then initial therapy should be intravenous (IV) and patients should be hospitalized. In mild cases, antimicrobials can be delivered orally in an outpatient setting. Antimicrobial therapy should include agents that are effective against streptococci and *S aureus*. Typical agents include penicillinase-resistant penicillins, first-generation cephalosporins, vancomycin, and clindamycin (the latter two agents typically are used for patients who have life-threatening penicillin allergies). If patients have a history of recent methicillin-resistant *S aureus* (MRSA) infection, ongoing IV drug abuse, or recent health care exposures, then initial therapy should include vancomycin, linezolid, daptomycin, or other agents that demonstrate in vitro activity against MRSA. If patients have purulent cellulitis, then community-acquired MRSA (CA-MRSA) should be considered a pathogen and should be treated with trimethoprim-sulfamethoxazole, vancomycin, clindamycin (if D-test negative), linezolid, or daptomycin. Typical courses of antimicrobial therapy range from 5 to 14 days, depending on severity of infection and clinical response [2]. If therapy is initiated IV, transition to oral therapy can be considered when patients' local and systemic symptoms improve clinically. Elevation of the affected area (eg, a lower extremity) helps to decrease edema by promoting lymph and venous drainage and can accelerate the time from treatment initiation to cure [2].

Prevention

Limiting the severity of edema through medications (such as diuretics) and medical stockings and by elevating affected extremities can prevent cellulitis. Treating macerated feet with topical antifungals also can prevent recurrent cellulitis. For patients who have multiple recurrent episodes of cellulitis, prophylactic antibiotics can be considered. Antibiotics typically used for prophylaxis include penicillin and erythromycin [2].

Necrotizing fasciitis

Overview, pathophysiology, and microbiology

Necrotizing fasciitis is a rare but severe infection of the subcutaneous tissue that tracks along the fascial layers, destroying the fascia (usually the superficial fascia). Necrotizing fasciitis usually develops after a superficial injury. The initial injury might be mild (such as insect bite, abrasion, or cut) and, in approximately 20% of cases, no primary lesion is identified [2].

There are two types of necrotizing fasciitis. Type 1 is a polymicrobial infection and usually follows a surgical procedure. Infection occurs most often in the lower extremities, abdominal wall, groin, or perianal region. Subsets of type 1 necrotizing fasciitis include Fournier's gangrene and cervical necrotizing fasciitis. Pathogens typically arise from the bowel and include a mix of aerobic and anaerobic gram-positive and gram-negative bacteria. Organisms commonly described as pathogens in type 1 infection, including those occurring in the elderly, are coliform bacteria, such as *E coli*, *Klebsiella pneumonia*, and *P aeruginosa*, and anaerobes [4]. Type 2 infection is a monomicrobial infection. Most commonly, type 2 infection is caused by *S pyogenes* (group A streptococcus) and represents a variant of toxic shock syndrome. Other pathogens that can cause type 2 necrotizing fasciitis include *S agalactiae* (group B streptococcus; particularly in those who have diabetes mellitus), *S aureus*, *V vulnificans*, *A hydrophila*, and anaerobic streptococci. Toxin production plays an important role in the pathophysiology of disease.

Risk factors, presentation, and diagnosis

Predisposing factors for type 1 necrotizing fasciitis include surgical procedures (typically involving the bowel or bladder), decubiti or pressure ulcers, perianal abscess, IV drug abuse, and presence of a Bartholin abscess or other vulvovaginal infection [2]. Frequently, patients have a history of diabetes mellitus. Type 2 necrotizing fasciitis usually occurs in the lower extremities. Predisposing factors for type 2 infection include diabetes mellitus, peripheral vascular disease (PVD), zoster, blunt trauma, IV drug abuse, exposure to another case of type 2 necrotizing fasciitis, childbirth, and surgery.

It may be difficult to diagnose necrotizing fasciitis when patients first present for medical evaluation. Local symptoms might be mild and unimpressive. Frequently, the affected area is extremely painful and the pain, toxicity, and discomfort are out of proportion to physical examination findings. An overlying cellulitis, typified by erythema, edema, and warmth, often can be identified. After the first few days of illness, the skin changes evolve to dark, reddish-purple lesions, then to blisters and bullae. Systemic toxicity is inevitable and usually prominent with fever, tachycardia, and sometimes hypotension present [2].

Clinical suspicion is necessary to diagnosis necrotizing fasciitis. If patients seem toxic or septic, if patients are not responding to antibiotics, or if patients are deteriorating despite appropriate antimicrobial therapy, necrotizing fasciitis must be considered. CT and MRI of affected areas often provide nonspecific results that might not be diagnostic. Leukocytosis often is present and blood cultures usually are positive. Direct observation of the fascial planes and subcutaneous tissue is critical for diagnosis and usually reveals swelling, dullness, and gray discoloration of the fascia. Often, a brownish exudate is present. Gram's stain and culture of affected tissue often demonstrates the pathogens (often multiple in type 1 and a single pathogen in type 2). Aspiration of fluid at the leading edge of the lesion can also provide good material for Gram's stain analysis and culture.

Treatment and outcomes

The hallmark of treatment is surgical intervention. Surgical drainage and exploration is warranted if local wounds demonstrate necrosis or easy dissection along fascial planes or if a soft tissue infection is accompanied by the presence of gas. Typically, patients have to return to an operating room frequently for additional débridement. Antimicrobial therapy is a useful adjuvant to surgical débridement and should be directed against suspected pathogens. For the mixed, type 1 infection, recommended therapies include (1) a β-lactam/β-lactamase inhibitor agent (eg, piperacillin-tazobactam) plus clindamycin plus ciprofloxacin; (2) carbapenem monotherapy; (3) cefotaxime plus metronidazole or clindamycin; or (4) clindamycin or metronidazole plus aminoglycoside or fluoroquinolone. For type 2 streptococcal infection, an important component of initial therapy is clindamycin, which helps to decrease toxin production and modulate cytokine production. Initial therapeutic regimens include (1) penicillin plus clindamycin; (2) vancomycin; (3) linezolid; (4) quinupristin/dalfopristin; or (5) daptomycin. For type 2 *S aureus* infection, therapeutic options include nafcillin, cefazolin, vancomycin, and clindamycin. For clostridial infection, clindamycin and penicillin are therapeutic options [2].

Furuncles, carbuncles, and boils

Overview, pathophysiology, and microbiology

A furuncle, or boil, is an infection of the hair follicle. Typically, a furuncle involves an inflammatory nodule overlying a pustule. When infection involves several adjacent follicles, a coalescent purulent mass or carbuncle forms. In adults, the most common pathogen causing furuncles and carbuncles is *S aureus*. Classically, among patients who do not have health care contact or other risk factors for MRSA, methicillin-susceptible *S aureus* has been the most common type of *S aureus* to cause infection. Recently, however, CA-MRSA has become a common cause of carbunculosis in many parts of the United States. In addition to causing endemic carbunculosis, CA-MRSA also is associated with outbreaks in diverse, previously healthy populations, including children, families, athletes, military recruits, and prisoners.

Risk factors, presentation, and diagnosis

Risk factors for infection include inadequate personal hygiene, exposure to other cases of carbunculosis, and skin injury. Fomites can harbor pathogens causing carbunculosis and can facilitate spread in families and in other populations. For example, among athletes, body shaving, sharing of razors and other personal equipment, and sports equipment itself (eg, wrestling mats) are important risk factors for infection. One might speculate that institutions with common equipment, such as rehabilitation facilities, might place older adults at similar risk, but no data have been generated specifically to answer this question. CA-MRSA seems to have a predilection for infecting younger individuals and occurs less frequently in persons 65 or older, but the reasons for this are unclear [5,6].

Treatment and outcomes

Drainage of purulent lesions is critical to cure carbunculosis. For small lesions, application of moist heat to promote drainage might be all that is required. For larger lesions, however, incision and drainage often are necessary. If carbuncles are small (eg, <5 cm) and not associated with cellulitis or systemic infection, then systemic antibiotics might not be needed [7]. If lesions are large or there is associated cellulitis, however, then antibiotics should be prescribed in addition to incision and drainage.

Prevention

If exposed to individuals who have carbuncles, practicing good hygiene, bathing with antibacterial soaps, and not sharing personal items all can help prevent the spread of boils, in particular those resulting from CA-MRSA. If individuals have repeated attacks of carbunculosis, abnormal host immune response should be ruled out as a predisposing cause. Attempts can be made to decolonize individuals. One approach involves applying mupirocin to the anterior nares twice daily for 5 days. This approach is reported to reduce recurrences by 50% [8]. This regimen often is conducted in conjunction with daily chlorhexidine gluconate showers for 5 days. This regimen should be used judiciously, however, as investigators report the rapid emergence of resistance of MRSA to mupirocin [9]. For recurrent attacks despite these approaches, some investigators report limited success with long courses of low-dose antibiotics, including rifampin, trimethoprim-sulfamethoxazole, or clindamycin [2]. If providers want to decolonize patients using long courses of systemic antibiotics, consultation with an infectious diseases expert should be considered.

Health care–associated skin and soft tissue infections

Decubiti or pressure ulcers

Overview, pathophysiology, and microbiology

Pressure ulcers are common yet often preventable and often occur in high-risk populations, such as patients who have physical impairments or older persons. In fact, more than two thirds of decubiti occur in persons older than 70 years of age. The incidence rate for pressure ulcers ranges from 2% to 24% in long-term care settings and 0.4% to 38% in acute care settings [10]. The majority of pressure ulcers occurring in hospitals develop during the initial 5 days of hospitalization. An estimated 2.5 million pressure ulcers are treated annually in the United States. In addition to having an adverse impact on patients clinically, pressure ulcers prolong duration of hospitalization and lead to excess health care costs.

Pressure ulcers occur when prolonged pressure and tissue compression cause local ischemia and the accumulation of toxic metabolites and cell death, eventually leading to ulceration and necrosis [11]. For example, excessive pressure on the heels of patients on an operating room table can lead to necrosis if the duration of pressure exceeds 2 hours. Moreover, ulcers might be quite small initially, but with continued pressure and ischemia, ulcers rapidly can get larger, deeper, and sometimes infected. Infectious complications of pressure ulcers include cellulitis, osteomyelitis, and bacteremia. Factors that increase susceptibility for developing pressure ulcers include external and host factors. External factors include pressure, friction, shear force, and moisture; host factors include malnutrition, anemia, and vascular disease.

Most pressure ulcer infections are polymicrobial. Pathogens isolated frequently include *Staphylococci, Enterococci,* Enterobacteriaciae, and *Pseudomonas* spp. Anaerobic bacteria, such as *Bacteroides fragilis, Peptostreptococcus,* and *Clostridium* spp, also are common pathogens.

Risk factors, presentation, diagnosis, and classification

The most common sites of pressure ulcers are the sacrum and hips (67%), but other sites, such as the occiput, elbows, lower extremities, and heels, also are affected commonly. Populations at increased risk for pressure ulcers include persons who are older, incontinent, unconscious, or paralyzed. As a result of immobilization, the postoperative period is an important risk period for the development of pressure ulcers. Several comorbid conditions also are associated with pressure ulcers, including contractures, spasticity, PVD, diabetes mellitus, and autonomic regulatory dysfunction. Furthermore, medications that cause immobility and devices that cause excessive heat can predispose patients to pressure ulcers. In general, patients who develop pressure ulcers usually have impaired mobility, mental status, and sensation [10,11].

Most pressure ulcers are diagnosed when they are observed directly by health care providers, nursing home staff, or family members. Sometimes, patients present with systemic signs of infection, such as fever, bacteremia, or declining cognitive status.

The system used most commonly for classifying pressure ulcers is the National Pressure Ulcer Advisory Panel. This system has four classification stages based on the depth of the ulcer. Stage I represents intact skin with early signs of impending ulceration including erythema, warmth, and induration. Stage II lesions present as shallow ulcers, involving the epidermis and often the dermis. Often, pigmentation changes are present. Stage III ulcers involve a full-thickness loss of skin with extension into the subcutaneous tissue but sparing of the fascia and may present as foul-smelling ulcerative lesions with pigmentation changes. Stage IV ulcers present with complete, full-thickness skin and subcutaneous tissue loss. There usually is ulcer penetration into the deep fascia and involvement of the muscle, tendon, joint capsule, or bone [11]. When the bone is involved, osteomyelitis invariably is present.

Treatment and outcomes

The general treatment of pressure ulcers is based on four modalities: pressure reduction, surgical intervention, nutrition, and wound management. Empiric antibiotic regimens should be focused on common pathogens, include *Staphylococci, Pseudomonas,* Enterobacteriaciae, and anaerobes

when pressure ulcers are complicated by infection. Culture data can be helpful in guiding therapy, particularly if specimens are obtained from the blood
or from operative tissue. In general, swab cultures do not provide useful information. Typically, 10- to 14-day antibiotic regimens are prescribed for
the treatment of infected ulcers, although no studies have studied antibiotic
duration systematically [12]. Infected stage III and stage IV ulcers and osteomyelitis usually require longer durations of treatment (eg, 4–6 weeks), and
surgical débridement, often in conjunction with flap placement, frequently is
required for definitive cure [11]. If definitive surgical cure cannot be at-
tained, then patients frequently have infectious relapses. The role of chronic,
suppressive antibiotics in the management of osteomyelitis complicating
stage IV ulcers remains unclear. Frequently, providers treat acute infectious
flares rather than chronically suppressing patients with systemic antibiotics.

Prevention

Several modalities exist for the prevention of pressure ulcers. Detailed review of recommended preventive practices is beyond the scope of this article.
The basic modalities for prevention include using support surfaces, reposi-
tioning patients routinely, optimizing nutritional status, and maintaining
moist sacral skin [10].

Surgical site infections

Epidemiology of surgical site infections in elderly

SSIs are a growing threat to the health of the aging population. SSIs are
a common complication of hospitalization, occurring in 2% to 5% of all
patients undergoing surgery in the United States [13]. Given the high number of surgical procedures performed in the United States, this translates
into 300,000 to 500,000 SSIs each year [14]. From 1980 to 1998, the percentage of operations performed for patients ages 65 years and older increased
from 19% to 43% of all surgical operations [15]. SSIs account for 11% of
nosocomial infections in patients ages 65 years and older [16], and as the
population of older persons increases over time, the number of SSIs in
this population likely will increase. Many aspects of SSIs are similar in
the elderly population and in the general population, including pathophysiology, risk factors, and associated poor outcomes. Several key differences
and important similarities are reviewed here.

SSIs remain a leading cause of morbidity and mortality in all populations, leading to increased length of hospitalization [14], costs [17], and mortality [18]. Overall, SSI is believed to account for up to $10 billion in health
care expenditure annually [19] and 77% of deaths in patients who have SSIs
are attributed directly to the SSI [20]. Outcomes for elderly patients are reported to be even worse. Compared with uninfected control patients ages 65
years and older, elderly patients who have SSI have 4 to 5 times higher
mortality, longer length of hospitalization, and at least twofold greater

hospital costs [21,22]. Elderly patients who have infection have worse outcomes compared with younger infected patients [23], and this holds true also with SSI. Compared with younger patients who have SSI, elderly patients who have SSI are 3 times more likely to die, have 4 more days of hospitalization, and have more than $40,000 extra attributable costs [22].

Definition and pathophysiology

The CDC has developed standardized surveillance criteria for defining SSIs that are used widely [24]; SSIs are classified as incisional or organ/space (Fig. 1). Incisional SSIs are classified further into superficial (involving only skin or subcutaneous tissue of the incision) or deep (involving fascia or muscular layers). Organ/space SSIs include infections occurring in any part of the body opened or manipulated during surgery. Definitions used for standardized surveillance criteria are described in Box 1.

The risk for developing a SSI is a balance between microbial contamination of the surgical wound and host immunity. Microbial contamination of surgical sites is universal. The period of greatest risk for infection is from the time of incision to the time of wound closure [19]. Pathogens that lead to SSI are acquired from a patient's endogenous flora or exogenously from an operating room environment. There is no evidence to suggest that wound

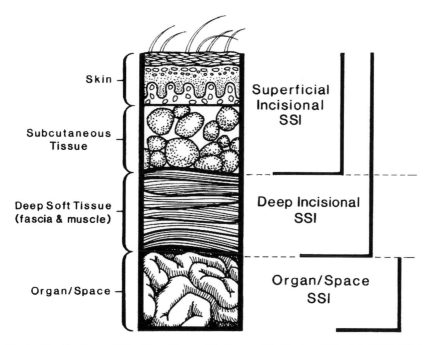

Fig. 1. Classification of SSIs. (*From* Horan TC, Gaynes RP, Martone WJ, et al. CDC definitions of nosocomial surgical site infections, 1992: a modification of CDC definitions of surgical wound infections. Infect Control Hosp Epidemiol 1992;13(10):606–8; with permission.)

Box 1. Criteria for defining a surgical site infection*

Incisional surgical site infection
Superficial infection involves skin or subcutaneous tissue of the
  incision and at least one of the following:
  1. Purulent drainage, with or without laboratory confirmation,
     from the superficial incision
  2. Organisms isolated from an aseptically obtained culture
     from the superficial incision
  3. At least one of the following signs or symptoms: pain,
     localized swelling, erythema, or heat; *and* superficial
     incision is opened deliberately by surgeon, unless incision is
     culture negative.
  4. Diagnosis of superficial incisional SSI by surgeon

Deep infection involves deep soft tissues (eg, fascial and muscle
  layers) of the incision and at least one of the following:
  1. Purulent drainage from the deep incision, excluding organ/
     space[a]
  2. A deep incision that dehisces spontaneously or is opened
     deliberately by a surgeon when a patient has one or more of
     the following signs or symptoms: fever (>38°C) or localized
     pain, unless site is culture negative.
  3. An abscess or other evidence of infection is found on direct
     examination, during repeat surgery, or by histopathologic or
     radiologic examination
  4. Diagnosis of a deep incisional SSI by surgeon

---

  * For all classifications, infection is defined as occurring within 30 days after
the operation if no implant is placed or within 1 year if an implant is in place and
the infection is related to the incision. For the sake of this classification, the CDC
defines "implant" as a nonhuman-derived implantable foreign body (eg, prosthetic
heart valve, nonhuman vascular graft, mechanical heart, or joint prosthesis) that
is placed permanently in a patient.
  [a] Report infection that involves both superficial and deep incision sites as a deep
incisional SSI.
  From Horan TC, Gaynes RP, Martone WJ, et al. CDC definitions of nosocomial
surgical site infections, 1992: a modification of CDC definitions of surgical
wound infections. Infect Control Hosp Epidemiol 1992;13(10):606–8; with
permission.

contamination is more frequent or more concentrated in patients age 65
years or older than in younger patients.

  Gram-positive cocci, such as *Staphylococci*, from endogenous host flora
located at or near an operative site, remain the leading cause of SSIs (Box 2)

Box 2. Ten most common pathogens in surgical site infections

Pathogen	Percent of infections
S aureus	20
Coagulase-negative staphylococci	14
Enterococcus spp	12
P aeruginosa	8
Escherichia coli	8
Enterobacter spp	7
Proteus mirabilis	3
Streptococcus spp	3
K pneumoniae	3
Candida albicans	2

Data from Mangram AJ, Horan TC, Pearson ML, et al. Guideline for prevention of surgical site infection, 1999. Hospital Infection Control Practices Advisory Committee. Infect Control Hosp Epidemiol 1999;20(4):250–78 [quiz: 279–80]; and National Nosocomial Infections Surveillance (NNIS) report, data summary from October 1986-April 1996, issued May 1996. A report from the National Nosocomial Infections Surveillance (NNIS) System. Am J Infect Control 1996; 24(5):380–8.

[20,25]. For surgeries involving the abdomen or genitourinary tract, gram-negative pathogens and anaerobes also are important pathogens. Pathogens that cause SSIs are similar in elderly and younger populations [26]. Modern methods of pre- and perioperative antisepsis can reduce but not eliminate the endogenous skin flora of surgical patients; 20% of bacterial skin flora reside in skin appendages, such as sebaceous glands, hair follicles, and sweat glands [27], and, thus, are difficult to eradicate completely. Rarely, inoculation of a surgical site with endogenous flora from remote sites of a patient may occur [28].

Exogenous sources of contamination, including surgical personnel, operating room environment, and surgical instruments, occasionally are implicated in SSIs. Infections resulting from exogenous sources most commonly occur sporadically, but several point source outbreaks are documented [29,30]. Finally, postsurgical inoculation of a surgical site secondary to a remote focus of infection, such as urinary tract infection or pneumonia, occurs rarely [31].

Risk factors for surgical site infection

Many risk factors for SSI are elucidated for the general surgical population (Box 3). Surprisingly few studies have examined specific risk factors specifically for patients age 65 years or older.

Box 3. Risk factors for surgical site infections

Perioperative characteristics	Operative characteristics
Age	Appropriate patient
Diabetes mellitus	skin preparation
and hyperglycemia	Appropriate hair removal
Tobacco use	Surgical team
Obesity	Appropriate
Malnutrition	surgical scrub
Immunosuppression	Operating room traffic
(steroids, HIV)	Surgical technique
Prolonged hospitalization	
Colonization with *S aureus*	Procedural
	Appropriate
	antimicrobial
	prophylaxis
	Hypothermia
	Oxygenation

From Mangram AJ, Horan TC, Pearson ML, et al. Guideline for prevention of surgical site infection, 1999. Hospital Infection Control Practices Advisory Committee. Infect Control Hosp Epidemiol 1999;20(4):250–78 [quiz: 279–80]; with permission.

Age is a complex but immutable risk factor for SSIs. Different groups of investigators report contradictory results concerning the relationship between increasing age and risk for SSIs. For example, several investigators conclude that increasing age is associated with a greater risk for all types for postoperative infections, including SSIs [32–34]. Some investigators speculate that factors indirectly related to age, such as increased prevalence of comorbid conditions, increased severity of acute illness, and decreased host response to bacterial invasion in older patients, are the reasons why older patients might have an increased risk for SSI [35,36]. In other studies, advanced age is associated with a decreased risk for SSI [33,37]. In a recent large cohort study of more than 144,000 surgical procedures, increasing age independently predicted an increased risk for deep and organ space SSI until age 65, but at ages 65 years and older, increasing age independently predicted a linear decrease in the risk for SSI [38]. The explanation for this finding of decreased risk after age 65 is unclear, and may be because of either selection bias (ie, frail elderly patients might be less likely to have surgical procedures) or a "hardy survivor" effect.

Many diseases and risk factors for SSI occur with increased frequency in older patients. Diabetes mellitus, which leads to 2 to 5 times higher rates of SSI than in patients who are not diabetic [39], is more prevalent with age.

Similarly, elderly patients have higher prevalence of PVD and resulting tissue ischemia. As with smoking, decreased tissue oxygenation increases the risk for wound infection and dehiscence by decreasing collagen synthesis [40] and affecting the oxidative killing mechanisms of host neutrophils [41]. Furthermore, advanced age is associated with poor nutritional intake, malnutrition, and hypoalbuminemia, known risk factors for SSI [42]. Studies concerning the usefulness of pre-, peri-, or postoperative total parenteral nutrition or total enteral nutrition for preventing postoperative complications and SSI, however, have provided inconsistent and generally unfavorable results [43–45].

Few specific risk factors for patients ages 65 years and older are described. One recent case-control study of 1158 patients ages 65 years and older undergoing surgical procedures shows that obesity (odds ratio [OR] 1.8) and chronic obstructive pulmonary disease (OR 1.7) were independent risk factors for SSI among elderly patients; elderly patients who had private insurance, perhaps a marker for higher socioeconomic status, had lower risk for SSI (OR 0.3) [46]. The investigators of another case-control study of 340 patients ages 65 years and older undergoing orthopedic surgery conclude that patients admitted from a health care facility (nursing home, outside hospital, or rehabilitation facility) were more than 4 times more likely to develop a SSI than patients admitted from home [21].

Although many other factors contribute to the risk for SSI, the burden of surgical wound inoculation remains one of the most well understood and accepted risks. That is, the higher the amount of surgical wound contamination, the higher the risk for infection. Even in the setting of appropriate antimicrobial prophylaxis, the risk for SSI increases as total bacterial burden of the surgical wound increases [47]. Generally, wound contamination with greater than 10^5 microorganisms is required to lead to SSI [48]. When foreign bodies are present, the inoculum may be much lower. When sutures are present, the required inoculum of organisms is decreased by 99.99% (from 10^6 to 10^2 organisms) [49]—as few as 10 colony-forming units of bacteria with polytetrafluoroethylene vascular grafts [50] or 1 colony-forming unit of bacteria with dextran beads is necessary to potentially cause SSI [51]. These findings are important particularly as orthopedic and vascular procedures with implants are common for patients age 65 years or older [15].

Prevention of surgical site infection in patients age 65 years or older

No studies have been performed to determine methods of preventing SSIs specifically in patients age 65 years or older. Thus, in addition to paying close attention to comorbid conditions (discussed previously) and encouraging glucose control (for patients who have diabetes mellitus) and cessation of tobacco use, standard techniques used in the general surgical population must be applied rigorously to elderly surgical patients. Several proved modalities to prevent SSIs in the general population exist and are incorporated into national quality improvement initiatives.

The Institute for Healthcare Improvement's 100,000 Lives Campaign, a nationwide campaign to improve patient outcomes by preventing medical errors, included prevention of SSI as one of their six major areas of focus [52]. Four specific interventions to prevent SSI have been targeted: appropriate selection, timing, and discontinuation of prophylactic antimicrobial agents; appropriate hair removal; postoperative glucose control; and maintaining postoperative normothermia.

The appropriate use of perioperative antimicrobial prophylaxis is accepted as a well-proved intervention to reduce the risk for SSI in elective procedures [20]. The Centers for Medicare and Medicaid Services created the Surgical Infection Prevention Project in 2002 to decrease the morbidity and mortality associated with postoperative SSI by promoting appropriate selection and timing of prophylactic antimicrobials. An expert panel identified proved performance measures for quality improvement: IV antimicrobial prophylaxis within 1 hour before incision (2 hours are allowed for the administration of vancomycin and fluoroquinolones) [53]; antimicrobial prophylactic agent consistent with guidelines [54]; and discontinued prophylactic antimicrobial agent within 24 hours after surgery end time. The Surgical Infection Prevention Project focuses on several procedures important for older populations: hip arthroplasty, knee arthroplasty, cardiothoracic surgery, vascular surgery, and colorectal surgery. When used together, these performance measures lead to decreased rates of SSI. A national collaborative of 56 hospitals participated in implementing these performance measures and, over a 1-year period, reported a mean reduction in the rate of SSI of 27% [55].

The use of razors for hair removal or hair removal the night before surgery leads to higher rates of SSI [56,57]. If hair removal is necessary, clippers or a depilatory method should be used on the day of surgery.

As discussed previously, diabetes and hyperglycemia are established as independent risk factors for SSI. In fact, elevated serum glucose in the pre- and postoperative periods are associated with increased risk for SSI [39,58]. Aggressive glycemic control, including postoperative IV insulin, can reduce the rate of SSI and the rate of death while in an intensive care unit [59]. A study of 1585 patients who had diabetes and underwent open heart surgery showed that aggressive postoperative glucose control with continuous IV insulin infusion reduced the rate of SSI from 2.4% to 1.5% ($P < .02$) [39].

Surgical patients may become hypothermic, defined as a core body temperature below 36°C, from exposure to cold operating room ambient temperatures, anesthesia, or changes in body heat distribution, or routinely during some types of cardiac surgeries [60]. Elderly patients, in particular, may become hypothermic more easily as a result of loss of fat with age. Hypothermia increases the risk for SSI through thermoregulatory vasoconstriction and impaired immunity. Vasoconstriction is universal in patients who have hypothermia [61] and leads to decreased partial pressure of oxygen in tissues [62], decreased microbial killing [63], impaired chemotaxis and phagocytosis of granulocytes, and decreased motility of macrophages [64].

A randomized, controlled trial evaluating 200 patients undergoing elective colorectal surgery demonstrated a threefold reduction in the rate of SSI by maintaining body temperature above 36°C [65].

Decreased tissue oxygenation leads to increased risk for SSI [66] by limiting the respiratory burst of neutrophils [67]. Increasing age may exacerbate this effect as aging leads to decreased levels of tissue oxygenation [68]. Thus far, three randomized, controlled trials on postoperative oxygenation have been published, with conflicting results [69–71]. Both studies in favor of supplemental oxygen included patients who underwent colorectal surgery, whereas the study reporting adverse effect of supplemental oxygen included patients undergoing various of types of surgery; when results of the three studies are pooled, the rate of SSI decreases from 15.2% in patients receiving 30% to 35% supplemental fraction of inspired oxygen (F_{IO_2}) to 11.5% in patients who received 80% F_{IO_2} during and 6 hours after surgery (3.7% absolute risk reduction; $P = .10$) [72]. Given the low cost of supplemental oxygen, plausible biologic rationale, and potential benefit, supplemental oxygen therapy should be considered strongly as a strategy to reduce the rate of SSI, particularly in colorectal surgery.

Surveillance for surgical site infection

The majority of SSIs are diagnosable within 21 days of surgery [73,74]. Surgical procedures have been shifting to outpatient settings during the past 3 decades [75]. Thus, postdischarge and outpatient SSI surveillance increasingly are becoming important. Currently, no one method of surveillance is proved more beneficial than others for the geriatric population. In particular, the diagnosis of SSI in the setting of an implanted device is challenging for clinicians, as signs and symptoms not always are uniform and can occur long after a surgical procedure [76]. Thus, surveillance for SSI should continue for at least 12 months for procedures in which an implant is placed. A recent analysis of 756 patients who had undergone insertion of a hip or knee prosthesis confirmed that all SSIs were detected within 12 months of the procedure [77]. Similarly, geriatric patients may not manifest typical symptoms of infection (eg, fever or elevated white blood cell count), but might present with cognitive or functional decline; thus, vigilance is necessary when evaluating older patients after surgery.

Treatment of surgical site infection

No specific guidelines exist for the treatment of SSI, but the principles for treatment of SSI are the same in elderly and younger populations. Superficial SSIs, including mild wound drainage and simple cellulitis, can be treated in an outpatient setting, usually with oral antibiotics. Serious SSIs (those classified as deep or organ space), however, generally require readmission to a hospital for further surgical débridement and IV antibiotics. In both situations, the key to curing the infection is removal of dead, necrotic tissue, with antibiotics used only as adjunctive therapy. Empiric antimicrobial choices should cover pathogens that cause SSI most commonly in a given anatomic site but should be tailored to culture results when available.

References

[1] Nicolle LE. Infection control in long-term care facilities. Clin Infect Dis 2000;31(3):752–6.

[2] Stevens DL, Bisno AL, Chambers HF, et al. Practice guidelines for the diagnosis and management of skin and soft-tissue infections. Clin Infect Dis 2005;41(10):1373–406.

[3] Laube S, Farrell AM. Bacterial skin infections in the elderly: diagnosis and treatment. Drugs Aging 2002;19(5):331–42.

[4] Laube S. Skin infections and ageing. Ageing Res Rev 2004;3(1):69–89.

[5] King MD, Humphrey BJ, Wang YF, et al. Emergence of community-acquired methicillin-resistant Staphylococcus aureus USA 300 clone as the predominant cause of skin and soft-tissue infections. Ann Intern Med 2006;144(5):309–17.

[6] Graham PL 3rd, Lin SX, Larson EL. A U.S. population-based survey of Staphylococcus aureus colonization. Ann Intern Med 2006;144(5):318–25.

[7] Lee MC, Rios AM, Aten MF, et al. Management and outcome of children with skin and soft tissue abscesses caused by community-acquired methicillin-resistant Staphylococcus aureus. Pediatr Infect Dis J 2004;23(2):123–7.

[8] Raz R, Miron D, Colodner R, et al. A 1-year trial of nasal mupirocin in the prevention of recurrent staphylococcal nasal colonization and skin infection. Arch Intern Med 1996; 156(10):1109–12.

[9] Miller MA, Dascal A, Portnoy J, et al. Development of mupirocin resistance among methicillin-resistant Staphylococcus aureus after widespread use of nasal mupirocin ointment. Infect Control Hosp Epidemiol 1996;17(12):811–3.

[10] Reddy M, Gill SS, Rochon PA. Preventing pressure ulcers: a systematic review. JAMA 2006; 296(8):974–84.

[11] Bansal C, Scott R, Stewart D, et al. Decubitus ulcers: a review of the literature. Int J Dermatol 2005;44(10):805–10.

[12] Livesley NJ, Chow AW. Infected pressure ulcers in elderly individuals. Clin Infect Dis 2002; 35(11):1390–6.

[13] Graves HJ. National hospital discharge survey: annual summary 1987. National Center for Health Statistics 1989;13:11.

[14] Cruse P. Wound infection surveillance. Rev Infect Dis 1981;3(4):734–7.

[15] Centers for Disease Control and Prevention. Advanced data no. 316. Washington, DC: National Center for Health Statistics; 2000.

[16] Emori TG, Banerjee SN, Culver DH, et al. Nosocomial infections in elderly patients in the United States, 1986–1990. National Nosocomial Infections Surveillance System. Am J Med 1991;91(3B):289S–93S.

[17] Kirkland KB, Briggs JP, Trivette SL, et al. The impact of surgical-site infections in the 1990s: attributable mortality, excess length of hospitalization, and extra costs. Infect Control Hosp Epidemiol 1999;20(11):725–30.

[18] Engemann JJ, Carmeli Y, Cosgrove SE, et al. Adverse clinical and economic outcomes attributable to methicillin resistance among patients with Staphylococcus aureus surgical site infection. Clin Infect Dis 2003;36(5):592–8.

[19] Wong ES. Surgical site infections. 3rd edition. Balitmore (MD): Lippincott, Williams, and Wilkins; 2004.

[20] Mangram AJ, Horan TC, Pearson ML, et al. Guideline for prevention of surgical site infection, 1999. Hospital Infection Control Practices Advisory Committee. Infect Control Hosp Epidemiol 1999;20(4):250–78, quiz 279–80.

[21] Lee J, Singletary R, Schmader K, et al. Surgical site infection in the elderly following ortho-
     paedic surgery. Risk factors and outcomes. J Bone Joint Surg [Am] 2006;88(8):1705–12.
[22] McGarry SA, Engemann JJ, Schmader K, et al. Surgical-site infection due to Staphylococcus
     aureus among elderly patients: mortality, duration of hospitalization, and cost. Infect Con-
     trol Hosp Epidemiol 2004;25(6):461–7.
[23] Strausbaugh LJ. Emerging health care-associated infections in the geriatric population.
     Emerg Infect Dis 2001;7(2):268–71.
[24] Horan TC, Gaynes RP, Martone WJ, et al. CDC definitions of nosocomial surgical site
     infections, 1992: a modification of CDC definitions of surgical wound infections. Infect Con-
     trol Hosp Epidemiol 1992;13(10):606–8.
[25] National Nosocomial Infections Surveillance (NNIS) report, data summary from October
     1986–April 1996, issued May 1996. A report from the National Nosocomial Infections Sur-
     veillance (NNIS) System. Am J Infect Control 1996;24(5):380–8.
[26] Kaye KS, Schmader KE, Sawyer R. Surgical site infection in the elderly population. Clin In-
     fect Dis 2004;39(12):1835–41.
[27] Tuazon CU. Skin and skin structure infections in the patient at risk: carrier state of Staph-
     ylococcus aureus. Am J Med 1984;76(5A):166–71.
[28] Wiley AM, Ha'eri GB. Routes of infection. A study of using "tracer particles" in the ortho-
     pedic operating room. Clin Orthop Relat Res 1979;139:150–5.
[29] Berkelman RL, Martin D, Graham DR, et al. Streptococcal wound infections caused by
     a vaginal carrier. JAMA 1982;247(19):2680–2.
[30] McIntyre DM. An epidemic of Streptococcus pyogenes puerperal and postoperative sepsis
     with an unusual carrier site–the anus. Am J Obstet Gynecol 1968;101(3):308–14.
[31] Edwards LD. The epidemiology of 2056 remote site infections and 1966 surgical wound
     infections occurring in 1865 patients: a four year study of 40,923 operations at Rush-Presby-
     terian-St. Luke's Hospital, Chicago. Ann Surg 1976;184(6):758–66.
[32] de Boer AS, Mintjes-de Groot AJ, Severijnen AJ, et al. Risk assessment for surgical-site
     infections in orthopedic patients. Infect Control Hosp Epidemiol 1999;20(6):402–7.
[33] Delgado-Rodriguez M, Gomez-Ortega A, Sillero-Arenas M, et al. Epidemiology of surgical-
     site infections diagnosed after hospital discharge: a prospective cohort study. Infect Control
     Hosp Epidemiol 2001;22(1):24–30.
[34] Scott JD, Forrest A, Feuerstein S, et al. Factors associated with postoperative infection. In-
     fect Control Hosp Epidemiol 2001;22(6):347–51.
[35] Pessaux P, Msika S, Atalla D, et al. Risk factors for postoperative infectious complications in
     noncolorectal abdominal surgery: a multivariate analysis based on a prospective multicenter
     study of 4718 patients. Arch Surg 2003;138(3):314–24.
[36] Raymond DP, Pelletier SJ, Crabtree TD, et al. Surgical infection and the aging population.
     Am Surg 2001;67(9):827–32 [discussion: 832–3].
[37] Byrne DJ, Lynch W, Napier A, et al. Wound infection rates: the importance of definition and
     post-discharge wound surveillance. J Hosp Infect 1994;26(1):37–43.
[38] Kaye KS, Schmit K, Pieper C, et al. The effect of increasing age on the risk of surgical site
     infection. J Infect Dis 2005;191(7):1056–62.
[39] Zerr KJ, Furnary AP, Grunkemeier GL, et al. Glucose control lowers the risk of wound in-
     fection in diabetics after open heart operations. Ann Thorac Surg 1997;63(2):356–61.
[40] Jorgensen LN, Kallehave F, Christensen E, et al. Less collagen production in smokers. Sur-
     gery 1998;123(4):450–5.
[41] Sorensen LT, Nielsen HB, Kharazmi A, et al. Effect of smoking and abstention on oxidative
     burst and reactivity of neutrophils and monocytes. Surgery 2004;136(5):1047–53.
[42] Klein JD, Hey LA, Yu CS, et al. Perioperative nutrition and postoperative complications in
     patients undergoing spinal surgery. Spine 1996;21(22):2676–82.
[43] Brennan MF, Pisters PW, Posner M, et al. A prospective randomized trial of total parenteral
     nutrition after major pancreatic resection for malignancy. Ann Surg 1994;220(4):436–41 [dis-
     cussion: 441–4].

[44] Perioperative total parenteral nutrition in surgical patients. The Veterans Affairs Total Parenteral Nutrition Cooperative Study Group. N Engl J Med 1991;325(8):525–32.

[45] Muller JM, Brenner U, Dienst C, et al. Preoperative parenteral feeding in patients with gastrointestinal carcinoma. Lancet 1982;1(8263):68–71.

[46] Kaye KS, Sloane R, Sexton DJ, et al. Risk factors for surgical site infections in older people. J Am Geriatr Soc 2006;54(3):391–6.

[47] Houang ET, Ahmet Z. Intraoperative wound contamination during abdominal hysterectomy. J Hosp Infect 1991;19(3):181–9.

[48] Krizek TJ, Robson MC. Evolution of quantitative bacteriology in wound management. Am J Surg 1975;130(5):579–84.

[49] Elek SD, Conen PE. The virulence of Staphylococcus pyogenes for man; a study of the problems of wound infection. Br J Exp Pathol 1957;38(6):573–86.

[50] Arbeit RD, Dunn RM. Expression of capsular polysaccharide during experimental focal infection with Staphylococcus aureus. J Infect Dis 1987;156(6):947–52.

[51] Froman G, Switalski LM, Speziale P, et al. Isolation and characterization of a fibronectin receptor from Staphylococcus aureus. J Biol Chem 1987;262(14):6564–71.

[52] Institute for Healthcare Improvement. 100K lives campaign: some is not a number. Soon is not a time. Available at: http://www.ihi.org. Accessed December 2, 2006.

[53] Classen DC, Evans RS, Pestotnik SL, et al. The timing of prophylactic administration of antibiotics and the risk of surgical-wound infection. N Engl J Med 1992;326(5):281–6.

[54] Antimicrobial prophylaxis in surgery. Med Lett Drugs Ther 2001;43(1116–1117):92–7.

[55] Dellinger EP, Hausmann SM, Bratzler DW, et al. Hospitals collaborate to decrease surgical site infections. Am J Surg 2005;190(1):9–15.

[56] Cruse PJ, Foord R. The epidemiology of wound infection. A 10-year prospective study of 62,939 wounds. Surg Clin North Am 1980;60(1):27–40.

[57] Mishriki SF, Law DJ, Jeffery PJ. Factors affecting the incidence of postoperative wound infection. J Hosp Infect 1990;16(3):223–30.

[58] Wilson SJ, Sexton DJ. Elevated preoperative fasting serum glucose levels increase the risk of postoperative mediastinitis in patients undergoing open heart surgery. Infect Control Hosp Epidemiol 2003;24(10):776–8.

[59] van den Berghe G, Wouters P, Weekers F, et al. Intensive insulin therapy in the critically ill patients. N Engl J Med 2001;345(19):1359–67.

[60] Sessler DI. Mild perioperative hypothermia. N Engl J Med 1997;336(24):1730–7.

[61] Sessler DI, Rubinstein EH, Moayeri A. Physiologic responses to mild perianesthetic hypothermia in humans. Anesthesiology 1991;75(4):594–610.

[62] Chang N, Mathes SJ. Comparison of the effect of bacterial inoculation in musculocutaneous and random-pattern flaps. Plast Reconstr Surg 1982;70(1):1–10.

[63] Hohn DC, MacKay RD, Halliday B, et al. Effect of O2 tension on microbicidal function of leukocytes in wounds and in vitro. Surg Forum 1976;27(62):18–20.

[64] van Oss CJ, Absolom DR, Moore LL, et al. Effect of temperature on the chemotaxis, phagocytic engulfment, digestion and O2 consumption of human polymorphonuclear leukocytes. J Reticuloendothel Soc 1980;27(6):561–5.

[65] Kurz A, Sessler DI, Lenhardt R. Perioperative normothermia to reduce the incidence of surgical-wound infection and shorten hospitalization. Study of Wound Infection and Temperature Group. N Engl J Med 1996;334(19):1209–15.

[66] Hopf HW, Hunt TK, West JM, et al. Wound tissue oxygen tension predicts the risk of wound infection in surgical patients. Arch Surg 1997;132(9):997–1004 [discussion: 1005].

[67] Allen DB, Maguire JJ, Mahdavian M, et al. Wound hypoxia and acidosis limit neutrophil bacterial killing mechanisms. Arch Surg 1997;132(9):991–6.

[68] Boyko EJ, Ahroni JH, Stensel VL, et al. Predictors of transcutaneous oxygen tension in the lower limbs of diabetic subjects. Diabet Med 1996;13(6):549–54.

[69] Greif R, Akca O, Horn EP, et al. Supplemental perioperative oxygen to reduce the incidence of surgical-wound infection. Outcomes Research Group. N Engl J Med 2000;342(3):161–7.

[70] Pryor KO, Fahey TJ 3rd, Lien CA, et al. Surgical site infection and the routine use of perioperative hyperoxia in a general surgical population: a randomized controlled trial. JAMA 2004;291(1):79–87.

[71] Belda FJ, Aguilera L, Garcia de la Asuncion J, et al. Supplemental perioperative oxygen and the risk of surgical wound infection: a randomized controlled trial. JAMA 2005;294(16): 2035–42.

[72] Dellinger EP. Increasing inspired oxygen to decrease surgical site infection: time to shift the quality improvement research paradigm. JAMA 2005;294(16):2091–2.

[73] Weigelt JA, Dryer D, Haley RW. The necessity and efficiency of wound surveillance after discharge. Arch Surg 1992;127(1):77–81 [discussion: 81–2].

[74] Sands K, Vineyard G, Platt R. Surgical site infections occurring after hospital discharge. J Infect Dis 1996;173(4):963–70.

[75] Burke JP. Infection control—a problem for patient safety. N Engl J Med 2003;348(7):651–6.

[76] Lentino JR. Prosthetic joint infections: bane of orthopedists, challenge for infectious disease specialists. Clin Infect Dis 2003;36(9):1157–61.

[77] Huenger F, Schmachtenberg A, Haefner H, et al. Evaluation of postdischarge surveillance of surgical site infections after total hip and knee arthroplasty. Am J Infect Control 2005;33(8): 455–62.

ELSEVIER
SAUNDERS

CLINICS IN
GERIATRIC
MEDICINE

Clin Geriatr Med 23 (2007) 615–632

Herpes Zoster and Postherpetic Neuralgia in Older Adults

Kenneth Schmader, MD[a,b],*

[a]Center for the Study of Aging and Human Development and Division of Geriatrics,
Department of Medicine, Duke University Medical Center, Box 3469,
Durham, NC 27710, USA
[b]Geriatric Research, Education and Clinical Center 182, Durham Veterans Affairs
Medical Center, 508 Fulton Street, Durham, NC 27705, USA

Herpes zoster (HZ) is caused by the reactivation of varicella-zoster virus (VZV) from a latent infection of dorsal sensory or cranial nerve ganglia. VZV is a double-stranded DNA herpesvirus with a genome that contains approximately 125,000 base pairs and encodes approximately 70 gene products [1]. VZV is intriguing because it establishes and maintains a latent infection for the lifetime of the host after primary infection (varicella), yet it emerges at unpredictable times to cause HZ decades after the establishment of latency. Competent cellular immunity is critical to containing VZV. With aging-related decline in T-cell immune responsiveness to VZV, however, the virus may escape cell-mediated immune containment, replicate fully, and spread in the affected ganglia and sensory nerves to the skin. This review focuses on older, immunocompetent patients.

Epidemiology

The probability of developing HZ increases strikingly with aging. Incidence rates in persons of all ages are 1.2 to 3.4 cases per 1000 persons per year, whereas the incidence of HZ in persons over 60 years old is 7.2 to 11.8 cases per thousand per year [2]. Nearly all HZ epidemiology studies determine HZ incidence using retrospective medical or administrative record review of clinically diagnosed cases. The zoster vaccine trial, a Veterans

This work was supported by the Durham VA Medical Center Geriatric Research, Education and Clinical Center (GRECC) and K24-AI-51324-03 from the National Institute of Allergy and Infectious Diseases.

* 182 GRECC, Durham Veterans Affairs Medical Center, Durham, NC 27705.
E-mail address: schma001@mc.duke.edu

Affairs Cooperative Trial, known as the Shingles Prevention Study, was prospective, used active surveillance in a community sample, and diagnosed HZ definitively via polymerase chain reaction (PCR) [3]. In the placebo group of the Shingles Prevention Study, the incidence of zoster was 11.8 cases per 1000 persons per year in adults 60 years of age and older. The incidence of HZ increases sharply at approximately 50 to 60 years old and continues an upward course in the decades older than 60. In the Duke Established Populations for Epidemiological Studies of the Elderly, the lifetime risk for HZ increased significantly with age even among elderly individuals (odds ratio 1.20 for every 5-year interval above 65 years old; 95% CI, 1.10–1.31) [4]. The lifetime incidence of HZ is estimated to be 20% to 30% in the general population and as high as 50% of a cohort surviving to age 85. HZ incidence data and current population figures yield estimates of up to 1 million new cases of HZ each year in the United States, with more than 500,000 occurring in persons age 60 or older [3,5].

Disease- and drug-related suppression of cellular immunity is the other major predictor of HZ [5]. The frequency of HZ in those who have HIV infection, hematologic malignancies, bone marrow and solid organ transplantation, systemic lupus erythematosus, or immunosuppressive therapy is 20 to 100 times greater than the frequency of HZ in immunocompetent individuals. Other risk factors include white race, psychologic stress, and physical trauma [4,6]. Studies conflict on whether or not female gender is a risk factor for HZ. There are no controlled studies indicating that exposure of latently infected individuals to HZ or varicella causes HZ.

Patients who have HZ and who have a vesicular rash may transmit VZV via direct contact or airborne or droplet nuclei to seronegative, nonimmune individuals. These individuals then may develop varicella. If a rash is only maculopapular or crusted, there is no danger of VZV transmission. Important groups at risk for varicella from contact with patients who have HZ include children who have not received the varicella vaccine or who have had an insufficient response to the vaccine and susceptible health care workers and staff in hospitals or in nursing homes, particularly if they are pregnant or immunocompromised. The exposure of latently infected individuals to HZ does not cause HZ or varicella. Nearly all older adults are latently infected with VZV.

Increasing age is the most powerful risk factor for developing postherpetic neuralgia (PHN) [2]. Increasing age also is associated with increased severity of PHN, so a large majority of persons who suffer from moderate to severe PHN are older adults. The other major risk factors for PHN are greater acute pain severity, presence of a prodrome, and greater rash severity [7]. The precise incidence and prevalence of PHN are not clear because of variable definitions and because data on PHN are not collected and reported routinely in large population groups. PHN is defined as any pain after rash healing or any pain 1 month, 3 months, 4 months, or 6 months after rash onset. Most recent definitions specify any pain 90 to 120 days after rash onset, which eliminates pain from acute inflammation and ensures a group of patients that has true chronic neuropathic pain [8,9]. Investigators estimate that the prevalence of PHN ranges from 500,000 to 1 million in the United States [10].

Clinical features

VZV reactivation and spread in the affected sensory ganglion and peripheral sensory nerve evoke a cellular immune response and neuronal inflammation and destruction. Before VZV reaches the skin, patients experience prodromal sensations in the affected dermatome, such as aching, burning, or lancinating pain; itching; or tingling. Prodromal symptoms baffle patients and physicians alike by imitating other painful conditions in older persons (migraine headaches, trigeminal neuralgia, myocardial infarction, cholecystitis, biliary or renal colic, appendicitis, lumbosacral strain, "pulled" muscles, and so forth). One clue to incipient HZ is sensitive skin in the affected dermatome before the rash breaks out. The prodrome usually lasts a few days. VZV may not reach the skin in some patients, which results in neuralgia without a rash. This condition is known as zoster sine herpete.

Once VZV invades the dermis and epidermis, the rash appears and reveals the reason for patient pain or discomfort. The rash is unilateral, dermatomal, red, maculopapular, and usually develops vesicles (Fig. 1). It is not uncommon for patients to develop lesions in adjacent dermatomes. The rash generally starts crusting over in a week to 10 days and heals within 2 to 4 weeks. Atypical rashes may occur in older persons. The rash may be limited to a small patch located within a dermatome or may remain maculopapular without ever developing vesicles. Conversely, vesicles may form for several days and involve several dermatomes.

VZV-induced acute neuritis produces dermatomal neuralgic pain in many older adults, although a few patients never develop pain whereas others may experience the delayed onset of pain days or weeks after rash onset. The

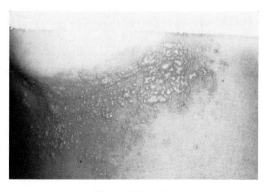

Fig. 1. HZ rash.

neuritis is described as burning, deep aching, tingling, itching, or stabbing. A subset of patients may develop severe pain, especially those who have trigeminal nerve involvement. Acute herpetic neuralgia has a profound negative impact on functional status and quality of life and usually results in substantial health service use [11].

In general, the number of older patients who have HZ who have pain decreases over weeks to months from rash onset. Unfortunately, a significant number of older persons who have HZ continue to experience pain for months after the acute phase of the illness and, therefore, develop PHN. Patients who have PHN may suffer from constant pain ("burning, aching, throbbing"), intermittent pain ("stabbing, shooting"), and stimulus-evoked pain, such as allodynia ("tender"). Allodynia, the experience of pain after a nonpainful stimulus, is a particularly disabling component of the disease. Patients who have allodynia suffer from severe pain after the lightest touch of the affected skin by things as trivial as a cold wind or a piece of clothing. These subtypes of pain may produce chronic fatigue, disordered sleep, depression, anorexia, weight loss, and social isolation. Furthermore, PHN can impair elderly patients' functional status by interfering with basic activities of daily living (such as dressing, bathing, and mobility) and instrumental activities of daily living (such as traveling, shopping, cooking, and housework).

HZ occurs in the ophthalmic division of the trigeminal nerve in 10% to 15% of patients and may cause ocular complications. The likelihood of inflammation of the eye seems higher when a rash is on the tip of the nose (nasociliary branch involvement) but in general the appearance and location of a facial rash does not predict the presence or extent of eye involvement. VZV-induced damage to the cornea and uvea and other eye structures can cause corneal anesthesia and ulceration, glaucoma, optic neuritis, eyelid scarring and retraction, visual impairment, and blindness in patients who did not receive antiviral therapy.

Other less frequent but important complications of HZ in older adults include stroke secondary to granulomatous arteritis of the internal carotid artery in ophthalmic HZ; focal motor paresis in muscles served by nerve roots of the corresponding affected dermatome; disordered balance, hearing, and facial paresis in cranial neuritis (Ramsay Hunt syndrome); meningoencephalitis; and secondary bacterial infection of the rash.

Diagnosis

HZ may be diagnosed clinically with high confidence when the characteristic unilateral, dermatomal, vesicular rash and neuralgic pain present in older patients. The main source of diagnostic error is herpes simplex virus (HSV) infection [5]. Features that may distinguish HSV from HZ include multiple recurrences, especially around the genitals or mouth, and the absence of chronic pain. It may be impossible, however, to distinguish the two conditions on clinical grounds because HSV presents with a unilateral, red, maculopapular, vesicular rash and acute pain similar to HZ. The differential diagnosis also includes contact dermatitis, burns, and vesicular lesions associated with fungal infections, but the history and examination usually make the distinction clear.

HZ should be diagnosed using laboratory diagnostic testing, when differentiating HZ from HSV infection is difficult, for suspected organ involvement and for atypical presentations, particularly in immunocompromised hosts. If patients say they have recurrent shingles, suspect HSV and do laboratory diagnostic testing on vesicle fluid when the patients next develop the rash. Available diagnostic tests include viral culture, immunofluorescence antigen (IFA) or enzyme immunoassay (EIA) antigen detection, PCR, and serology (Table 1). The best specimen is vesicle fluid, which contains abundant VZV. Lacking vesicle fluid, acceptable specimens include lesion scrapings, crusts, tissue biopsy, or cerebrospinal fluid for the first three techniques. Crusts cannot be used for VZV culture.

Treatment

Acute herpes zoster

General principles

The main goal of the treatment of HZ in older adults is the reduction or elimination of acute pain and the prevention of PHN. The impact of HZ on functional status, mood, and quality of life in older adults is related directly to pain intensity. Education and counseling about HZ reduce anxiety and misunderstandings about the disease. Questions about the duration of pain and transmission of VZV are common. Social support, mental and physical activity, adequate nutrition, and a caring attitude help patients cope with HZ. Treatment adherence and response may be altered in older adults who are living alone, cognitively impaired, frail, or coping with recent negative life events. Management of HZ is discussed in more detail in recently published guidelines [12].

Antiviral therapy

Acyclovir, famciclovir, valacyclovir, and brivudin are nucleoside analogs that treat VZV infections effectively (Table 2) [5]. These agents are phosphorylated by viral thymidine kinase and cellular kinases to a triphosphate form that interferes with viral DNA synthesis by inhibiting viral DNA polymerase. Valacyclovir and famciclovir are prodrugs that are absorbed better than acyclovir after oral administration, which results in much higher blood levels of antiviral activity. Brivudin is highly active against VZV and licensed to treat HZ outside of the United States, but it is not licensed in the United States partly because of a potentially lethal interaction with 5-fluorouracil.

Table 1
Laboratory tests for detecting varicella-zoster virus and diagnosing herpes zoster

Test	Detects	Sensitivity	Specificity	Turnaround	Pros	Cons
Culture	Whole VZV	Low (approximately 40%)	Very high (near 100%)	Days	Whole virus isolation is the standard for diagnosis; only method that yields infectious VZV for further analysis; readily available	Slow, insensitive, VZV difficult to grow on tissue culture
Immunoassays (IFA, EIA)	VZV antigen	High (90%)	High (90%)	Hours	Readily available; good sensitivity and specificity	Must be done in experienced laboratory; careful interpretation to avoid false positive and negatives
PCR	VZV DNA	Very high (near 100%)	Very specific (near 100%)	Hours	Superb sensitivity and specificity; valuable for unusual specimens or when clinicians suspect that IFA or culture has yielded false-negative test results	Expensive; not as readily available; must be done by experienced laboratory to avoid false positives
Serology (ELISA, FAMA, LA)	IgG, IgM antibody	High for antibody detection; unknown for HZ diagnosis	High for antibody detection; unknown for HZ diagnosis	Hours	Can be used to diagnose zoster sine herpete or HZ, retrospectively, using acute and convalescent VZV IgG titers	Not clinically useful for diagnosing HZ at time of presentation; requires acute and convalescent (6 weeks later) samples

Abbreviations: FAMA, fluorescent antibody to membrane antigen; LA, latex agglutination.

Table 2
Oral anti–varicella-zoster virus medications for herpes zoster (United States)

Characteristic	Acyclovir	Valacyclovir	Famciclovir
Structure	Deoxyguanosine analog	Valine ester of acyclovir	Diacetyl 6-deoxy analog of penciclovir, a deoxyguanosine analog
Active agent	Acyclovir	Acyclovir	Penciclovir
Oral bioavailability	10%–20%	54%	77%
Standard dosing	800 mg every 4 h (5 times a day) for 7 days	1 g every 8 h (3 times a day) for 7 days	500 mg every 8 h (3 times a day) for 7 days
Renal dosing	CrCl ≥25 mL/min: no adjustment CrCl 10–24 mL/min: 800 mg every 8 h CrCl < 10 mL/min: 800 mg every 12 h	CrCl ≥ 50 mL/min: no dosage adjustment CrCl 30–49 mL/min: 1 g every 12 h CrCl 10–29 mL/min: 1 g every 24 h CrCl <10 mL/min: 500 mg every 24 h	CrCl ≥60 mL/min: no dosage adjustment CrCl 40–59 mL/min: 500 mg every 12 h CrCl 20–39 mL/min: 500 mg every 24 h CrCl <20 mL/min: 250 mg every 24 h
Benefit: pain median days to resolution, drug versus control [8,11,12]	41 versus 101 (placebo)	38 versus 51 (acyclovir)	63 versus 163 (placebo)
Adverse events	Nausea/vomiting, headache, diarrhea	Nausea/vomiting, headache, diarrhea	Nausea/vomiting, headache, diarrhea
How supplied	200-mg capsules; 200-, 400-, 800-mg tablets; 200-mg/5-mL solution	500-mg, 1-g tablets	125-, 250-, and 500-mg tablets

Abbreviation: CrCl, creatinine clearance.

Many randomized controlled trials demonstrate that oral acyclovir, famciclovir, and valacyclovir reduce acute pain and the duration of chronic pain in older patients who have HZ and who are treated within 72 hours of rash onset [12]. No head-to-head study shows superiority of one of these agents over another so all three agents are acceptable. Because of their superior pharmacokinetics and simpler dosing schedule, famciclovir or valacyclovir are preferred to acyclovir for oral therapy for VZV infections. The benefits of treating patients who have HZ and who present more than 72 hours after rash onset are unknown. Some experts recommend antiviral therapy for patients presenting more than 72 hours after rash onset with continued new vesicle formation or when there are cutaneous, motor, neurologic, or ocular complications. Unfortunately, 20% to 30% of treated patients in antiviral trials had pain 6 months from HZ onset. These data indicate that even optimally treated patients can develop PHN.

Ophthalmic HZ is important in older patients because of the risk for visual impairment or blindness in persons who already may have compromised vision from other age-related pathology, such as glaucoma, macular degeneration, cataracts, or diabetic neuropathy. Oral acyclovir, famciclovir, and valacyclovir are effective for the prevention of ocular complications from ophthalmic HZ. Ophthalmologist consultation is recommended in older patients who have ophthalmic HZ to determine the presence and extent of ocular involvement and to determine the usefulness of local treatments, such as mydriatics, glucocorticoids, or topical antivirals.

Analgesics

Although no clinical trials have been conducted to determine the effect of analgesic therapy on the risk for developing PHN, relief of acute pain clearly is important. Acute HZ pain management requires the same principles as managing any pain: use of standardized pain measures, scheduled analgesia, and consistent and frequent follow-up to adjust dosing to the needs of patients. The choice of treatment is contingent on patients' comorbidities, concurrent medications, pain intensity, and preferences.

Patients who have mild pain may be managed with acetaminophen or nonsteroidal agents. Patients who have moderate to severe pain usually require treatment with a strong opioid analgesic (eg, oxycodone). There are several approaches to using short- or long-acting opioids in the treatment of HZ pain. One approach commonly used is to start with a short-acting medication at an oxycodone equianalgesic dosage (5 mg 4 times daily) and titrating the dose until pain reduction or intolerable adverse effects [12]. If an effective and tolerable dose is found, then treatment can be switched from a short-acting to a long-acting medication depending on cost and patient preference. Long-acting medications are more convenient and may provide a more consistent level of pain relief. Rescue doses of a short-acting opioid can be used for exacerbations of pain as needed with the long-acting opioid. Opioids have multiple adverse effects, including nausea, constipation, and sedation, which may be intolerable in some older adults. In most cases, constipation should be anticipated and managed with laxative therapy.

Adjuvant agents

If antiviral and analgesic therapy does not adequately control patients' pain, then clinicians can consider the addition of corticosteroids, gabapentin or pregabalin, a tricyclic antidepressant (TCA), or a neural blockade [12]. None of these approaches are shown to prevent PHN, but they may be useful in reducing acute pain.

Randomized controlled trials of corticosteroids versus placebo or acyclovir with or without corticosteroids in older patients who have HZ show equal rates of PHN [13–15]. These findings argue against the routine use of corticosteroids in older patients who have HZ. In most trials, corticosteroids reduced acute HZ pain although that beneficial effect was not sustained. In the a trial of acyclovir and prednisone, time to uninterrupted sleep, return to daily activity, and cessation of analgesic therapy was accelerated significantly in patients who received corticosteroids [15]. The patients in the trial were an average age of 60 years old, however, and had no relative contraindications to corticosteroids, such as hypertension, diabetes mellitus, or osteoporosis. The most common adverse effects of short-term prednisone use are gastrointestinal symptoms (dyspepsia, nausea, or vomiting), edema, and granulocytosis. Some clinicians use corticosteroids for VZV-induced facial paralysis and cranial polyneuritis to improve motor outcomes, reduce peripheral nerve damage from foraminal compression, and reduce pain. If corticosteroid treatment is considered, it always should be used with antiviral therapy.

A single dose (900 mg) of gabapentin is shown to reduce acute HZ pain over a 6-hour period [16]. This study provides proof of concept that gabapentin may be useful in reducing HZ pain [16]. A 900-mg starting dose of gabapentin, however, is too high for older adults. Neither gabapentin nor pregabalin is shown to prevent PHN or provide significant acute HZ pain relief in randomized controlled trials. If used, gabapentin and pregabalin can cause sedation, dizziness, ataxia, and peripheral edema. It is best to give starting doses at bedtime and increase subsequent doses carefully to 3 times daily for gabapentin and twice daily for pregabalin.

Low-dose amitriptyline used during acute HZ is associated with lower rates of pain at 6 months from rash onset but not 1 month or 3 months in one clinical trial [17]. The trial was unbalanced with regards to antiviral use, however, and amitriptyline has high rates of adverse events in older adults because of its high anticholinergic effects. If TCA therapy is considered, low-dose nortriptyline or desipramine is a better option. Baseline and follow-up EKGs are mandatory when using TCAs in older adults. Other TCA adverse effects include cognitive impairment, visual impairment, urinary retention, constipation, and dry mouth.

If pain control from antiviral agents and analgesics with or without any of the adjuvant drugs (discussed previously) is inadequate, then anesthetic nerve blocks should be considered. This intervention requires referral to a pain specialist. Although a single epidural injection of anesthetic and corticosteroid does not prevent PHN, these techniques can reduce severe acute pain [18].

Postherpetic neuralgia

General principles

The main goal of the treatment of PHN in older adults is the reduction of pain and associated symptoms, including depression, insomnia, and functional impairment. No one treatment is uniformly and completely effective in all older patients who have PHN. It is important, therefore, to set realistic goals with patients. Specifically, patients need to know that it is unlikely that any intervention will take the pain away completely but some interventions are likely to reduce pain at the risk for potential adverse effects. They need to understand that the natural history of PHN is one of improvement over weeks, months, and even years, regardless of the underlying treatment in many patients. The same comments in the section on HZ treatment regarding pain management apply to patients who have PHN, as do comments regarding social support, mental and physical activity, adequate nutrition, and a caring attitude.

Pharmacotherapy

The topical lidocaine patch, gabapentin, nortriptyline (a TCA), opioids, pregabalin, and tramadol are considered first-line therapies, as one or more high-quality, randomized controlled trials demonstrated efficacy with these agents. The topical lidocaine patch, gabapentin, and pregabalin are approved by the Food and Drug Administration (FDA) for the treatment of PHN. Opioids and TCAs are not approved by the FDA partly because the manufacturers of these products have not sought approval. Pharmacotherapy for PHN is discussed in more detail in recently published guidelines [19,20]. In general, these agents produce clinically significant reduction in pain in approximately 30% to 60% of patients. Unfortunately, there is no good way to predict which patients will respond or not respond to a given drug. Furthermore, there are few head-to-head comparisons of these drugs, so it is unknown if one agent clearly is superior in efficacy to another. Clinical information about these drugs is summarized in Table 3 [21]. Starting doses and maximum doses of drugs generally are lower in frail older adults. The upward titration of drug doses also often needs to be slower in frail older adults.

The initial choice of agent depends on patient comorbidities and preferences and cost and formulary restrictions. The topical lidocaine patch, gabapentin, and pregabalin generally are better tolerated than opioids and TCAs in older adults. The topical lidocaine patch is easy to use and gives initial pain relief in hours to days when effective (2 weeks for an adequate trial) but can produce a skin rash that prevents use of the patch. Gabapentin has few drug interactions and gives initial pain relief in days to weeks when effective (adequate trial requires 3–8 weeks for titration plus 1–2 weeks at maximum tolerated dosage) but can produce somnolence, dizziness, and peripheral edema. These adverse effects require monitoring and possibly dosage adjustment but usually not treatment discontinuation. Gabapentin may cause or exacerbate gait and balance problems and cognitive impairment in the frail elderly, which can require discontinuation of therapy. Pregabalin has few drug interactions, has a more rapid onset of action than gabapentin, and gives initial pain relief within 1 to 2 days when effective but also produces the same adverse effects as gabapentin.

Opioids give initial pain relief in hours to days when effective (adequate trial requires 4 weeks) but the well-known adverse effects of opioids preclude their use in some older adults. Opioid analgesics must be used cautiously in patients who have a history of substance abuse. The risk that substance abuse develops in patients who do not have a history of substance abuse is believed low in older patients who have PHN. Tramadol gives initial pain relief in hours to days when effective (adequate trial requires 4 weeks) but has similar adverse effects as opioids because a major metabolite is a mu-opioid agonist. Tramadol is associated with an increased risk for seizures in patients who have a history of seizures or use drugs that can reduce the seizure threshold and serotonin syndrome in patients who use serotonergic medications, especially selective serotonin reuptake inhibitors (SSRIs).

Nortriptyline gives initial pain relief in several days to weeks when effective (adequate trial requires 6–8 weeks with at least 1–2 weeks at maximum tolerated dosage) but has several potentially significant anticholinergic and cardiac adverse effects in older adults. A screening EKG to check for cardiac conduction abnormalities is recommended before beginning any TCA treatment in the elderly. TCAs are contraindicated in patients who have QT prolongation or familial histories of long QT syndromes, with atrioventricular block or bundle-branch block and with a recent acute myocardial infarction. Although amitriptyline was tested in many PHN trials, it often is tolerated poorly in older adults because of its much higher anticholinergic activity. Nortriptyline has equivalent efficacy compared with amitriptyline in PHN but is better tolerated [22]. Desipramine is a reasonable alternative to nortriptyline. In a crossover study of PHN comparing opioid analgesics, TCAs, and placebo, controlled-release morphine and TCAs provided significant benefits on pain [23]. In this trial, patients preferred treatment with opioid analgesics compared with TCAs and placebo but there was a greater incidence of adverse effects and dropouts during opioid treatment.

Nonresponse to single drug therapy often leads to combination therapy with one or more of the agents described previously, but there are few data regarding the additive or synergistic benefits of combination treatment. The potential advantages of combination therapy include augmentation of a partial response to a single drug, more rapid effect when a medication that requires titration to reach an effective dosage also is used, and better analgesia at lower doses of drug. The potential disadvantages of combination therapy in older adults include an increased risk for adverse effects as the number of medications is increased, the difficulty determining which medication is responsible for adverse effects, and increased cost. In a randomized, double-blind, active placebo-controlled, 4- to 5-week crossover trial including 22 patients who had PHN, investigators studied the effects of morphine alone, gabapentin alone, and morphine-gabapentin combination on neuropathic pain [24]. The results showed that gabapentin and morphine combined achieved modestly better pain relief at lower doses of each drug than either as a single agent. The combination, however, was associated with higher levels of sedation, dry mouth, and cognitive dysfunction than the maximal tolerated dose of each single agent.

Table 3
Oral medications for postherpetic neuralgia

Characteristic	Lidocaine patch	Gabapentin	Nortriptyline	Opioids	Pregabalin	Tramadol
Structure	Amino amide anesthestic	γ-aminobutyric acid (GABA) analog	Dibenzocycloheptene TCA	Mu-opioid receptor agonist	GABA analog	Mu-opioid agonist and serotonin and norepinephrine reuptake inhibitor
Kinetics	Very little systemic absorption	Renal elimination; prolonged half-life with renal impairment	Hepatic metabolism; higher levels of active metabolites in the elderly	Hepatic metabolism and renal elimination	Renal elimination; prolonged half-life with renal impairment	Hepatic metabolism and renal elimination
Standard dosing	Up to 3 patches applied over the affected area for 12 hours a day	Start at 100–300 mg at night; increase by 100–300 mg/d every 1–7 days as tolerated in three-times-a-day dosing; maximum dose 3600 mg/d	Start 10 mg at night; increase by 10 mg every 4–7 days by the same amount until reduction in pain; maximum dose 75–150 mg/d	In morphine equivalents start 2.5–15 mg every 4 hours; after 1–2 weeks, convert total daily dosage to long-acting opioid analgesic and continue short-acting medication as needed	150 mg/d given in 2 or 3 divided doses; may increase to 300 mg/d, given in 2 or 3 divided doses, within 1 week; maximum dosage 600 mg/d	Start 50 once daily; increase by 50 mg daily in divided doses every 3–7 days as tolerated; maximum dose 400 mg daily; in patients over 75 years of age, 300 mg/d in divided doses
Benefit: % significant improvement	≥50% reduction in pain scores: 31% lidocaine patch versus 8% placebo patch	Moderate or much pain improvement: 41%–43% gabapentin versus 12%–23% placebo	Moderate to good pain relief: 44%–67% TCAs versus 5%–19% placebo or control drug	Masked preference: 67% oxycodone versus 11% placebo	≥50% reduction in pain scores: 50% pregabalin versus 20% placebo	≥50% reduction in pain scores 77% tramadol versus 56% placebo

Adverse events	Skin redness or rash	Somnolence, dizziness, ataxia, peripheral edema	Arrhythmia, cardiac conduction block, orthostatic hypotension, urinary retention, constipation, cognitive impairment	Constipation, sedation, nausea/vomiting, respiratory depression, nervous system symptoms, pruritis	Somnolence, dizziness, ataxia, peripheral edema	Constipation, sedation, nausea/vomiting, respiratory depression, nervous system symptoms, seizures
Main drug-drug interactions	Class I antiarrythmics	Opioids	Antipsychotics, anticholinergics, SSRIs, sedative-hypnotics, antiarrhythmics, monoamine oxidase inhibitors	Anticholinergics, sedative-hypnotics, anxiolytics, CYP2D6 inhibitors, TCAs, muscle relaxants	Opioids	Anticholinergics, sedative-hypnotics, anxiolytics, CYP2D6 inhibitors, SSRIs, TCAs, muscle relaxants
Main drug-disease interactions	None	Dementia, ataxia, falls	Myocardial infarction, QT prolongation, atrioventricular block, bundle-branch block, ileus, prostatic hypertrophy, seizure disorder, glaucoma, dementia	Ileus, chronic obstructive pulmonary disease, dementia, prostatic hypertrophy	Dementia, ataxia, falls	Ileus, chronic obstructive pulmonary disease, dementia, prostatic hypertrophy, seizure disorder
How supplied	10- by 14-cm lidocaine patch contains 5% lidocaine base on polyester backing	100-mg, 300-mg, 400-mg capsules; 600-mg, 800-mg tablets	10-mg, 25-mg, 50-mg, 75-mg capsules; 10-mg/5 mL solution	Multiple drugs and dosage forms	25-mg, 50-mg, 75-mg, 100-mg, 150-mg, 200-mg, 225-mg, 300-mg capsules	50-mg tablet

Data from Schmader KE, Dworkin RH. Clinical features and treatment of postherpetic neuralgia and peripheral neuropathy in older adults. In: Gibson SJ, Weiner DK, editors. Pain in older persons. Progress in Pain Management and Research, vol. 35. Seattle, WA: International Association for the Study of Pain/IASP Press, 2005.

Other treatments

Some older patients who have PHN do not have an adequate response to any of the frontline medications. For these patients, other drug and nondrug treatments deserve consideration. Patients who require complex drug combinations, risky second-line medications, or invasive treatments should be referred to a pain management center. A detailed review of these interventions is beyond the scope of this article, but nondrug, noninvasive, and invasive treatments are summarized briefly.

Noninvasive treatments include physical modalities, such as cold application or transcutaneous electrical nerve stimulation, percutaneous electrical nerve stimulation, psychologic treatments, and acupuncture. These interventions have little risk and may be useful in some patients but whether or not they are effective in a population of patients that has PHN is unknown and needs to be tested in controlled clinical trials. Some patients who have PHN may have associated myofascial pain in addition to neuropathic pain [25]. The presence of myofascial pathology is indicated by taut muscle bands (ie, a group of tense muscle fibers extending from a trigger point to the muscle attachments) and trigger points (ie, a hyperirritable spot in skeletal muscle that is painful on compression) in the affected dermatome. These patients are good candidates for a trial of percutaneous electrical nerve stimulation.

Invasive treatments may be considered when patients fail to obtain adequate relief from noninvasive treatment approaches. Invasive treatments include peripheral and central neural blockade, central nervous system drug delivery, spinal cord stimulation, and neurosurgical techniques. Neural blockade techniques include sensory nerve, plexus, and sympathetic nerve blocks and epidural and intrathecal blockade with lidocaine-like drugs or corticosteroids. Many patients who have PHN note initial relief of pain with nerve blocks but few experience long-lasting relief. Central nervous system drug delivery attempts to place a drug (eg, morphine) as close as possible to central pain receptors in the spinal cord corresponding to the affected dermatomes. Spinal cord stimulation requires implantation of an electrode in the thoracic or lumbar epidural space and the placement of a percutaneous electrical stimulator. These interventions represent rational approaches to pain relief but they are not proved effective in controlled trials, partly because the design and conduct of such trials are difficult, and they carry procedural risks in the elderly. In general, these interventions have a limited role in PHN treatment and should be contemplated in patients who have failed all other treatments and continue to have disabling pain.

Prevention

A live, attenuated varicella-zoster vaccine was developed by isolating VZV from a child who had varicella and passing the isolate in human embryonic lung fibroblasts and guinea pig embryo cells. The varicella vaccine is safe, well tolerated, and highly effective in preventing varicella in seroneg-ative nonimmune individuals. Widespread use of the varicella vaccine has produced a marked decrease in the incidence of varicella in the United States [26]. Although the vaccine virus can establish a latent infection and reactivate, vaccine virus–associated HZ probably is less frequent and severe in older adults than natural HZ because the vaccine virus is highly attenu-ated. Some experts speculate that the incidence of HZ could increase in younger adults in the near future because a decline in the incidence of var-icella may reduce the population's exposure to VZV, prevent immune boost-ing to VZV, and increase the risk for VZV reactivation.

Almost all adults are latently infected with VZV and at risk for HZ for the foreseeable future. The zoster vaccine essentially is the same as the var-icella vaccine but it is formulated to yield much higher concentrations of live attenuated VZV and antigen than the varicella vaccine. The zoster vaccine induces significant increases in VZV-specific T lymphocytes and humoral immunity in older adults that is not achieved by the varicella vaccine. Given that cellular immunity to VZV declines with age and the zoster vaccine boosts immunity in older adults, the Shingles Prevention Study tested the hypothesis that vaccination against VZV would decrease the incidence or severity of HZ and PHN among older adults.

The Shingles Prevention Study was a randomized, double-blind, placebo-controlled trial in 38,546 community-dwelling persons 60 years old and older followed for a median of 3 years [3]. A total of 957 confirmed cases of HZ (315 among vaccine recipients and 642 among placebo recipients) and 107 cases of PHN (27 among vaccine recipients and 80 among placebo recipients) were included in the efficacy analysis. The zoster vaccine reduced the burden of illness (a pain severity by duration measure) resulting from HZ by 61.1% ($P < .001$), reduced the incidence of HZ by 51.3% ($P < .001$) (Fig. 2), and reduced the incidence of PHN by 66.5% ($P < .001$) (Fig. 3). The zoster vaccine reduced the incidence of neuralgic pain signifi-cantly at all time points from zoster rash onset (ie, 30, 60, 120, and 180 days). The zoster vaccine maintained its efficacy for HZ burden of illness and for the incidence of PHN (see Fig. 3) regardless of the age of the sub-jects. Efficacy in the 60- to 70-year-old group was mediated mostly by pre-venting HZ, whereas efficacy in the greater-than-70-year-old group was mediated mostly by attenuating HZ, because the vaccine was less effective in preventing HZ in that age group (see Fig. 2). Reactions at the injection site were more frequent among vaccine recipients but generally were mild. This landmark study showed that the zoster vaccine reduced morbidity from HZ and PHN markedly in older adults. Based on these findings, the FDA licensed the zoster vaccine for the prevention of HZ in immunocom-petent adults 60 years of age and older in 2006. The Advisory Committee on Immunization Practices (ACIP) of the CDC unanimously recommended the vaccine for the prevention of HZ and PHN in immuncompetent adults 60 years of age and older in 2006.

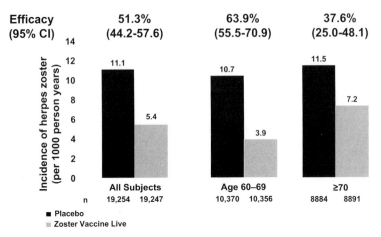

Fig. 2. Effect of zoster vaccine on the incidence of HZ in the Shingles Prevention Study [3]. The figure shows the incidence of HZ per 1000 person-years in zoster vaccine recipients (*gray bars*) and placebo recipients (*black bars*) for all subjects and for subjects in prespecified strata of 60 to 69 years old and subjects 70 years old and older. In all subjects, the incidence of zoster was 11.1 versus 5.4 in the placebo and zoster vaccine groups, respectively, which yields a vaccine efficacy of 51.3% (95% CI, 44.2–57.6). Vaccine efficacy was higher in the 60-to-69-year-old group compared with the 70-years-and-older group.

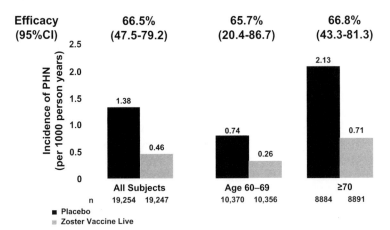

Fig. 3. Effect of zoster vaccine on the incidence of PHN in the Shingles Prevention Study [3]. The figure shows the incidence of PHN per 1000 person-years in zoster vaccine recipients (*gray bars*) and placebo recipients (*black bars*) for all subjects and for subjects in prespecified strata of 60 to 69 years old and subjects 70 years old and older. In all subjects, the incidence of PHN was 1.38 versus 0.46 in the placebo and zoster vaccine groups, respectively, which yields a vaccine efficacy of 66.5% (95% CI, 47.5–79.2). Vaccine efficacy was maintained equally in the 60-to-69-year-old group and the 70-years-and-older group.

The use of the zoster vaccine raises several important clinical questions. The long-term duration of the protective effect of the vaccine is unknown but the Shingles Prevention Study data indicate that vaccine efficacy persists for at least 4 years. A subset of study vaccine recipients are being followed long term to determine the durability of the zoster vaccine's efficacy and the possible need for and timing of booster vaccination. The effectiveness of the vaccine in persons more than 80 years old is unclear. These individuals, however, are at highest risk for HZ and PHN and reduction of HZ pain severity and duration seems to occur in the "old-old" even when HZ is not prevented. Neither the FDA nor the ACIP sets an upper age limit on the use of the vaccine. The efficacy of the zoster vaccine in individuals who already have had HZ is unknown because these individuals were excluded from the Shingles Prevention Study. Persons who have had recent episodes (within 3–5 years) of HZ may not benefit from the zoster vaccine, because the boost in immunity from reactivated wild-type VZV is as strong or better than that obtained from the zoster vaccine. Other individuals, however, who have a history of HZ may benefit because HZ can recur. The ACIP recommends the zoster vaccine for persons over 60 years of age whether or not they report a prior episode of HZ.

It is not necessary to ask patients about a history of varicella or HZ before administration of the zoster vaccine or to conduct serologic testing for varicella immunity. If negative VZV IgG test results are presented, then patients should be offered varicella vaccine according to current recommendations. The zoster vaccine can be administered with other vaccines (eg, influenza, tetanus, or pneumococcal polysaccharide) but each vaccine should be administered using a separate syringe at a different anatomic site. Currently, the zoster vaccine is not recommended for use in immunocompromised individuals or persons under 60 years old. With the development of the zoster vaccine, antiviral therapy, acute pain management, and neuropathic pain treatments, clinicians now have multiple effective tools to reduce the suffering of older adults from HZ and PHN markedly.

References

[1] Cohen JI, Brunell PA, Straus SE, et al. Recent advances in varicella-zoster virus infection. Ann Intern Med 1999;130:922–32.
[2] Dworkin RH, Schmader KE. Epidemiology and natural history of herpes zoster and postherpetic neuralgia. In: Watson CPN, Gershon AA, editors. Herpes zoster and postherpetic neuralgia. 2nd edition. New York: Elsevier Press; 2001. p. 39–64.
[3] Oxman MN, Levin MJ, Johnson GR, et al. A vaccine to prevent herpes zoster and postherpetic neuralgia in older adults. N Engl J Med 2005;352:2271–84.
[4] Schmader KE, George LK, Hamilton JD. Racial differences in the occurrence of herpes zoster. J Infect Dis 1995;171:701–5.
[5] Gnann JW Jr, Whitley RJ. Herpes zoster. N Engl J Med 2002;347:340–6.
[6] Thomas SL, Hall AJ. What does epidemiology tell us about risk factors for herpes zoster? The Lancet Infect Dis 2004;4:26–33.

[7] Jung BF, Johnson RW, Griffin DR, et al. Risk factors for postherpetic neuralgia in patients with herpes zoster. Neurology 2004;62:1545–51.

[8] Cunningham AL, Dworkin RH. The management of post-herpetic neuralgia. BMJ 2000; 321:778–9.

[9] Desmond RA, Weiss HL, Arani RB, et al. Clinical applications for change-point analysis of herpes zoster pain. J Pain Symptom Manage 2002;23:510–6.

[10] Bennett GJ. Neuropathic pain: an overview. In: Borsook D, editor. Molecular neurobiology of pain. Seattle (WA): IASP Press; 1997. p. 109–13.

[11] Katz J, Cooper EM, Walther RR, et al. Acute pain in herpes zoster and its impact on health-related quality of life. Clin Infect Dis 2004;39:342–8.

[12] Dworkin RH, Johnson RW, Breuer J, et al. Recommendations for the management of herpes zoster. Clin Infect Dis 2007;44:S1–26.

[13] Esmann V, Geil JP, Kroon S, et al. Prednisolone does not prevent postherpetic neuralgia. Lancet 1987;2:126–9.

[14] Wood MJ, Johnson RW, McKendrick MW, et al. A randomized trial of acyclovir for 7 days or 21 days with and without prednisolone for treatment of acute herpes zoster. N Engl J Med 1994;330:896–900.

[15] Whitley RJ, Weiss H, Gnann JW, et al. Acyclovir with and without prednisone for the treatment of herpes zoster: a randomized, placebo-controlled trial. Ann Intern Med 1996;125: 376–83.

[16] Berry JD, Petersen KL. A single dose of gabapentin reduces acute pain and allodynia in patients with herpes zoster. Neurology 2005;65:444–7.

[17] Bowsher D. Acute herpes zoster and postherpetic neuralgia: effects of acyclovir and outcome of treatment with amitriptyline. Br J Gen Pract 1992;42:244–6.

[18] Van Wijck AJM, Opstelten W, Moons KG, et al. The PINE study of epidural steroids and local anaesthetics to prevent postherpetic neuralgia: a randomised controlled trial. Lancet 2006;367:219–24.

[19] Dworkin RH, Allen RR, Argoff CR, et al. Guidelines for the pharmacologic management of chronic neuropathic pain. Arch Neurol 2003;60:1524–34.

[20] Dubinsky RH, Kabbani H, El-Chami Z, et al. Practice parameter: treatment of postherpetic neuralgia. Neurology 2004;63:959–65.

[21] Schmader KE, Dworkin RH. Clinical features and treatment of postherpetic neuralgia and peripheral neuropathy in older adults. In: Gibson SJ, Weiner DK, editors. Pain in older persons. Prog Pain Res Management 2005;35:355–77.

[22] Watson CPN, Vernich L, Chipman M, et al. Nortriptyline versus amitriptyline in postherpetic neuralgia: a randomized trial. Neurology 1998;51:1166–71.

[23] Raja SN, Haythornthwaite JA, Pappagallo M, et al. Opioids versus antidepressants in postherpetic neuralgia: a randomized, placebo-controlled trial. Neurology 2002;59:1015–21.

[24] Gilron I, Bailey JM, Tu D, et al. Morphine, gabapentin, or their combination for neuropathic pain. N Engl J Med 2005;352:1324–34.

[25] Weiner DK, Schmader KE. Postherpetic pain: more than sensory neuralgia? Pain Med 2006; 7:243–9.

[26] Seward JF, Watson BM, Peterson CL, et al. Varicella disease after introduction of varicella vaccine in the United States, 1995–2000. JAMA 2002;287:606–11.

ELSEVIER
SAUNDERS

CLINICS IN
GERIATRIC
MEDICINE

Clin Geriatr Med 23 (2007) 633–647

Bacteremia and Sepsis in Older Adults

Timothy D. Girard, MD, MSCI[a,*],
E. Wesley Ely, MD, MPH[a,b]

[a]*Division of Allergy, Pulmonary, and Critical Care Medicine, Center for Health Services Research, Vanderbilt University School of Medicine, 6th Floor Medical Center East, Suite 6100, Nashville, TN 37232-8300, USA*
[b]*VA Tennessee Valley Geriatric Research, Education, and Clinical Center (GRECC), VA Service, Department of Veteran0s Affairs Medical Center, 1310 24th Avenue South, Nashville, TN 37212-2637, USA*

For many years, clinicians used different terms for similar but overlapping clinical disorders of infection, such as *bacteremia*, *septicemia*, and *sepsis*. To standardize terminology and "to provide a conceptual and a practical framework to define the systemic inflammatory response to infection," the American College of Chest Physicians and the Society of Critical Care Medicine convened a Consensus Conference in 1991 and published definitions the following year [1]. The term *bacteremia* denotes the presence of bacteria in the blood (Table 1); the designation provides no information regarding the host response to infection. Alternatively, the term *sepsis* is a syndrome of systemic inflammation in response to infection. Both bacteremia and sepsis can result from a variety of infections.

Although not every patient with bacteremia has sepsis, the syndrome is underrecognized in patients with bacteremia, especially in older patients who may not exhibit the typical manifestations of the systemic inflammatory response syndrome (SIRS) (see Table 1). In a study of 238 episodes of bacteremia in patients aged 65 years or more, 75% of patients met the definition of sepsis, but only 11% of patients were admitted with a diagnosis of sepsis [2]. In another study of 842 episodes of bacteremia in adult inpatients, 26% were complicated by severe sepsis and 15% by septic shock [3]. Forty-three percent of patients with severe sepsis in the same study had documented bacteremia.

Dr. Girard receives support from the Hartford Geriatrics Health Outcomes Research Scholars Award Program. Dr. Ely receives support from the VA Clinical Science Research and Development Service (VA Merit Review Award) and the National Institutes of Health (AG0727201).

* Corresponding author.
E-mail address: timothy.girard@vanderbilt.edu (T.D. Girard).

doi:10.1016/j.cger.2007.05.003

geriatric.theclinics.com

Table 1
Definitions of sepsis, bacteremia, and related disorders*

Disorder	Definition
Infection	A pathologic process caused by the invasion of normally sterile tissue or fluid or body cavity by pathogenic or potentially pathogenic microorganisms
Bacteremia	Presence of bacteria in the blood
SIRS	The systemic inflammatory response to a variety of clinical insults exhibited by at least two of the following: (1) temperature $>38°C$ or $<36°C$, (2) heart rate >90 beats/min, (3) respiratory rate >20 breaths/min with a $PaCO_2$ <32 mm Hg, and (4) WBC $>12,000/$ mm^3 or $<4000/mm^3$ or $>10\%$ immature (band) forms
Sepsis	SIRS and documented or suspected infection
Severe sepsis	Sepsis complicated by organ dysfunction
Septic shock	Sepsis complicated by hypotension (ie, SBP <90 mm Hg or MAP <60 mm Hg) despite adequate fluid resuscitation

Abbreviations: MAP, mean arterial pressure; SBP, systolic blood pressure; SIRS, systemic inflammatory response syndrome; WBC, white blood cells.
    * American College of Chest Physicians/Society of Critical Care Medicine Consensus Conference definitions [1].

Because the epidemiology, prognosis, and treatment of bacteremia in older patients are dependent on the source of infection (ie, pneumonia versus urinary tract infection versus other sources) and the host response (ie, the presence or absence of sepsis), this review article focuses primarily on sepsis in older patients and highlights features of bacteremia when appropriate. The reader should refer to the other articles in this issue for information regarding other infectious disorders that may be complicated by bacteremia in older patients.

Epidemiology

Each year in the United States nearly 2500 cases of sepsis occur per 100,000 persons aged 85 years or older, with older persons being much more likely to acquire sepsis and bacteremia than younger persons [4,5]. Using data from the National Hospital Discharge Survey, Martin and colleagues [5] determined that patients 65 years of age or older were 13 times more likely to have sepsis during the 24-year study period than younger adults (relative risk [RR], 13.1; 95% confidence interval [CI], 12.6–13.6). In fact, this disparity in risk increased over time. Incidence rates of sepsis increased 20.4% faster among older patients than among younger patients from 1979 to 2002 (mean increase per year, 11.5% versus 9.5%; $P<.001$; Fig. 1). Other large studies have also reported that the incidences of sepsis and bacteremia increase with older age [3,4,6].

In addition to sepsis and bacteremia being more common among older persons, the microbiology of these infectious disorders varies with age.

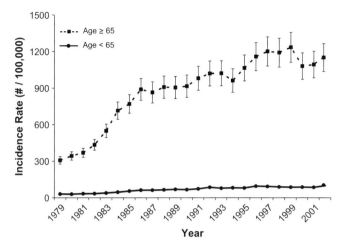

Fig. 1. Age-adjusted incidence rates of sepsis among hospitalized patients stratified by age 65 years and older (*dashed line*) or less than 65 years (*solid line*). Points are mean values; I-bars represent the SEM. (*From* Martin GS, Mannino DM, Moss M. The effect of age on the development and outcome of adult sepsis. Crit Care Med 2006;34(1):17; with permission.)

Older patients are more likely than younger patients to experience infections due to gram-negative organisms. Martin and colleagues [5] found that patients 65 years of age or older with sepsis were 1.31 times more likely to have gram-negative infections than younger septic patients (95% CI, 1.27–1.35). Similarly, in a study of 25,745 bloodstream infections reported from 1997 to 2000, *Escherichia coli* was the most frequently isolated pathogen among older patients with community-acquired bacteremia [7]. In contrast, *Staphylococcus aureus* was the most frequently isolated pathogen among younger adults with community-acquired bacteremia. Although *S aureus* was the most common pathogen causing nosocomial bacteremia in this study regardless of age, other studies suggest that older age affects the microbiology of nosocomial bacteremia. McClelland and colleagues [8] studied 385 patients with *S aureus* bacteremia and found that older patients were more likely than younger patients to have infections with methicillin-resistant *S aureus* (MRSA).

Age-related differences in the microbiology of bacteremia and sepsis are, in part, a result of differences in the source infections leading to these disorders among older patients when compared with younger patients. For example, urinary tract infections, which are typically due to gram-negative organisms, are more frequently the source of bacteremia and sepsis in older patients than in younger patients. In a study of community-acquired bacteremia, Lark and colleagues [9] found that bacteremic patients 65 years of age or older were more likely than younger patients to have a urinary tract source of infection (odds ratio [OR], 2.5; *P* < .001). In a study limited to patients over 59 years of age, Leibovici and colleagues [10] observed that the urinary tract was the source of bacteremia in 50% of patients 80 years of age or older compared with 34% of patients aged 60 to 79 years. Similarly, Martin and colleagues [5] found that genitourinary infections were more frequently the cause of sepsis among older patients when compared with younger patients (RR, 1.38; 95% CI, 1.32–1.44).

Other factors likely contribute to age-related differences in the microbiology of bacteremia and sepsis in addition to differences in source infections. In a comparison of older and younger patients who all had respiratory infections as the cause of sepsis, Martin and colleagues [5] found that gram-negative infections accounted for 34.1% of cases in patients aged 65 years and older compared with 20.5% of cases in younger patients (RR, 1.66; 95% CI, 1.63–1.69). This finding suggests that older persons may be exposed to gram-negative pathogens more frequently than younger persons or may be more susceptible to infection with gram-negative pathogens due to changes in immune function associated with aging.

Risk factors

Indeed, older persons are at increased risk for bacteremia and sepsis owing to multiple factors, including exposure to instrumentation and procedures, institutionalization, comorbid illnesses, immunosenescence, malnutrition, and poor performance status. Studies of bacteremia and sepsis have demonstrated that older patients have higher rates of comorbid illness [5,10,11]. In the Protein C Worldwide Evaluation of Severe Sepsis (PROWESS) trial, septic patients aged 75 years or older more frequently had a history of coronary artery disease, chronic obstructive pulmonary disease, malignancy, and recent surgery when compared with younger patients [11]. The management of such conditions often necessitates instrumentation that creates a portal of entry for infection. For instance, older patients in the community and in health care institutions often have urinary catheters, and urinary tract infections—the most common source of bacteremia and sepsis in older patients—are frequently attributable to the presence of indwelling urinary catheters in older patients. Lark and colleagues [9] found that 44% of older patients with community-acquired bacteremia had indwelling urinary catheters. In a study of 533 chronically institutionalized older patients, indwelling urinary catheters were the leading risk factor for bacteremia (OR, 39; 95% CI, 16–97) [12].

Both short- and long-term institutionalization carry with them multiple risks for infection. Hospitalized patients as well as those residing in long-term care facilities are at high risk for complications, such as decubitus ulcers (a common source of bacteremia [13]), and for colonization or infection with antibiotic-resistant organisms. One study of 297 patients with S aureus bacteremia at the time of hospital admission found that patients aged more than 60 years were more likely than younger patients to be infected with MRSA [14]. Further analysis using multivariable logistic regression revealed that age was not an independent risk factor for MRSA infection, but that the increased risk observed in older patients was attributable to the higher likelihood of exposure to factors that were independently associated with MRSA infection, including nursing home residence (OR for MRSA versus methicillin-sensitive *S aureus* bacteremia, 9.89; 95% CI, 3.87–25.58), hospitalization in the past 6 months (OR, 4.38; 95% CI, 1.95–9.84), antimicrobial use in the past 3 months (OR, 5.62; 95% CI, 2.64–11.92), and indwelling urinary catheters (OR, 7.26; 95% CI, 2.51–20.9).

Older patients are also at increased risk for colonization with gram-negative organisms that may lead to bacteremia and sepsis. Nursing home residence and hospitalization are each associated with oropharyngeal colonization with gram-negative bacilli, as are respiratory disease and poor functional status [15]. Nearly one third of persons 80 years of age and older live in long-term care facilities where antibiotic resistance is a growing problem. Wiener and colleagues [16] evaluated 39 patients at a nursing home involved in an outbreak of drug-resistant gram-negative infections and determined that 46% had antibiotic-resistant *Escherichia coli.*

Among patients with bacteremia or other infections, older patients are more likely to experience sepsis. Studying 832 patients with bacteremia, Brun-Buisson and colleagues [3] found that older age was independently associated with an increased likelihood of severe sepsis, although the relationship was nonlinear. Specifically, bacteremic patients 50 years of age and older were at higher risk for severe sepsis than were younger patients, but the risk plateaued above 50 years of age instead of continuing to rise. In addition to age, the source of bacteremia had an important role in determining the risk for severe sepsis. Patients with abdominal, respiratory tract, and neuromeningeal infections were at highest risk, as were those with multiple sources of infection. Alternatively, patients with urinary tract infections were at lowest risk for severe sepsis.

Despite the fact that life-sustaining treatments typically administered in ICUs are often withheld from older patients [17], bacteremia in such patients more frequently results in severe illness requiring ICU admission when compared with bacteremia in young patients. A large population-based study in Calgary determined that patients 65 years of age or older were seven times more likely than younger patients to sustain bacteremia requiring ICU admission (95% CI, 5.6–8.7). Other risk factors included hemodialysis, diabetes mellitus, alcoholism, cancer, and lung disease [18]. Owing to the increased frequency of these comorbid conditions among older persons as well as other factors described herein, these patients are at increased risk for bacteremia, sepsis, and severe sepsis.

Immune function and the pathophysiology of sepsis

Changes in the immune system that occur with age (ie, immunosenescence) clearly contribute to the increased susceptibility of older persons to infection [19]. Adaptive immunity is significantly impaired with increasing age such that cell-mediated immune responses are diminished, as are elements of humoral immunity, rendering older individuals more susceptible to pathogens [20,21]. Additionally, although the cytokine response in older persons is complex and difficult to interpret, studies have clearly demonstrated that cytokine and chemokine signaling networks are altered with increasing age. These changes are believed to predispose older patients to sepsis. Higher levels of proinflammatory cytokines, such as tumor necrosis factor-α and interleukin-6, have been observed in older patients with sepsis when compared with younger septic patients [22,23]. In sepsis, these cytokines and others that are generated in response to toxic microbial stimuli (eg, lipopolysaccharides, peptidoglycans, or other pattern-recognition molecules) activate leukocytes, promote leukocyte-vascular endothelium adhesion, and induce endothelial damage [24]. Tissue factor, expressed from activated immune cells (especially macrophages) and from damaged endothelium, activates a clotting cascade that ultimately leads to microvascular thrombosis, impaired capillary blood flow, and decreased oxygen delivery to local tissues [25]. A prothrombotic state, which contributes to the increased risk of sepsis and death in infected patients, exists in older persons, as evidenced by increased concentrations of D-dimer, activated factor VII, and other coagulation factors [26,27].

Diagnostic challenges

Older patients with bacteremia or sepsis often present a diagnostic challenge to clinicians because nonspecific clinical manifestations of infection are common in such patients [28]. Altered mental status (eg, delirium, somnolence, or coma) is common in acutely ill older persons and does not necessarily herald central nervous system infection; likewise, tachypnea does not always indicate a respiratory infection. Nevertheless, these signs are common harbingers of infection in older patients. One study of 811 septic patients found that tachypnea and altered mentation were more common among patients aged more than 75 years than among younger patients, whereas tachycardia and hypoxemia were less common among older patients [29]. Other nonspecific expressions of infection in the elderly may include anorexia, malaise, generalized weakness, falls, and urinary incontinence [30]. Clinicians should have a heightened suspicion for infection when evaluating older patients with such symptoms.

Although fever is a classic sign of infection that is present in most patients with bacteremia or sepsis, studies examining the clinical manifestations of bacteremia and sepsis in older patients have almost uniformly found that they are less likely to develop fever than younger patients. Among 320 bacteremic patients, Gleckman and Hibert [31] noted that fever was absent in 25 (13%) of the 192 elderly patients compared with 5 (4%) of the 128 younger patients ($P<.01$). In another study of nearly 1000 episodes of bacteremia in patients 60 years of age and older, those 80 years of age and older had lower temperatures than patients aged 60 to 79 years [10]. Knowledge of an older person's basal temperature may be helpful when evaluating for infection, because some patients without significant fever during infection do demonstrate a noticeable change from baseline. In one study of nursing home residents, a "blunted" fever response (maximum temperature <101°F) was noted in 47% of infectious episodes, but an adequate change in temperature from baseline (change ≥2.4°F) was observed in one quarter of the episodes without robust fever (temperature <101°F) [32].

The atypical symptoms exhibited by older patients with infection, especially the increased prevalence of delirium, and the high frequency of comorbid conditions such as cerebrovascular disease and dementia often pose challenges during a diagnostic work-up. Specifically, it may be more difficult to obtain samples of blood, sputum, body fluids, or tissue from patients who are delirious, demented, debilitated, dehydrated, or frail [30].

Prognostic differences between older and younger patients

Although the severity of illness (as indicated by organ dysfunction and acute physiologic abnormalities) has more prognostic importance than age, older patients are at higher risk of death due to bacteremia and sepsis than are younger patients. Brun-Buisson and colleagues [3] evaluated 832 patients with bacteremia and found that increasing age was associated with high mortality. After adjusting for relevant covariates, bacteremic patients 80 years of age and older were 2.4 times more likely to die in the hospital when compared with those aged less than 50 years (95% CI, 1.6–3.7). Patients aged 60 to 69 years (RR, 1.5; 95% CI, 1.0–2.4) and those aged 70 to 79 years (RR, 2.1; 95% CI, 1.4–3.3) were also at increased risk for death. Other factors independently associated with increased mortality were severe sepsis, shock, infection with a gram-positive organism, and a poor prognosis of pre-existing disease. The urinary tract as the source of bacteremia was the only factor associated with improved survival. Other studies of bacteremia have similarly reported that increasing age is a risk factor for death [8,33], although some investigations have found no association between age and death [2,9,10]. Often, these studies compared octogenarians with younger geriatric patients (60–79 years of age), and their findings may be attributable to a lack of statistical power.

Similar to studies of bacteremia, many prospective studies of patients with sepsis have found that older age is a risk factor for death. In a study of nearly 200,000 cases of severe sepsis in the United States, Angus and colleagues [4] found that the mortality rate increased with age from 10% in children to 38.4% in patients 85 years of age and older. Likewise, Knaus and colleagues [34] studied 1195 patients with sepsis and determined that older age was independently associated with increased 28-day mortality; severity of illness, however, was a more important determinant of the risk of death (Table 2). In another study, the case fatality rate for sepsis in the United States from 1979 to 2002 was consistently higher among older patients when compared with younger patients; septic patients 65 years of age and older were 1.56 times more likely to die than septic patients aged less than 65 years (95% CI, 1.52–1.61) [5]. Even after adjusting for gender, the source of infection, comorbid conditions, and the severity of illness, an age of 65 years or greater was an independent predictor of death (OR, 2.26; 95% CI, 2.17–2.36). Of note, the case fatality rate declined most rapidly during the 24-year study period in the older cohort ($P < .001$) (Fig. 2).

Although specific data regarding the impact of age on quality of life and functional outcomes in survivors of bacteremia and sepsis are lacking, numerous studies have evaluated these outcomes in broader populations of older survivors of critical illness. The results of these studies are inconsistent owing to the heterogeneity of the patient populations studied and the variety of instruments used to measure outcomes. Nevertheless, many investigations demonstrate that some functional decline is evident among older survivors of critical illness, whereas quality of life is often maintained [35–37]. At least one study suggests that a significant number of older patients who survive sepsis require long-term care. Of the 222 PROWESS patients aged 75 years and older who were discharged from the hospital, only 42% were discharged home; 45% were transferred to a nursing home, and 11% were transferred to another hospital [11].

Table 2
Association of acute physiology score and age with 28-day mortality in patients with sepsis

Parameter	Number	28-Day mortality (%)	ARLL	Confidence interval
Acute physiology score[a]				
0–40	152	12	1.0	1.0
41–60	330	22	1.99	1.14–3.45
61–80	348	36	4.27	2.48–7.37
81–100	218	45	5.88	3.31–10.43
101–120	75	64	15.67	7.90–31.08
120+	72	85	42.93	21.25–86.71
Age, years				
0–44	184	26	1.0	1.0
45–54	116	34	1.33	0.75–2.36
55–64	203	33	1.59	0.97–2.62
65–74	315	35	1.61	1.01–2.55
75–84	285	41	2.31	1.45–3.70
85+	100	42	2.29	1.27–4.11

Abbreviations: APACHE, Acute Physiology and Chronic Health Evaluation; ARLL, adjusted ratio of life length (multivariate results: larger ARLLs associated with shorter expected survival time; similar to odds ratio).

[a] Acute physiology score of APACHE III.

Adapted from Knaus WA, Harrell FE, Fisher CJ, Jr, et al. The clinical evaluation of new drugs for sepsis: a prospective study design based on survival analysis. JAMA 1993;270(10):1237; with permission. Copyright © 1993 American Medical Association. All rights reserved.

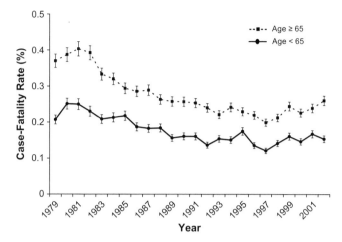

Fig. 2. Fatality rates of sepsis among hospitalized patients longitudinally from 1979 to 2002 stratified by age 65 years and older (*dashed line*) or less than 65 years (*solid line*). (*From* Martin GS, Mannino DM, Moss M. The effect of age on the development and outcome of adult sepsis. Crit Care Med 2006;34(1):18; with permission.)

Society may use studies evaluating the association between increasing age and undesirable outcomes due to critical illness to guide health care policy. In contrast to those who would use age as a criterion for health care rationing due to rising health care costs and limited resources [38,39], the authors suggest an alternative approach. If an older patient, their family, and the health care team conclude that the patient has the right mix of baseline health, an individual preference for aggressive care, and reversible acute illness, the health care team should treat that patient just as they would a younger patient with such preferences [40].

Management

Successful management of older patients with bacteremia requires elimination of the offending pathogen through the timely administration of antibiotics and removal of the source of infection. Other articles in this issue provide detailed information regarding appropriate treatment of pneumonia, urinary tract infection, skin and soft tissue infections, and other infections that may be complicated by bacteremia, and the principles of management are often determined by the source of infection. The host response to infection also has a significant role in influencing treatment. Specifically, patients with sepsis, severe sepsis, and septic shock require careful management that eliminates infectious pathogens and minimizes the detrimental effects of the inflammatory prothrombotic state that occurs in sepsis. Although there are some differences between older and younger patients regarding the management of sepsis, most of the strategies reviewed herein should be employed for all septic patients regardless of age. Some therapies actually provide larger absolute benefits for older patients compared with younger patients.

Empiric antibiotic therapy should be initiated as quickly as possible after samples of blood and other suspected sites of infection have been obtained for culture; antibiotic administration should not be delayed more than 1 hour after sepsis is suspected [41]. The antibiotics chosen should have a broad spectrum of activity so that all probable pathogens are empirically treated because delayed or inadequate antibiotic therapy is associated with reduced survival for patients with sepsis or bacteremia [42–45]. The selection of antimicrobial agents in older patients with sepsis is similar to that in younger patients, but attention should be directed toward unique aspects of antibiotic use in older patients that make prescribing complicated and monitoring unpredictable (reviewed in the article by Williamson elsewhere in this issue) [46]. When possible, diagnostic studies should be performed without delay to identify the source of infection, and source control measures should be instituted when indicated [41]. Often, the source of infection can be removed, such as infected catheters or devices, abscesses or empyemas, and necrotic skin, lung, or other tissue.

All patients with severe sepsis or septic shock should receive fluid resuscitation without delay; blood pressure, urine output, central venous pressure, and central venous or mixed venous oxygen saturation provide measures of adequate tissue perfusion [41]. In one randomized controlled trial, an early goal-directed therapy protocol guided by these measures improved survival in patients with severe sepsis [47]. Although care should be taken to avoid excess fluid accumulation in older patients, liberal amounts of crystalloid or colloid fluids should be used initially because underresuscitation is more likely than overresuscitation owing to the increased capacitance of the vasculature in patients with sepsis. If initial resuscitation efforts do not restore adequate tissue perfusion in a patient with shock, vasopressor therapy with norepinephrine or dopamine may be needed. Vasopressin can be used as an adjunct to catecholamines for refractory shock, but recent evidence suggests this drug does not improve survival when compared with norepinephrine alone [48].

After antibiotics and early resuscitation have been initiated, recombinant human activated protein C (rhAPC) (drotrecogin alfa [activated], Xigris) should be administered to septic patients at high risk of death (as indicated by an Acute Physiology and Chronic Health Evaluation [APACHE] II score greater than or equal to 25 or dysfunction of two or more organs) [41]. The drug is contraindicated in patients with active bleeding, platelet counts less than 30,000/μL, or other risks of uncontrollable bleeding. In the PROWESS trial, 1690 patients with severe sepsis were randomized to treatment with rhAPC or placebo. Treatment with rhAPC resulted in a 6.1% reduction in the absolute risk of death by 28 days ($P = .005$) [49]. A planned subgroup analysis evaluated the efficacy and safety of rhAPC among the 386 patients aged 75 years and older and revealed a larger benefit from rhAPC in this population. Among older patients, rhAPC resulted in a 15.5% reduction in the absolute risk of death by 28 days ($P = .002$) [11]. This survival benefit extended to 2 years (Fig. 3). Serious bleeding events occurred in 3.9% of older patients on rhAPC compared with 2.2% on placebo ($P = .34$), whereas thrombotic events were less common in older patients on rhAPC compared with placebo (1.0% versus 5.0%, $P = .02$).

Although replacement-dose hydrocortisone has been recommended recently for patients with septic shock who require treatment with vasopressors [41], the use of steroids in such patients remains a source of controversy because steroids may result in immunosuppression (at high doses), poor glucose control, poor wound healing, alterations in mental status, and myoneuropathy. The largest randomized trial to evaluate the efficacy of replacement-dose steroids for septic shock was recently completed. The Corticosteroid Therapy of Sepsis and Septic Shock (CORTICUS) trial found no difference in the 28-day mortality rate based on treatment group (33.5% for hydrocortisone patients versus 31.0% for placebo patients) [50]; therefore, steroids cannot be recommended for the broad population of older patients with septic shock.

Red blood cell transfusion is frequently considered for older patients with sepsis or bacteremia because chronic anemia is common in this population and acute infection may drive counts lower. A large randomized trial that compared a conservative transfusion strategy (hemoglobin levels were maintained between 7.0 and 9.0 g/dL) with a more liberal approach found a trend

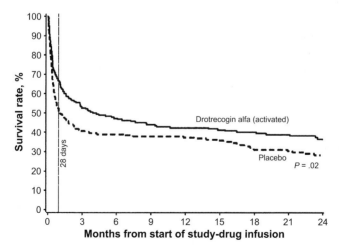

Fig. 3. Twenty-four month Kaplan-Meier survival curves for patients aged 75 years and older enrolled in PROWESS, according to treatment group. Patients aged 75 years and older who were treated with drotrecogin alfa (activated) had significantly higher survival rates sustained throughout the 2-year follow-up period when compared with older patients treated with placebo ($P = .02$). (*From* Ely EW, Angus DC, Williams MD, et al. Drotrecogin alfa (activated) treatment of older patients with severe sepsis. Clin Infect Dis 2003;37(2):192; with permission.)

toward improved outcomes in the group transfused conservatively [51]; many eligible older patients, however, were not enrolled in this trial, and another study found that older patients with active myocardial ischemia (not infection) had higher survival rates when a more liberal transfusion strategy was used (targeting a hemoglobin level at 10–11 g/dL) [52]. Older septic patients with known coronary artery disease and uncorrected coronary anatomy may benefit from a liberal approach to red blood cell transfusion, but the default threshold for transfusion for other patients with sepsis or bacteremia should be a hemoglobin level less than 7 g/dL [41].

Respiratory failure in the form of the acute respiratory distress syndrome (ARDS) is common among patients with severe sepsis, and mechanical ventilation is the mainstay of treatment [53]. All adult patients with ARDS, regardless of age, should be ventilated with low tidal volume ventilation (< 6 mL/kg predicted body weight) and managed with a conservative fluid strategy. In a randomized controlled trial that enrolled 861 patients, the National Heart, Lung, and Blood Institute ARDS Network found that low tidal volume ventilation reduced in-hospital mortality to 31% (compared with 40% in the control group) [54]. Among patients aged 70 years and older in this trial, ventilation with low tidal volumes resulted in an absolute risk reduction of 9.9% in mortality at 28 days [55]. The ARDS Network recently completed another randomized controlled trial that compared two fluid strategies. That trial found that ARDS patients managed with the conservative strategy spent fewer days receiving mechanical ventilation and fewer days in the ICU compared with those managed with the liberal strategy [56]. Patients receiving mechanical ventilation (as well as other septic patients with recognized risk factors) should also receive prophylactic therapy of proven efficacy, including low-dose unfractionated heparin, low-molecular-weight heparin, or mechanical prophylactic devices to prevent deep vein thrombosis; H2-receptor blockers or proton pump inhibitors to prevent stress ulcers; and elevation of the head of the bed to reduce the risk of ventilator-associated pneumonia [57].

Because older patients with sepsis or bacteremia are at high risk for anxiety, pain, and delirium, sedation and analgesia should be administered as needed. The majority of older inpatients, including those at high risk for delirium owing to sedative administration, pre-existing cognitive impairment, and a high severity of illness, should be monitored routinely with a validated sedation scale and delirium instrument [58–60]. Mechanically ventilated older patients should be managed with a sedation protocol that uses a standardized sedation scale, a sedation goal, and daily interruption of sedatives, because these strategies have been proven to reduce the duration of mechanical ventilation [61–63].

Summary

Despite the increasing incidence of bacteremia and sepsis in older patients and the high risk of death associated with these infectious disorders, many elderly patients respond remarkably well to the evidence-based diagnostic and management strategies reviewed herein. Clinicians must maintain a high index of suspicion to quickly diagnosis bacteremia or sepsis in older patients and initiate appropriate interventions in a timely manner.

References

[1] Bone RC, Balk RA, Cerra FB, et al. Definitions for sepsis and organ failure and guidelines for the use of innovative therapies in sepsis: The ACCP/SCCM Consensus Conference Committee, American College of Chest Physicians/Society of Critical Care Medicine. Chest 1992; 101(6):1644–55.

[2] Greenberg BM, Atmar RL, Stager CE, et al. Bacteraemia in the elderly: predictors of outcome in an urban teaching hospital. J Infect 2005;50(4):288–95.

[3] Brun-Buisson C, Doyon F, Carlet J. Bacteremia and severe sepsis in adults: a multicenter prospective survey in ICUs and wards of 24 hospitals. French Bacteremia-Sepsis Study Group. Am J Respir Crit Care Med 1996;154(3):617–24.

[4] Angus DC, Linde-Zwirble WT, Lidicker J, et al. Epidemiology of severe sepsis in the United States: analysis of incidence, outcome, and associated costs of care. Crit Care Med 2001; 29(7):1303–10.

[5] Martin GS, Mannino DM, Moss M. The effect of age on the development and outcome of adult sepsis. Crit Care Med 2006;34(1):15–21.

[6] Baine WB, Yu W, Summe JP. The epidemiology of hospitalization of elderly Americans for septicemia or bacteremia in 1991-1998: application of Medicare claims data. Ann Epidemiol 2001;11(2):118–26.

[7] Diekema DJ, Pfaller MA, Jones RN. Age-related trends in pathogen frequency and antimicrobial susceptibility of bloodstream isolates in North America: SENTRY Antimicrobial Surveillance Program, 1997–2000. Int J Antimicrob Agents 2002;20(6):412–8.

[8] McClelland RS, Fowler VG Jr, Sanders LL, et al. Staphylococcus aureus bacteremia among elderly vs younger adult patients: comparison of clinical features and mortality. Arch Intern Med 1999;159(11):1244–7.

[9] Lark RL, Saint S, Chenoweth C, et al. Four-year prospective evaluation of community-acquired bacteremia: epidemiology, microbiology, and patient outcome. Diagn Microbiol Infect Dis 2001;41(1–2):15–22.

[10] Leibovici L, Pitlik SD, Konisberger H, et al. Bloodstream infections in patients older than eighty years. Age Ageing 1993;22(6):431–42.

[11] Ely EW, Angus DC, Williams MD, et al. Drotrecogin alfa (activated) treatment of older patients with severe sepsis. Clin Infect Dis 2003;37(2):187–95.

[12] Rudman D, Hontanosas A, Cohen Z, et al. Clinical correlates of bacteremia in a Veterans Administration extended care facility. J Am Geriatr Soc 1988;36(8):726–32.

[13] Bryan CS, Dew CE, Reynolds KL. Bacteremia associated with decubitus ulcers. Arch Intern Med 1983;143(11):2093–5.

[14] Rezende NA, Blumberg HM, Metzger BS, et al. Risk factors for methicillin-resistance among patients with Staphylococcus aureus bacteremia at the time of hospital admission. Am J Med Sci 2002;323(3):117–23.

[15] Valenti WM, Trudell RG, Bentley DW. Factors predisposing to oropharyngeal colonization with gram-negative bacilli in the aged. N Engl J Med 1978;298(20):1108–11.

[16] Wiener J, Quinn JP, Bradford PA, et al. Multiple antibiotic-resistant Klebsiella and Escherichia coli in nursing homes. JAMA 1999;281(6):517–23.

[17] Hamel MB, Teno JM, Goldman L, et al. Patient age and decisions to withhold life-sustaining treatments from seriously ill, hospitalized adults: SUPPORT Investigators, Study to Understand Prognoses and Preferences for Outcomes and Risks of Treatment. Ann Intern Med 1999;130(2):116–25.

[18] Laupland KB, Gregson DB, Zygun DA, et al. Severe bloodstream infections: a population-based assessment. Crit Care Med 2004;32(4):992–7.

[19] Opal SM, Girard TD, Ely EW. The immunopathogenesis of sepsis in elderly patients. Clin Infect Dis 2005;41(Suppl 7):S504–12.

[20] Fry TJ, Mackall CL. Current concepts of thymic aging. Springer Semin Immunopathol 2002;24(1):7–22.

[21] Weksler ME, Goodhardt M, Szabo P. The effect of age on B cell development and humoral immunity. Springer Semin Immunopathol 2002;24(1):35–52.

[22] O'Mahony L, Holland J, Jackson J, et al. Quantitative intracellular cytokine measurement: age-related changes in proinflammatory cytokine production. Clin Exp Immunol 1998; 113(2):213–9.

[23] Marik PE, Zaloga GP, NORASEPT II Study Investigators. The effect of aging on circulating levels of proinflammatory cytokines during septic shock. J Am Geriatr Soc 2001; 49(1):5–9.

[24] Wheeler AP, Bernard GR. Treating patients with severe sepsis. N Engl J Med 1999;340(3): 207–14.

[25] Opal SM, Esmon CT. Bench-to-bedside review: functional relationships between coagulation and the innate immune response and their respective roles in the pathogenesis of sepsis. Crit Care 2003;7(1):23–38.

[26] Mari D, Mannucci PM, Coppola R, et al. Hypercoagulability in centenarians: the paradox of successful aging. Blood 1995;85(11):3144–9.

[27] Cohen HJ, Harris T, Pieper CF. Coagulation and activation of inflammatory pathways in the development of functional decline and mortality in the elderly. Am J Med 2003;114(3): 180–7.

[28] Chassagne P, Perol MB, Doucet J, et al. Is presentation of bacteremia in the elderly the same as in younger patients? Am J Med 1996;100(1):65–70.

[29] Iberti TJ, Bone RC, Balk R, et al. Are the criteria used to determine sepsis applicable for patients > 75 years of age? Crit Care Med 1993;21:S130.

[30] Rajagopalan S, Yoshikawa TT. Antimicrobial therapy in the elderly. Med Clin North Am 2001;85(1):133–47.

[31] Gleckman R, Hibert D. Afebrile bacteremia: a phenomenon in geriatric patients. JAMA 1982;248(12):1478–81.

[32] Castle SC, Norman DC, Yeh M, et al. Fever response in elderly nursing home residents: are the older truly colder? J Am Geriatr Soc 1991;39(9):853–7.

[33] Jensen AG, Wachmann CH, Espersen F, et al. Treatment and outcome of *Staphylococcus aureus* bacteremia: a prospective study of 278 cases. Arch Intern Med 2002;162(1): 25–32.

[34] Knaus WA, Harrell FE, Fisher CJ Jr, et al. The clinical evaluation of new drugs for sepsis: a prospective study design based on survival analysis. JAMA 1993;270(10):1233–41.

[35] Kleinpell RM, Ferrans CE. Quality of life of elderly patients after treatment in the ICU. Res Nurs Health 2002;25(3):212–21.

[36] Udekwu P, Gurkin B, Oller D, et al. Quality of life and functional level in elderly patients surviving surgical intensive care. J Am Coll Surg 2001;193(3):245–9.

[37] Hurel D, Loirat P, Saulnier F, et al. Quality of life 6 months after intensive care: results of a prospective multicenter study using a generic health status scale and a satisfaction scale. Intensive Care Med 1997;23(3):331–7.

[38] Shaw AB. Age as a basis for health care rationing: support for against policies. Drugs Aging 1996;9(6):403–5.

[39] Bowling A. Health care rationing: the public's debate. BMJ 1996;312(7032):670–4.

[40] Girard TD, Opal SM, Ely EW. Insights into severe sepsis in older patients: from epidemiology to evidence-based management. Clin Infect Dis 2005;40(5):719–27.

[41] Dellinger RP, Carlet JM, Masur H, et al. Surviving Sepsis Campaign guidelines for management of severe sepsis and septic shock. Crit Care Med 2004;32(3):858–73.

[42] Garnacho-Montero J, Garcia-Garmendia JL, Barrero-Almodovar A, et al. Impact of adequate empirical antibiotic therapy on the outcome of patients admitted to the intensive care unit with sepsis. Crit Care Med 2003;31:2742–51.

[43] Leibovici L, Shraga I, Drucker M, et al. The benefit of appropriate empirical antibiotic treatment in patients with bloodstream infection. J Intern Med 1998;244(5):379–86.

[44] Valles J, Rello J, Ochagavia A, et al. Community-acquired bloodstream infection in critically ill adult patients: impact of shock and inappropriate antibiotic therapy on survival. Chest 2003;123(5):1615–24.

[45] Kumar A, Roberts D, Wood KE, et al. Duration of hypotension before initiation of effective antimicrobial therapy is the critical determinant of survival in human septic shock. Crit Care Med 2006;34(6):1589–96.

[46] Williamson J. Principles of antibiotic use in older adults. Clin Geriatr Med 2007;23(3).

[47] Rivers E, Nguyen B, Havstad S, et al. Early goal-directed therapy in the treatment of severe sepsis and septic shock. N Engl J Med 2001;345(19):1368–77.

[48] Russell JA, Walley KR, Singer J, et al. A randomised controlled trial of low dose vasopressin versus norepinephrine infusion in patients who have septic shock [abstracts issue]. Am J Respir Crit Care Med 2007;175:A508.

[49] Bernard GR, Vincent JL, Laterre PF, et al. Efficacy and safety of recombinant human activated protein C for severe sepsis. N Engl J Med 2001;344(10):699–709.

[50] Sprung CL, Annane D, Briegel J, et al. Corticosteroid therapy of septic shock (CORTICUS) [abstracts issue]. Am J Respir Crit Care Med 2007;175:A507.

[51] Hebert PC, Wells G, Blajchman M, et al. A multicenter, randomized, controlled clinical trial of transfusion requirements in critical care. N Engl J Med 1999;340:409–17.

[52] Wu W, Rathore SS, Wang Y, et al. Blood transfusion in elderly patients with acute myocardial infarction. N Engl J Med 2001;345:1230–6.

[53] Girard TD, Bernard GR. Mechanical ventilation in ARDS: a state-of-the-art review. Chest 2007;131(3):921–9.

[54] The Acute Respiratory Distress Syndrome Network. Ventilation with lower tidal volumes as compared with traditional tidal volumes for acute lung injury and the acute respiratory distress syndrome. N Engl J Med 2000;342(18):1301–8.

[55] Ely EW, Wheeler AP, Thompson BT, et al. Recovery rate and prognosis in older persons who develop acute lung injury and the acute respiratory distress syndrome. Ann Intern Med 2002;136(1):25–36.

[56] The National Heart Lung and Blood Institute Acute Respiratory Distress Syndrome (ARDS) Clinical Trials Network. Comparison of two fluid-management strategies in acute lung injury. N Engl J Med 2006;354(24):2564–75.

[57] Drakulovic MB, Torres A, Bauer TT, et al. Supine body position as a risk factor for nosocomial pneumonia in mechanically ventilated patients: a randomised trial. Lancet 1999;354(9193):1851–8.

[58] Inouye SK. Delirium in older persons. N Engl J Med 2006;354(11):1157–65.

[59] Inouye SK, van Dyck CH, Alessi CA, et al. Clarifying confusion: the confusion assessment method. A new method for detection of delirium. Ann Intern Med 1990;113(12):941–8.

[60] Ely EW, Inouye SK, Bernard GR, et al. Delirium in mechanically ventilated patients: validity and reliability of the confusion assessment method for the intensive care unit (CAM-ICU). JAMA 2001;286(21):2703–10.

[61] Brook AD, Ahrens TS, Schaiff R, et al. Effect of a nursing-implemented sedation protocol on the duration of mechanical ventilation. Crit Care Med 1999;27(12):2609–15.

[62] Kress JP, Pohlman AS, O'Connor MF, et al. Daily interruption of sedative infusions in critically ill patients undergoing mechanical ventilation. N Engl J Med 2000;342(20):1471–7.

[63] Girard TD, Kress JP, Fuchs BD, et al. The Awakening and Breathing Controlled (ABC) Trial: a randomized controlled trial of the efficacy and safety of protocolized spontaneous breathing trials (SBTs) with or without daily spontaneous awakening trials (SATs) [abstracts issue]. Am J Respir Crit Care Med 2007;175:A508.

ELSEVIER
SAUNDERS

CLINICS IN
GERIATRIC
MEDICINE

Clin Geriatr Med 23 (2007) 649–668

Fever of Unknown Origin in Older Adults

Sari Tal, MD, MHA*, Vladimir Guller, MD, Alexander Gurevich, MD

Subacute Department, Harzfeld Geriatric Hospital, Kaplan Medical Center, Gedera, Israel

What is fever of unknown origin?

Fever of unknown origin (FUO) means fever that does not resolve itself in the period expected for self-limited infection and whose cause cannot be ascertained despite considerable diagnostic effort [1]. In 1961, Petersdorf and Beeson [2] introduced the definition that subsequently became standard—namely, illness of more than 3-week duration, fever higher than 38.3°C on several occasions, and diagnosis uncertain after 1 week of study in hospital. Recently, Durack and Street [3] have proposed a new system for classification of FUO: (1) classic FUO, (2) nosocomial FUO, (3) neutropenic FUO, and (4) FUO associated with HIV infection. Because hospital admission is so expensive and thorough diagnostic testing now can be performed in outpatient settings, the definition recently was modified to remove the requirement that a hospital be the setting for 1 week of evaluation. The revised criteria require an evaluation of at least 3 days in the hospital, three outpatient visits, or 1 week of logical and intensive outpatient testing without determining the fever's cause [1,3–5].

Based on these criteria, studies of FUO in the general population show that infections are the most common cause of FUO; intra-abdominal abscesses, endocarditis, and tuberculosis predominate [6]. Neoplasms and multisystem or collagen vascular diseases comprise the remaining major etiologies of FUO. The proportion of undiagnosed causes is 30% [7]. The applicability of research literature on FUO to everyday medical practice may be limited by several factors, which could include the geographic location of cases, differences in diagnostic facilities between hospitals and countries, and individual experience of the investigators and the specific subpopulations of patients who had FUO who were studied [8,9].

* Corresponding author.
E-mail address: mail@tal.org.il (S. Tal).

0749-0690/07/$ - see front matter © 2007 Elsevier Inc. All rights reserved.
doi:10.1016/j.cger.2007.03.004   *geriatric.theclinics.com*

Studies of FUO in the elderly show that unlike in the young, a precise diagnosis can be made 87% to 95% of the time (Table 1) [10]. Often, FUO in the elderly is the result of atypical presentation of common disease. Infection is the cause in 25% to 35% of cases, with tuberculosis occurring much more commonly in elderly than young patients who have FUO. Connective tissue diseases, such as temporal arteritis (TA), rheumatoid arthritis, and polymyalgia rheumatica (PMR), account for 25% to 31% of causes in elderly patients, and malignancy accounts for 12% to 23% of all cases [10]. As many of these diseases are treatable, etiology of FUO in the elderly should be investigated further.

Medical evaluation of elderly persons requires a different perspective from that needed of younger persons. The range of symptoms is different, the manifestations of distress are less apparent, improvement sometimes is slower and less dramatic, and the implication of maintenance of function is more important. The differential diagnosis varies with age, and presentation of disease frequently is nonspecific and symptoms difficult to interpret. FUO in the elderly is an example of a classic medical syndrome that requires a specific approach.

The four categories of potential etiology of FUO in the elderly are related to patient subtype—classic, nosocomial, neutropenic, and HIV associated. Each group needs a different process of evaluation based on its characteristics and vulnerabilities. This article reviews common causes and approaches to elderly patients who have classic FUO.

Causes of fever of unknown origin

Notwithstanding that many diseases that previously caused FUO now are diagnosed easily as a result of recent advances in diagnostic tools and

Table 1
Diagnosis of fever of unknown origin in elderly patients (more than 65 years old) compared with the diagnosis in younger patients

Diagnoses	Elderly (n = 47)	Young (n = 152)
Infections	12 (25.5%)	33 (21.7%)
Abscess	2	6
Endocarditis	1	2
Tuberculosis	6	4
Viral infections	1	8
Multisystem disease	15 (31.9%)	27 (17.7%)
Tumors	6 (12.8%)	8 (5.3%)
Miscellaneous	5 (10.6%)	24 (15.8%)
Drug-related fever	3 (6.4%)	3 (2.0%)
Habitual hyperthermia	0	5 (3.3%)
Factitious	0	7 (4.6%)
No diagnosis	6 (12.8%)	45 (29.6%)

Percentages represent pooled data from Knockaert DC, Vanneste LJ, Bobbaers HJ. Fever of unknown origin in the elderly patients. J Am Geriatr Soc 1993;41:1187–92.

techniques, FUO remains a challenging clinical problem. The proportion of infections and neoplasms as causes of FUO has decreased over the past 40 years.

The causes of FUO traditionally have been divided into five categories: infectious, malignant, noninfectious inflammatory disease (NID), miscellaneous, and undiagnosed. The NID group has been designated differently by investigators as "rheumatic" diseases, autoimmune diseases, systemic diseases, multisystem diseases, collagen vascular disease, or vasculitides [2,7,9,10].

The lack of a uniform classification of disease hampers comparison between different series [2,5–7,11,12]. Several investigators use a separate category, namely granulomatous diseases, which also are inflammatory disorders that can be included in the NID group. In addition to classical granulomatous disorders, such as sarcoidosis and granulomatous hepatitis, they include TA, Crohn's disease, and de Quervain's thyroiditis in this category [11,12]. Other investigators suggest including sarcoidosis and TA in the NID category and classifying Crohn's disease and thyroiditis in the miscellaneous group [9]. In this case, granulomatous hepatitis is not considered a disease, because it represents a histologic reaction to infections, neoplastic, and other causes. Some diseases included in the miscellaneous group have been moved to another category. A typical example is Whipple's disease, an infection caused by *Tropheryma whippelii* [13]. Another example, cardiac myxoma, is a benign neoplastic disease often classified in the miscellaneous group. Moreover, Knockaert and colleagues [9,14] believe that such nonmalignant lymphoproliferative disorders as Castelman disease will be moved to another group because of evidence of the causative role of human herpes virus 8.

Infections

Infection is the most common diagnosis in most published series of FUO in the general population, as described in the published series of FUO in the elderly [10,15–17]. Compared with the younger population, the elderly have increased susceptibility to infection and are at significantly increased risk for morbidity and mortality resulting from many common infections.

Two earlier studies, published in 1978 [16] and 1982 [17], reported that infections (37% and 41%, respectively) and multisystem or collagen vascular disease (23% and 30%, respectively) were the leading causes of extended fevers in the elderly. In a more recent study, by Knockaert and colleagues [10], infections were less common than multisystem diseases (Table 2). This trend was even more pronounced in patients older than 70 years. Although the overall frequency of infections was the same in older and younger patients, some important differences were noted. Tuberculosis (especially in extrapulmonary sites) and abdominal or pelvic abscesses are the most common infectious diseases associated with FUO in the elderly [5].

Table 2
Causes of fever of unknown origin

Diagnosis	Knockaert et al, 1993 [10]	Barrier et al, 1982 [17]	Esposito 1978 [16]
Infections	25.5%	41.3%	36.9%
Tumors	12.8%	13.0%	23.4%
Multisystem	31.9%	30.3%	25.2%
Miscellaneous	10.6%	2.1%	7.0%
No diagnosis	12.8%	13.0%	5.4%
Others	6.4%	0.3%	2.1%

Percentages represent pooled data from three studies in the elderly: Knockaert DC, Vanneste LJ, Bobbaers HJ. Fever of unknown origin in the elderly patients. J Am Geriatr Soc 1993;41:1187–92; Barrier J, Schneebeli S, Peltier P. Les fièvres prolongées inexpliquées chez les personnes, âgées [French]. Concours Med 1982;104:4679–89; and Esposito AL, Gleckman RA. Fever of unknown origin in the elderly. J Am Geriatr Soc 1978;26:498–505.

Tuberculosis was found in 12% of elderly who had FUO, compared with only 2% of the diagnoses in younger patients, in the study by Knockaert and colleagues [10]. In this study, tuberculosis accounted for 50% of the infections in the elderly (see Table 1). In two earlier series of FUO in the elderly, tuberculosis caused 20% of the infections [16,17]. Elderly individuals seem to be at increased risk for infection, mainly because of reactivation of earlier disease. Nursing home patients are at the highest risk for this disease. Some studies show the differing presentations of tuberculosis between the elderly and younger adults. The clinical presentation often is insidious and nonspecific, as is the radiologic presentation. Symptoms, such as weakness, unexplained weight loss, failure to thrive, fever, or a change in cognitive status, may be the only manifestation of the disease [18]. Symptoms, such as hemoptysis, night sweats, and a positive purified protein derivative (PPD) test response, are less common in the elderly. Pleural effusion may be the sole manifestation of the disease. There is no difference in bacteriologically proved disease or radiologic findings between the two groups. Occurrence of miliary tuberculosis in the elderly is more common, and disseminated disease to lymph nodes, bones, kidneys, gastrointestinal tract, and skin may cause diagnostic confusion and delay [19]. The elderly who account for a large proportion of TB cases discovered at autopsy illustrate the difficulty of clinical diagnosis in this age group [18].

Intra-abdominal abscesses were found in 4% of the elderly patients who had FUO in the study by Knockaert and colleagues [10], with the same proportion as in the younger group (see Table 1). Previous studies showed more abscesses than in Knockaert and colleagues' study [16,17]. This can be explained by the widespread use of ultrasonography and CT that allows early detection of what had been a common cause of FUO. The locations of intra-abdominal abscesses give rise to different clinical features. Symptoms, such as abdominal pain, nausea, vomiting, or diarrhea, are common in liver or intraperitoneal abscesses or chronic cholecystitis. Reporting of tenderness on examination is common in most cases of liver, splenic, or intraperitoneal abscesses. Elderly patients typically have a longer illness and a more subacute course with fewer signs and symptoms than younger patients [1]. It is suggested that the elderly do not feel pain as acutely as younger individuals or that they have less discomfort on average with a similar intra-abdominal mass, but neither of these assumptions has been proved definitively. Elderly patients who have serious, even life-threatening, intra-abdominal pathology (such as emphysematous cholecystitis, leaking abdominal aortic aneurysm, or perforated viscous) may report minimal abdominal pain. Neuropathy—especially when linked to diabetes, a common age-associated disease—and the chronic use of certain medications (such as corticosteroids or pain relievers) also may contribute to less perception of pain. Loss of abdominal wall muscle mass in the elderly patients makes guarding either impossible or less apparent [20].

Osteomyelitis is a rare cause of FUO in elderly patients. Infection reaches through the blood stream or is spread from adjacent tissue. Hematogenous osteomyelitis affects mainly the vertebrae but also may affect the long bones (eg, femur, tibia, and humerus). Hematogenous osteomyelitis almost always is a monomicrobial infection affecting predominantly the older population. *Staphylococcus aureus* is the microorganism isolated most commonly; other common pathogens include group β streptococci. Gram-negative aerobic bacilli also may be found, however, most likely caused by genitourinary tract infection or instrumentation [21]. Vascular insufficiency (eg, diabetes mellitus, atherosclerosis, or vasculitis) and neuropathy (eg, diabetes mellitus) are common factors contributing to osteomyelitis of the foot in elderly patients, involving mostly the small bones of the feet and toes. Pressure sores may be associated with underlying osteomyelitis that is difficult to differentiate clinically from infection or colonization of adjacent soft tissue. *S aureus* is a pathogen in more than 50% of the cases of contiguous-focus osteomyelitis. In contrast to hematogenous osteomyelitis, however, these infections often are polymicrobial and more likely to involve gram-negative and anaerobic bacteria. Although several bacteria often are cultured, not all of them necessarily are pathogenic. Cultures of bone specimens frequently are contaminated with organisms present in adjacent soft tissue [22]. The bacteria that are found commonly include *S aureus*, *S epidermidis*, streptococci, gram-negative aerobic bacilli, and anaerobic organisms. Isolation of common pathogens other than *S aureus* from sinus tracts does not reflect the pathogen isolated from bone and, therefore, a bacteriologic diagnosis of chronic osteomyelitis must be based on appropriate operative bone culture [23]. Vertebral osteomyelitis may occur through hematogenous dissemination from distant infected sources. Less commonly, in men who have urinary tract infections, aerobic gram-negative bacilli may ascend through Batson's plexus and reach the lumbar spine. Pyogenic vertebral osteomyelitis must be differentiated from tuberculous spinal osteomyelitis, which also is common among elderly patients [24]. The typical symptoms of osteomyelitis in the general population and in the elderly are pain and fever. Pain may be absent in some of the debilitated patients who have osteomyelitis, however, because of an overlying pressure sore that does not heal and in diabetic patients who have osteomyelitis of the foot [25].

Although the frequency of infective endocarditis as a cause of FUO is low, it has become more common in the elderly. Epidemiologic studies show an upswing in the average age of patients who have infective endocarditis. Recently, 50% these of patients were found to be above 60 years of age, with a higher prevalence in men [26]. Prevalence has risen as a result of the increasing number of elderly persons who have prosthetic valves; hospital-acquired bacteremia also has become more prevalent and patients who have valvular heart disease have a longer survival rate. *Streptococci* and *Staphylococci* are the leading organisms, which are isolated from approximately 80% of elderly patients who have endocarditis. Studies show a higher prevalence of enterococci in the elderly. In addition, *Streptococcus bovis*, an organism associated with colonic malignancy, is more common in elderly patients who have endocarditis [27,28]. No significant difference in the appearance of the various pathogens within the overall general population, however, was seen in a recent study [29,30]. Endocarditis occurs more frequently on the mitral valve than it does on the aortic valve in older patients [26]. Sites of primary infection include the mouth, the genitourinary tract (particularly after procedures involving instrumentation), the skin, decubitus ulcers, surgical wound, catheters, and, rarely, the gastrointestinal tract [30]. A digestive tract portal of entry is more frequent in the elderly, however, because of the higher incidence of colonic lesions. Urologic disorders, such as prostatic or vesical diseases, also are seen more frequently in the elderly. The high incidence of these two specific portals of entry has implications for diagnosis and emphasizes the importance of prophylactic procedures during endoscopic procedures, which frequently are performed on these patients. Finally, pacemaker endocarditis is seen most often in older patients with the accompanying difficulties in diagnosis and poor prognosis [31]. The presenting symptoms of infective endocarditis in older patients may be nonspecific, such as lethargy, fatigue, malaise, anorexia, and weight loss. Heart murmurs in elderly may be attributed wrongly to the underlying valvular calcification and, therefore, overlooked. Sometimes, endocarditis in the elderly may be present with a stroke syndrome, rheumatologic complaints, or peripheral nervous system abnormalities [32,33]. Studies using the Duke criteria for diagnosis of endocarditis—frequency of fever, heart failure, embolic events, neurologic symptoms, distribution of causative organisms, and cerebral deficit—have not found any relevant differences between old and young patients at time of discharge from the hospital. Renal insufficiency and malignancy at admission, however, is found significantly more common in elderly patients who have infective endocarditis [29,30].

Viral diseases as a cause of FUO are rare in elderly patients. A few viruses, however, such as cytomegalovirus (CMV), Epstein-Barr virus (EBV), and HIV, may cause FUO. Herpes viruses, CMV, and EBV, can cause prolonged febrile illnesses with constitutional symptoms and no prominent organ manifestations, particularly in the elderly. Each of these viruses usually causes lymphadenopathies, which may be missed on physical examination if the lymph nodes are not very enlarged. Even though CMV and EBV virus infections are typical diseases of children, adolescents, and young adults, it should not be forgotten that mononucleosis also occurs in elderly patients [34]. When patients present with lymphocytosis with atypical lymphocytes, serologic testing can confirm the diagnosis. As these initially tests can be negative, it is recommended to repeat them in suspected cases 2 to 3 weeks after the onset of illness.

HIV infection is considered mainly a disease of young sexually active people and rarely was found in the elderly population. More recent studies, however, show that older persons increasingly are affected by HIV. In 1996, the Centers for Disease Control and Prevention reported that 12% of all AIDS cases were age 65 years or older [35]. Older adults may be considered at risk for HIV infection for the same reasons as the younger population: sexual activity, intravenous drug use, and blood transfusions. In addition, the elderly already may have a compromised immune system as a result of other age- and health-related conditions [36]. Primary HIV infection, disseminated *Mycobacterium avium* infection, *Pneumocystis carinii* pneumonia, CMV infection, disseminated histoplasmosis, and lymphoma are the causes of fever in HIV-infected patients reported most commonly. The various infections account for HIV-associated FUO change according to their prevalence in the different global locations [37]. HIV and AIDS may be overlooked in many cases of elderly patients even though they seem to present with the same opportunistic infections as younger patients [38]. Symptoms in this group can mimic symptoms of other diseases prevalent among them making the diagnosis difficult. Elderly patients who have AIDS and who present with symptoms of opportunistic infection often undergo the work-up and treatment for other disease processes, such as cerebrovascular disease, bacterial or viral pneumonia, malnutrition, and occult malignancy. For example, the symptoms of HIV dementia can mimic Alzheimer's or Parkinson's disease. Similarly, pneumocystic pneumonia may be mistaken for heart failure in the elderly who have chronic heart disease. Thus, the diagnosis of HIV infection in many cases is made late in the course of disease in older patients [37,39].

Noninfectious inflammatory diseases

The general term, NID, applies to systemic rheumatologic or vasculitic disease, such as TA, PMR, rheumatoid arthritis, systemic lupus erythematosus, Wegener's disease, polyartheritis nodosa, and adult Still's disease, and granulomatous disease, such as sarcoidosis and Crohn's and granulomatous hepatitis [7]. This group of immune-mediated injury disorders forms the most important disease category in the study by Knockaert and colleagues

[10], and as age increases, this trend is more pronounced. TA and PMR represent 60% of cases in this category. PMR and TA are closely related conditions and frequently occur together, affecting persons of middle age and older. Some investigators consider them to be different phases of the same disease [40]. TA is less frequent than PMR and represents 17% of the cases of FUO in the elderly patients [10]. The disease almost always is confined to Caucasians. The incidence is higher in Scandinavia and north Europe (between 17 and 18 cases per 100 000 population ages over 50 years) [41]. In Olmsted County, Minnesota, which has a high population of Scandinavian descent, the average annual incidence was 17.8 cases per 100 000 persons 50 years of age and older [42]. Autopsy studies show that giant cell arteritis may be more common than is apparent clinically [40].

The American College of Rheumatology study determined highly sensitive parameters for diagnosis of TA [43]. These parameters include (1) age at onset of disease 50 years or older, (2) new localized headache, (3) temporal artery abnormality (eg, decreased pulse, tenderness, or nodules), (4) erythrocyte sedimentation rate (ESR) greater than or equal to 50 mm per hour according to the Westergren method, and (5) abnormal temporal artery biopsy (eg, necrotizing arteritis or multinucleated giant cells). Three of five parameters are necessary for diagnosis for the purposes of classification. TA affects many arteries throughout the body, producing symptoms and signs that mimic other medical and surgical conditions. Although the fever usually is low grade in approximately 15% of patients, it can reach 39°C to 40°C and may be the presenting clinical manifestation [44]. A systemic illness with malaise, anorexia, night sweats, weight loss, and depression is common. These symptoms often are confused with infection and malignancy, resulting in delayed diagnosis that can lead to blindness or stroke developing in the meantime [45]. Arteritic involvement by inflammation is noticed most frequently in superficial temporal arteries, which may stand out and are tender when brushing hair. Atherosclerosis may be responsible for reduced or absence of pulsation; therefore, the value of the presentation of the pulsation of temporal artery is limited. Histologic detection of giant cell arteritis remains the only diagnostic investigation in TA. Normal biopsy appearances do not exclude the diagnosis because of possible skip lesions [40,41,45].

PMR appears in certain populations, with a prevalence of one case for every 133 people over the age 50 [46]. Similar to TA, the incidence of PMR increases after age 50 and peaks between 70 and 80 years of age. Population surveys show higher frequencies of PMR at higher latitudes and in Scandinavian countries and United States communities that have a strong Scandinavian ethnic background [40,42,46]. Synovitis in proximal joints and periarticular structures is shown in arthroscopic, radioisotopic, and MRI studies of patients who have PMR [40,47]. PMR is a painful condition that presents typically with pain and stiffness in the shoulders, neck, and hips that may appear suddenly. Morning or late evening stiffness is common in both, muscles and joints. Headache, fatigue, depression, and generalized weakness may be confused with other diseases. Although tenderness on palpation of axial muscles or pain on motion of joints may be seen, physical findings usually are unremarkable. A markedly elevated sedimentation rate commonly is associated with PMR but its absence should not rule out this disease [48]. In several reports, up to 22% of patients who had PMR had an ESR that either was normal or slightly increased at diagnosis, supporting the notion that an increased ESR should not be necessary for its diagnosis. In these studies, the diagnosis was based on an otherwise typical presentation and a rapid response to a corticosteroid given in a low dose [49,50].

Tumors

Tumors are considered a common cause of FUO in the elderly. In the study by Knockaert and colleagues [10], tumors were slightly more prevalent in elderly than in younger patients but clearly less common than indicated in previous reports [16]. These tumors mainly were leukemia, Hodgkin's disease, multiple myeloma, and colon cancer. Lymphoma was the most common neoplastic cause of geriatric FUO, followed by renal cell carcinoma, atrial myxoma, hepatoma, and carcinoma of colon in previous studies by Esposito and Gleckman [16]. In the recent study by Knockaert and colleagues [10], however, colon cancer emerged as an important cause (17% of all tumors).

Many consider paraneoplastic fever more common in primary tumors, such as renal cell carcinomas and lymphomas, but some data suggest that it occurs in tumors of diverse primary sites [51]. Among the assumed causes of tumor fever are hypersensitivity reactions, pyrogen production, primary cytokine production, and tumor necrosis with secondary cytokine production [52].

Multiple myeloma rarely causes fever and is an insignificant cause of FUO. In a series of 5523 patients who had final diagnosis of multiple myeloma who were seen at Mayo Clinic, only 9 (0.2%) had FUO caused by multiple myeloma itself [53]. Nevertheless, multiple myeloma should be included in the differential diagnosis of FUO, thereby reducing unnecessary testing, rapidly establishing the diagnosis, and initiating effective treatment.

The easy detection of solid tumors and enlarged lymph nodes by ultrasonography and CT has reduced the relative importance of tumors as a cause of FUO.

Miscellaneous group

Pulmonary embolism is an important cause of FUO in the elderly, particularly in bedridden patients, and represents 4% of the cases of FUO in this population [10]. The clinical presentations can be classified into three large groups. The first and most common presentation is dyspnea with or without pleuritic chest pain and hemoptysis. The second presentation is hemodynamic instability and syncope, which usually is associated with massive embolism; the third and least common presentation mimics indolent pneumonia or heart failure, especially in the elderly [54,55]. Fever generally higher than 38.3°C is observed in patients who have extensive pulmonary infarction or who have secondary pneumonitis developed distal to the embolus [56].

Subacute thyroiditis with thyrotoxicosis may manifest as FUO. Although it is not a common cause of FUO, it is found consistently across several series of FUO and, together with hyperthyroidism, is the most common endocrinologic cause [57,58].

Thyrotoxicosis and the inflammation of subacute thyroiditis may cause fever. Hyperthyroidism is common in elderly individuals, although in the study by Knockaert and colleagues [10] only one patient had hyperthyroidism. In some cases, the symptoms are typical and include nervousness, palpitations, sweating, tremors, and weight loss, but often the most striking characteristic of hyperthyroidism in older patients is the lack of symptoms. They frequently do not have enlarged thyroids and do not complain of nervousness or heat intolerance. In contrast to the typical picture of weight loss despite an increased appetite, older patients may lose their desire for food and weight loss is common. Apathetic thyrotoxicosis is used to relate to patients in whom cardiovascular, myopathic, and neuropsychiatric symptoms are predominant [59]. In fact, many older patients who have hyperthyroidism are evaluated for depression or cancer before the correct diagnosis is made. Therefore, it is apparent that hyperthyroidism easily can be overlooked in the elderly, as the presenting features may not conform to the usual findings in younger people. Thus, subacute thyroiditis and hyperthyroidism should be considered in elderly patients who have FUO and elevations of ESR and alkaline phosphatase levels, even in the absence of symptoms suggestive of thyroid disease.

Drug fever

Drug-induced fever tends to be a difficult diagnosis, because it is confirmed only after other causes are eliminated. Diagnosis should include demonstration of the link between initiation of the drug and the start of the fever and resolution of fever within a few days of stopping the causative agent. Any pattern of fever may be seen in drug-induced fever; the mechanisms by which it occurs are numerous; and many drugs are implicated. Antibiotics are the most frequent cause of drug fever. Other classes of medication used most commonly by the elderly that cause the fever include cardiovascular drugs, nonsteroidal anti-inflammatory drugs and salicylates, histamine type 2 blockers, anticonvulsants, and psychotropic drugs. Typically, drug fever occurs 5 to 10 days after the start of treatment but it also may occur after the first dose. Although most patients are surprisingly well while febrile, some are profoundly septic. Drugs always should be considered in the differential diagnosis of FUO [1,10,60,61].

Habitual hyperthermia

Habitual hyperthermia never has been reported as a cause of FUO in the elderly and only rarely meets the criteria of FUO, because most patients who have this entity have a body temperature lower than 38°C [62].

Factitious fever

Factitious fever is a rare cause of FUO; it is more prevalent in young female patients allied with health professions and is not a cause of FUO in the elderly population in most previous studies [10,16].

Approach to elderly patients who have fever of unknown origin

Several algorithms and approaches to elderly patients who have FUO have been proposed with a staged diagnostic protocol [8–10,63,64]. The investigation of elderly patients, who have low tolerance to the long and exhausting FUO investigation, should be directed by the spectrum of underlying diseases rather than by reported results of selected diagnostic tests [10]. A reasonable approach to FUO in the elderly is to perform a thorough history and physical examination, focusing on symptoms and signs of intra-abdominal diseases, cardiac disorders, tuberculosis, musculoskeletal disorders, and cancers (Table 3). After chest radiograph and basic laboratory studies are repeated as indicated, imaging studies of the abdomen, repeated blood cultures, and echocardiography should be performed [64]. Elderly patients are more likely to have predisposing valvular conditions (eg, degenerative and calcified lesions) and prosthetic valves, which reduce the sensitivity of transthoracic echocardiography to 45%. Transesophageal echocardiography has increased the diagnostic yield of infective endocarditis in the elderly patients by 45% [27]. Early detection and treatment require a high index of suspicion and an aggressive diagnostic approach.

All nonessential drugs patients take should be discontinued immediately as should other essential drugs if fever persists. Persistence of fever beyond 72 hours after the suspected drug is removed allows the conclusion that the drug is not the cause for producing the fever [65].

Abdominal ultrasonography is a first-choice technique in investigation of FUO because of its low cost and the wealth of information it yields. CT scan of the chest and the abdomen forms the next step [10,63]. Abdominal CT scan has a major role in the detection of intra-abdominal pathology, because it has a high diagnostic value and is likely to reveal two of the most common causes of FUO: intra-abdominal abscesses and lymphoproliferative disorders [65]. These tests not only are beneficial for patients who have signs and symptoms suggesting an abdominal process but also occasionally can be useful for cases with no indication of disease elsewhere. Although this study rarely establishes a definitive diagnosis, it can help to identify abnormal tissue.

Table 3
Suggested approach to FUO in the elderly

Recommended actions	Clinical	Laboratory	Imaging	Intervention
Confirm fever by serial measures	*			
Through meticulous history and complete physical examination; blood count with differential, ESR, a chemistry panel, urinalysis, multiple cultures of urine and blood, TSH. Consider HIV, EBV, CMV, and antinuclear antibody in specific cases; chest radiographs.	*	*	*	
Discontinue all nonessential drugs	*			
Abdominal ultrasonography			*	
Echocardiography, transesophageal echocardiography			*	*
Search for tuberculosis	*	*	*	*
CT of abdomen and chest			*	
Consider temporal artery biopsy, particularly if the ESR exceeds 40 mm/h	*			*
Search for pulmonary embolism, particularly in bedridden patients	*	*	*	
Scanning with gallium-67, indium-111 labeled autologous leucocytes or FDG-PET			*	
Consider liver and bone marrow biopsy				*
Laparoscopy				*

This directs clinicians to identify sites where invasive procedures, such as needle biopsy, aspiration, or catheter placement, are likely to be helpful [66]. Because of the usefulness of abdominal CT and occasionally ultrasound scanning of the gallbladder and hepatobiliary system, these tests are applied to virtually all cases of FUO. MRI should be used only for clarifying conditions found through the use of other techniques or when a diagnosis remains obscure. There is limited value in imaging techniques, such as CT and MRI, that concentrate on one area of the body if there are no localizing sign or symptoms.

Due consideration should be given to the possibility of pulmonary embolism, particularly in bedridden patients. The ventilation-perfusion lung scan is the diagnostic test used most frequently for pulmonary embolism. Nondiagnostic scans are common, however, because of the frequency of underlying cardiopulmonary disease in the elderly. A spiral or helical CT scan of the chest with intravenous contrast is sensitive and specific for diagnosis of pulmonary embolism [55].

A total body inflammation tracer scintigraphy is a valuable tool in the localization of the cause of fever. Gallium-67-citrate, labeled leucocytes (indium-111, technetium-99), labeled polyclonal human immunoglobulins (indium-111, technetium-99), and [^{18}F] fluorodeoxyglucose–positron emission tomography (FDG-PET) represent the radiopharmaceuticals investigated most intensely in the field of FUO. Newer radiopharmaceuticals, such as avidin-labeled biotin, radiolabeled liposomes, labeled cytokines, labeled specific monoclonal antibodies (specific for endothelial or leucocyte ligands), and labeled antibiotics, are under clinical development [9,67,68]. The role of the scintigraphic technique in FUO is to localize a potential cause, which then can be investigated further by ultrasonography, classical x-ray studies, CT, MRI, endoscopy, and eventually biopsy [67]. Nuclear imaging studies are helpful in localizing a potential infectious or inflammatory focus because of their minimal toxicity and overall good test characteristics [65].

The need for additional diagnostic studies should be based on abnormalities found in the initial noninvasive work-up and only when clinical suspicion shows that these tests are indicated or when the source of the fever remains unidentified after extensive evaluation should more invasive testing be performed.

High pretest probability of TA suggests that the diagnostic yield of temporal artery biopsy in older patients who have FUO (with initial negative evaluations for other causes) would be high. In particular, FUO patients older than 60 who have anemia, elevated sedimentation rate, and an elevated alkaline phosphatase level should generate a high index of suspicion for TA. A markedly elevated sedimentation rate is considered a hallmark of TA, but a sedimentation rate of less than 30 mm h is found in 10% of patients [69,70]. A positive temporal artery biopsy result confirms the diagnosis, but a negative result does not exclude it because of possible skip lesions. TA biopsy samples are positive only in 60% to 80% of patients [41]. The biopsy may exclude other systemic vasculitides, such as polyarteritis nodosa and Wegener's granulomatosis [71]. When a biopsy is negative but clinical suspicion remains high, a contralateral biopsy should be considered even though a low diagnostic yield has been found [45,72]. Recent studies suggest that at some centers, color duplex ultrasonography may be a useful noninvasive technique for the diagnosis of TA [40,73]. A role for FDG-PET in the diagnosis of TA is proposed by Blockmans and colleagues [68,74]. As a delay in diagnosis of TA may lead to catastrophic results, such as blindness or stroke, it is essential to maintain a high index of suspicion when managing older patients at risk. Corticosteroid therapy should begin soon after obtaining initial investigations and even before performing a temporal artery biopsy in elderly patients who have FUO where there is a strong clinical suspicion of TA and serious complications, such as imminent visual loss or other vascular events. A dramatic response to glucocorticoid therapy can confirm the diagnosis [40,75].

A routine search for tuberculosis is recommended, because the presentation of tuberculosis in the elderly often is uncharacteristic in terms of symptoms and chest radiographic features [19]. Diagnosis may be difficult or even missed, hindering further treatment and cure. Because of the wide variation in presentation of the disease in the elderly, clinicians should perform the appropriate diagnostic tests at an early stage in the disease process. The Mantoux tuberculin test is the preferred method for diagnosis of tuberculosis. The tuberculin skin tests require, however, careful interpretation because healthy elderly individuals may have positive test results as a consequence of previous infection, whereas severely ill elderly patients who have tuberculosis may be anergic and, therefore, have a negative test result. Two-step tuberculin skin test is recommended for elderly patients at high risk who have not been skin tested for many years or who never have been tested [18]. In one study, skin test responses to 5TU PPD were positive in 86.2% of young adults who had tuberculosis and only in 67.6% of elderly patients tested [19]. The lower frequency of positive tuberculin skin tests in older patients can be explained by the impairment of the immunologic responses of T lymphocytes [76]. The tests always should include sputum for smear and culture; in some cases bronchoscopy with lavage and biopsy may be needed and, rarely, open lung biopsy. Three sputum specimens, collected in the morning, should be submitted for microscopic examination. The sputum smears may be positive for acid-fast bacilli in only 50% of the cases. The use of specimens of urine and gastric lavage fluid may be hampered by the presence of mycobacterial commensals, which can cause false-positive results [18]. If disease is suspected at an extrapulmonary site, appropriate specimens should be taken for histology and culture. Two potentially useful tests often are unhelpful: the tuberculin skin test frequently is negative in the miliary and peritoneal forms, and the chest radiograph is normal in approximately 50% of most extrapulmonary tuberculosis [19]. Lung and liver biopsy each demonstrate granulomas in 80% to 90% of cases of miliary tuberculosis, and bone marrow biopsy is likely to show granulomas in only half the cases [1]. DNA amplification techniques, such as polymerase chain reaction and gene probes, may have an increasing part to play in the diagnosis of tuberculosis in the elderly [76]. The importance of tuberculosis as a cause of FUO in the elderly warrants empiric treatment with antituberculous agents if a rapid deterioration of the clinical condition occurs. Many patients are diagnosed on the basis of response to therapy alone; therefore, treatment should be started before diagnosis can be confirmed in those who have severe symptoms [63,76].

If this initial approach reveals no clues, colonoscopy, bone marrow examination, and liver biopsy should be the next steps to consider [64]. Colonoscopy, which may be uncomfortable for elderly patients, usually entails intravenous sedation and has a perforation rate of up to 0.5% [77]. The diagnostic yield from liver biopsy is 14% to 17% [78,79]. For patients in whom elevated levels of alkaline phosphatase or transaminases, or both, are documented, liver biopsy can provide evidence for a variety of malignancies and granulomatous processes. Physical examination findings of hepatomegaly or abnormal liver profile, however, are not helpful in predicting which patients will have an abnormal liver biopsy result [65]. The most common biopsy finding is granulomas, and there may be histologic evidence of a specific cause (eg, caseation of tuberculosis, schistosomiasis, fungal organisms, or primary biliary cirrhosis) [78,79].

In immunocompetent individuals who have FUO, the diagnostic yield of bone marrow cultures is found to be 0% to 2% [80,81]. Because of the low diagnostic yield for bone marrow cultures in FUO, bone marrow cultures are not recommended in the diagnostic work-up [65]. Patients who have pancytopenia should undergo a bone marrow biopsy for histologic testing and culture. Histoplasmosis and mycobacterial infections often cause fever and pancytopenia. Bone marrow biopsy is a useful procedure for the diagnosis of FUO in patients who have advanced HIV disease, particularly in areas where tuberculosis is prevalent. Involvement of the marrow may be the first indication of the existence of extranodal lymphomas [82].

Aggressive interventions, such as explorative laparotomy, no longer are recommended if a patient's condition remains stable. Laparotomy as a final diagnostic method for FUO cases may contribute to the diagnosis if noninvasive and invasive diagnostic measures fail. The role of surgery, however, in post-CT era remains unclear [65,68]. Laparoscopy, including laparoscopic liver biopsy, is a less traumatic alternative. It is most helpful when other features point to abdominal disease. Should such features be absent, however, the yield is only 20% [1]. Alternatively, if patients are clinically stable, it is preferable, especially in elderly patients who are more frail, to observe the patients in an ambulatory setting and repeat all noninvasive diagnostic studies at a later time or when more specific manifestations appear. After all diagnostic studies are completed, a trial of 10 to 14 days of broad-spectrum antibiotics is recommended in elderly patients who are deteriorating clinically (Fig. 1) [9,63,64]. The response to therapy is seldom proof of a single disease, as many undiagnosed FUO patients experience spontaneous resolution of fever. Alternatively, the unpredictable and often sluggish response to therapy, well known in cases of tuberculosis and endocarditis, may cause clinicians to doubt the efficacy of the therapy [9].

Summary

Elderly patients who have FUO have a different spectrum of underlying conditions. NIDs have emerged as the most frequent cause of FUO in the elderly, and TA is the most frequent specific diagnosis. Infections, in particular tuberculosis, remain an important diagnostic category. The number of cases that remain without an identified cause is significantly lower in elderly patients who have FUO compared with younger individuals. Evaluation of FUO in the elderly is complex and challenging. Atypical disease presentation is complicated further by the fact that multiple diseases commonly exist. Further, investigative procedures may be tolerated less well by older people, with decision making dependent on clinical presentation, sensitivity

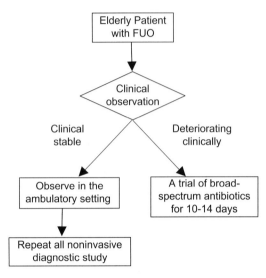

Fig. 1. Proposed algorithm for therapeutic trial.

and specificity of specific tests, and side effects and discomfort resulting from testing. Each patient who has FUO requires an individual approach; the use of the same algorithm in every patient is inappropriate. It is preferable to investigate the abnormalities already uncovered by others or to focus on the most likely conditions identified by unique epidemiology, age, or exposure.

FUO often is associated with treatable conditions in the elderly, and an accelerated evaluation is warranted because of the lack of physiologic reserve and risk for functional deterioration. A delay in diagnosis and initiation of appropriate treatment, therefore, may lead to increased morbidity and mortality. Early recognition and prompt initiation of appropriate empiric therapy in elderly patients, who are deteriorating clinically, are the cornerstones of the management strategy.

Finally, the physiology of thermoregulation and pathogenesis of fever is altered with advancing age, and elderly patients who have serious infections may have blunted febrile response, which may delay diagnosis and treatment. FUO in the elderly may be considered at a body temperature less than 38.3°C (at least the interval of 37.5°C –38.3°C). Within the modified definition of FUO, the relative proportion of the various etiologies in this population might change. Although there is no consensus, the authors believe that a redefinition of FUO in the elderly is required and that further studies are warranted to define the most appropriate temperature for FUO in the elderly and the causes of FUO in this group of vulnerable adults.

References

[1] Arnow PM. Fever of unknown origin. Review article. Lancet 1997;350:575–80.

[2] Petersdorf RG, Beeson PB. Fever of unexplained origin: report on 100 cases. Medicine 1961; 40:1–30.

[3] Durack DT, Street AC. Fever of unknown origin—reexamined and redefined. Curr Clin Top Infect Dis 1991;11:35–51.

[4] Petersdorf RG. Fever of unknown origin: an old friend revisited. Arch Intern Med 1992;152: 21–2.

[5] Kanzanjian P. Fever of unknown origin: review of 86 patients treated in community hospitals. Clin Infect Dis 1992;15:968–73.

[6] Knockaert DC, Vanneste LJ, Vanneste SB. Fever of unknown origin in 1980s. An update of the diagnostic spectrum. Arch Intern Med 1992;152:51–5.

[7] DeKleijn EM. Fever of unknown origin (FUO): I. A prospective multicenter study of 167 patients with FUO, using fixed epidemiologic entry criteria. Medicine 1997;76: 392–400.

[8] Roth AR, Basello GM. Approach to the adult patient with fever of unknown origin. Am Fam Physician 2003;68:2223–8.

[9] Knockaert DC, Vanderschueren S, Blockmans D. Fever of unknown origin in adults: 40 years on. J Intern Med 2003;253:263–75.

[10] Knockaert DC, Vanneste LJ, Bobbaers HJ. Fever of unknown origin in the elderly patients. J Am Geriatr Soc 1993;41:1187–92.

[11] Larson EB, Featherstone HJ, Petersdorf R. Fever of undetermined origin: diagnosis and follow-up of 105 cases, 1970–1980. Medicine 1982;61:269–92.

[12] Shoji S, Imamura A, Imai Y. Fever of unknown origin: a review of 80 patients from shin'etsu area of Japan from 1986–1992. Intern Med 1994;33:74–6.

[13] Dobbins WO. The diagnosis of Whipple's disease. N Engl J Med 1995;332:390–2.

[14] Moore PS. The emergence of Kaposi's sarcoma-associated herpes virus (human herpes virus 8). N Engl J Med 2000;343:1411–3.

[15] Norman DC. Fever in the elderly. Clin Infect Dis 2000;31:148–51.

[16] Esposito AL, Gleckman RA. Fever of unknown origin in the elderly. J Am Geriatr Soc 1978; 26:498–505.

[17] Barrier J, Schneebeli S, Peltier P. Les fièvres prolongèes inexpliquèes chez les personnes, âgèes [French]. Concours Med 1982;104:4679–89.

[18] Zevallos M, Justman JE. Tuberculosis in the elderly. Clin Geriatr Med 2003;19:121–38.

[19] Korzeniewska-Kosela M, Krysl J, Muller N, et al. Tuberculosis in young adults and the elderly. Chest 1994;106:28–32.

[20] Burg BM, Francis L. Acute abdominal pain in the elderly. Emerg Med 2005;8:8–12.

[21] Sapico FL. Microbiology and antimicrobial therapy of spinal infections. Orthop Clin North Am 1996;27:9–13.

[22] Darouiche RO, Landon GC, Klima M, et al. Osteomyelitis associated with pressure sores. Arch Intern Med 1994;154:753–8.

[23] Mackowiak PA, Jones SR, Smith JW. Diagnostic value of sinus-tract cultures in chronic osteomyelitis. JAMA 1978;239:2772–5.

[24] Cunha BA. Osteomyelitis in elderly patients. Clin Infect Dis 2002;35:287–93.

[25] Mader JT, Shirtliff ME, Bergquist S, et al. Bone and joint infections in the elderly: practical treatment. Drugs Aging 2000;16:67–80.

[26] Dhawan VK. Infective endocarditis in elderly patients. Clin Infect Dis 2002;34:806–12.

[27] Werner GS, Shulz R, Fuchs JB. Infective endocarditis in the elderly in era of transesophageal echocardiography: clinical features and prognosis compared with younger patients. Am J Med 1996;100:90–7.

[28] Leport C, Bure A, Leport J, et al. Incidence of colonic lesions in Streptococcus bovis and enterococcal endocarditis. Lancet 1987;1:748.

[29] Gagliardi JP, Nettles RE, Sanders LL, et al. Native valve infective endocarditis in elderly and younger adult patients: comparison of clinical features and outcomes with use of the Duke criteria and the Duke Endocarditis Database. Clin Infect Dis 1998;26:1165–8.

[30] Netzer RO, Zollinger E, Seiler C, et al. Native valve infective endocarditis in elderly and younger patients: comparison of clinical features and outcomes with Duke criteria. Clin Infect Dis 1999;28:1165–8.

[31] Di Salvo G, Rosenberg V, Pergola V, et al. Endocarditis in the elderly: clinical, echocardiographic, and prognostic features. Eur Heart J 2003;24:1575–82.

[32] Terpenning MS, Buggy BP, Kauffman CA. Infective endocarditis: clinical features in young and elderly patients. Am J Med 1987;83:626–34.

[33] Cantrell M, Yoshikawa TT. Infective endocarditis in the aging patient. Gerontology 1984; 30:316–26.

[34] Axelrod P, Finestone AJ. Infectious mononucleosis in older patients. Am Fam Physician 1990;42:1599–606.

[35] Centers for Disease Control and Prevention. AIDS among persons aged $\geq$ 50 years—United States, 1991–1996. MMWR Morb Motral Wkly Rep 1998;47:21–7.

[36] Whipple B, Scura K. HIV and the older adult. J Gerontol Nurs 1989;15:15–9.

[37] Armstrong WS, Katz J, Kazanjian PH. Human immunodeficiency virus-associated fever of unknown origin: a study of 70 patients in the United States and review. Clin Infect Dis 1999; 28:341–5.

[38] Chiao EY, Ries KM, Sande MA. AIDS and the elderly. Clin Infect Dis 1999;28:740–5.

[39] Linsk H. HIV and the elderly. Fam Soc 1994;75:362–72.

[40] Salvarani C, Cantini F, Boiardi L, et al. Polymyalgia rheumatica and Giant-Cell arteritis. N Engl J Med 2002;347:261–71.

[41] Swannell AJ. Polymyalgia rheumatica and temporal arteritis: diagnosis and management. BMJ 1997;314:1329–32.

[42] Salvarani C, Gabriel SE, O'Fallon WM, et al. The incidence of giant cell arteritis in Olmsted County, Minnesota: apparent fluctuations in a cyclic pattern. Ann Intern Med 1995;123: 192–4.

[43] Hunder GG, Bloch DA, Michel BA, et al. The American College of Rheumatology 1990 criteria for the classification of giant cell arteritis. Arthritis Rheum 1990;33:1122–8.

[44] Calamia KT, Hunder GG. Giant cell arteritis (temporal arteritis) presenting as fever of undetermined origin. Arthritis Rheum 1981;24:1414–8.

[45] Lee AG, Brazis PW. Temporal arteritis: a clinical approach. J Am Geriatr Soc 1999;47: 1364–70.

[46] Salvarani C, Gabriel SE, O'Fallon WM, et al. Epidemiology of polymyalgia rheumatica in Olmsted County, Minnesota, 1970–1991. Arthritis Rheum 1995;38:369–73.

[47] Salvarani C, Cantini F, Olivieri I, et al. Proximal bursitis in active polymyalgia rheumatica. Ann Intern Med 1997;127:27–31.

[48] Salvarani C, Macchioni P, Boiardi L. Polymyalgia rheumatica. Lancet 1997;350:437–9.

[49] Martinez-Taboada VM, Blanco R, Rodriguez-Valverde V. Polymyalgia rheumatica with normal erythrocyte sedimentation rate, clinical aspects. Clin Exp Rheumatol 2000;18: 34–7.

[50] Gonzalez-Gay MA, Rodriguez-Valverde V, Blanco R, et al. Polymyalgia rheumatica without significantly increased erythrocyte sedimentation rate. A more benign syndrome. Arch Intern Med 1997;157:317–20.

[51] Dinarello CA, Bunn PA. Fever. Semin Oncol 1977;24:288–98.

[52] Cleary JF. Fever and sweats: including the immunocompromised hosts. In: Berger A, Portenoy RK, Weissman DE, editors. Principles and practice of supportive oncology. Philadelphia: Lippincott-Raven Publishers; 1998. p. 119–31.

[53] Mueller PS, Terrell CL, Gertz MA. Fever of unknown origin caused by multiple myeloma. Arch Intern Med 2002;162:1305–9.

[54] Hyers TM. Venous thromboembolism. Am J Respir Crit Care Med 1999;159:1–14.

[55] Berman AR, Arnsten JH. Diagnosis and treatment of pulmonary embolism in the elderly. Clin Geriatr Med 2003;19:157–75.

[56] Stein PD, Afzal A, Henry JW, et al. Fever in acute pulmonary embolism. Chest 2000;117: 39–42.

[57] Weiss BM, Hepburn MJ, Mong DP. Subacute thyroiditis manifesting as fever of unknown origin. South Med J 2000;93:926–9.

[58] Hoffmann HS. Subacute thyroiditis as fever of unknown origin. Conn Med 1996;60:438–9.

[59] Gambert SR. Hyperthyroidism in the elderly. Clin Geriatr Med 1995;11:181–8.

[60] Mackowiak PA, LeMastre CF. Drug fever: a critical appraisal of conventional concepts. An analysis of 51 episodes in the Dallas hospitals and 97 episodes reported in the English literature. Ann Intern Med 1987;106:728–33.

[61] Hall RC, Appleby B. Atypical neuroleptic malignant syndrome presenting as fever of unknown origin in the elderly. South Med J 2005;98:114–7.

[62] Kauffman CA, Jones PG. Diagnosing fever of unknown origin in older patients. Geriatrics 1984;39:46–51.

[63] Tal S, Guller V, Gurevich A, et al. Fever of unknown origin in the elderly. J Intern Med 2002; 252:295–304.

[64] Yoshikawa TT, Norman DC. Fever in the elderly. Infect Med 1998;15:704–6.

[65] Mourad O, Palda V, Detsky AS. A comprehensive evidence-based approach to fever of unknown origin. Arch Intern Med 2003;163:545–51.

[66] Rowland MD, Del Bene VE. Use of body computed tomography to evaluate fever of unknown origin. J Infect Dis 1987;156:409.

[67] Peters AM. Nuclear medicine imaging in fever of unknown origin. Q J Nucl Med 1999;43: 61–73.

[68] Blockmans D, Knockaert D, Maes A, et al. Clinical value of [18F] fluoro-deoxyglucose positron emission tomography for patients with fever of unknown origin. Clin Infect Dis 2001; 32:191–6.

[69] Martinez-Taboada VM, Blanco R, Armona J, et al. Giant cell arteritis with an erythrocyte sedimentation rate low than 50. Clin Rheumatol 2000;19:73–5.

[70] Salvarani C, Hunder GG. Giant cell arteritis with low erythrocyte sedimentation rate: of occurrence in a population-based study. Arthritis Rheum 2001;45:140–5.

[71] Chakravarty K, Elgabani HS, Scott DRI, et al. A district audit on management of polymyalgia rheumatica and giant cell arteritis. Br J Rheumatol 1994;33:152–6.

[72] Danesh-Meyer HV, Savino PJ, Eagle RC Jr, et al. Low diagnostic yield with second biopsies in suspected giant arteritis. J Neuroophthalmol 2000;20:213–5.

[73] Schmitt WA, Kraft HE, Worpol K. Color duplex ultrasonography in the diagnosis of temporal arteritis. N Engl J Med 1997;337:1336–42.

[74] Blockmans D, Stroobants S, Maes A, et al. Positron emission tomography in giant cell arteritis and polymyalgia rheumatica: evidence for inflammation of the aortic arch. Am J Med 2000;108:246–9.

[75] Dwolatzky T, Sonnenblick M, Nesher G. Giant cell arteritis and polymyalgia rheumatica: clues to early diagnosis. Geriatrics 1997;52:38–44.

[76] Davies PDO. Tuberculosis in the elderly: epidemiology and optimal management. Drugs Aging 1996;6:436–44.

[77] Yoong KKY, Heymann T. Colonoscopy in the very old: why bother? Postgrad Med J 2005; 81:196–7.

[78] Holtz T, Moseley RH, Scheiman JM. Liver biopsy in fever of unknown origin. A reappraisal. J Clin Gastroenterol 1993;17:29–32.

[79] Paez-Rodriguez O, Garcia-Tsao G, Sifuentes J. Usefulness of the histologic and microbiologic study of liver biopsy in the diagnosis of fever of unknown origin. Rev Gastroenterol Mex 1990;55:1–6.

[80] Volk E, Miller ML, Kirskley BA, et al. The diagnostic usefulness of bone marrow cultures in patients with fever of unknown origin. Am J Clin Pathol 1998;110:150–3.

[81] Riley U, Crawford S, Barrett SP, et al. Detection of mycobacteria in bone marrow biopsy specimens taken to investigate pyrexia of unknown origin. J Clin Pathol 1995;48:706–9.
[82] Benito N, Nunez A, de Gorgolas M, et al. Bone marrow biopsy in the diagnosis of fever of unknown origin in patients with acquired immunodeficiency syndrome. Arch Intern Med 1997;157:1577–80.

CLINICS IN
GERIATRIC
MEDICINE

ELSEVIER
SAUNDERS

Clin Geriatr Med 23 (2007) 669–685

Immunizations in Older Adults

Kevin High, MD, MSc

Sections on Infectious Diseases, Hematology/Oncology, and Molecular Medicine,
Wake Forest University Health Sciences, 100 Medical Center Boulevard,
Winston Salem, NC 27157-1042, USA

The Advisory Council for Immunization Practices (ACIP) of the Centers for Disease Control and Prevention (CDC) provides age-defined recommendations for adult immunization (Fig. 1) [1]. Despite significant public health efforts, immunization rates for vaccines indicated in older adults continue to lag behind national goals (Fig. 2) [2]. Many factors have contributed to this failure. Poor reliability of vaccine production, particularly for influenza vaccine, has led to several years of vaccine shortages reducing the number of subjects immunized. Complex recommendations regarding re-immunization and its safety have plagued efforts to provide simple approaches to pneumococcal immunization. Both influenza and pneumococcal vaccines have suffered from the lack of universal medical record keeping for immunizations in adults, and reimbursement systems are usually perceived as providing negative incentives for vaccines and other preventive care. These important issues strongly contribute to a greater risk of vaccine-preventable illness in older adults. Solutions to these problems are broad in scope and require changes at a national level. This review focuses on patient-provider interaction and outlines the reasons for and clinical predictors of decreased vaccine efficacy in older adults, emphasizes that vaccine efficacy in older adults must be defined differently than in children or even young adults, reviews the evidence supporting the use and cost-effectiveness of vaccines indicated in the elderly, and outlines current and future strategies to reduce vaccine-preventable illnesses in older adults.

Dr. High is a member of the Vaccine Advisory Board for Merck and on the Speaker's Bureau for Merck and Wyeth Pharmaceuticals.

E-mail address: khigh@wfubmc.edu

Recommended adult immunization schedule, by vaccine and age group

Vaccine ▼ / Age group (yrs) ►	19–49 years	50–64 years	≥65 years
Tetanus, diphtheria, pertussis (Td/Tdap)[1*]	1-dose Td booster every 10 yrs / Substitute 1 dose of Tdap for Td		
Human papillomavirus (HPV)[2*]	3 doses (females)		
Measles, mumps, rubella (MMR)[3*]	1 or 2 doses	1 dose	
Varicella[4*]	2 doses (0, 4–8 wks)	2 doses (0, 4–8 wks)	
Influenza[5*]	1 dose annually	1 dose annually	
Pneumococcal (polysaccharide)[6,7]	1–2 doses		1 dose
Hepatitis A[8*]	2 doses (0, 6–12 mos, or 0, 6–18 mos)		
Hepatitis B[9*]	3 doses (0, 1–2, 4–6 mos)		
Meningococcal[10]	1 or more doses		

Fig. 1. Immunization schedule for adults by age group. (*From* Centers for Disease Control National Immunization Program. Recommended adult immunization schedule, United States, October 2006–September 2007. Available at: http://www.cdc.gov/nip/recs/adult-schedule.pdf. Accessed January 1, 2007.)

Causes for vaccine failure in older adults and clinical predictors of nonresponse

Poor administration rates

Obviously, vaccines can only work if they are administered. As shown in Fig. 2, administration rates for pneumococcal and influenza vaccine lag far behind year 2010 goals. Over the last 10 years, an inconsistent supply of influenza vaccine has contributed to the flattening of the curve between 1997 and 2004. Because influenza and pneumococcal vaccine are often administered at the same time, the unavailability of influenza vaccine likely contributes to the flattening of pneumococcal immunization rates over this time.

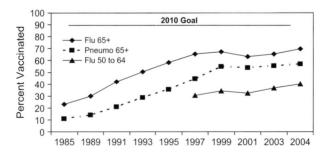

Fig. 2. Percent of adults aged 65 years and over immunized with influenza or pneumococcal polysaccharide (PPS) over the last 2 decades. The year 2010 goal for both vaccines is 90%. Data from the CDC. (*Data from* Advisory Committee on Immunization Practices. Prevention and control of influenza. MMWR Morb Mortal Wkly Rep 2005;54(RR08):1–40.)

Interestingly, childhood immunization rates are far superior to adult immunization, exceeding 95% for most vaccines [3]. Although there are many reasons why childhood immunization rates are superior to rates in adults, one contributor is a lack of perceived vaccine efficacy by patients and providers for adult vaccines. Unlike childhood vaccines that frequently prevent clinical illness altogether, most adult vaccines do not prevent illness but lessen the severity of a given infection. For example, it is rare to experience measles or polio after one is immunized as a child. In contrast, older adults often still experience influenza or zoster following immunization. Even if it is less severe, such episodes are usually viewed by the public as vaccine "failures." Misrepresentation of vaccines given to adults also contributes to this problem. The pneumococcal vaccine is often represented to patients as a "pneumonia shot" yet this vaccine has never been clearly shown to prevent pneumonia, only invasive pneumococcal disease (IPD) [4]. Because there are so many non-pneumococcal causes of pneumonia, it is unlikely that a vaccine directed at any pathogen, even the most common pathogen to cause pneumonia requiring hospitalization, is likely to reduce overall pneumonia risk. Similarly, many influenza-like illnesses may suggest vaccine failure to those who have received the influenza vaccine when their illness is commonly due to another respiratory virus. This perceived lack of efficacy results in patient and provider apathy regarding adult vaccines. The question as to which factor is more important was addressed by a study nearly 20 years ago that examined patient and provider attitudes regarding influenza vaccine. Table 1 demonstrates that the provider attitude is by far the most important factor contributing to vaccine uptake [5]. If providers strongly recommend adult immunization, patient apathy is likely to be overcome.

Immune senescence and vaccine nonresponse

An important factor allowing clinicians to become stronger advocates for adult immunization is to clearly outline the data regarding limitations of vaccine responses in older adults and the reasons for failure, allowing providers to identify those at risk for vaccine failure to employ alternate

Table 1
Influence of patient and provider attitudes on immunization status in older adults

Patient attitude	Provider attitude	Percent vaccinated
Yes	Yes	87
No	Yes	70
Yes	No	8
No	No	7

Yes indicates support for the vaccine; no indicates no support for the vaccine.
Data from CDC. Adult immunization: knowledge, attitudes, and practices—DeKalb and Fulton Counties, Georgia, 1988. MMWR 1988;37(43):657–61.)

strategies. Age is associated with a decline in vaccine efficacy, presumably owing to waning immunity with advanced age, termed *immune senescence*. Immune senescence results in reduced responses to new antigens and re-duced memory/booster responses to antigens previously encountered, but the effect is much greater for new antigens. A good example of this can be found in determining age-related response rates for hepatitis A and B vaccines [6–8]. Although adequate responses are nearly universal before age 35 years, less than half of persons aged 65 years and over respond with antibody titers that correlate with protection (Fig. 3). Waning re-sponses to other vaccine antigens also occurs, but the age at which nonre-sponse becomes a major issue varies for any given vaccine. Most data reveal little to no protection provided by pneumococcal vaccine if given af-ter the age of 85 years [9–12]. The specific causes for immune senescence have not been identified, and an extensive discussion of the basic science in this field is beyond the scope of this article. The reader is referred to the article by Castle elsewhere in this issue for more information.

Comorbidity is strongly associated with vaccine nonresponse, and spe-cific comorbidities are notable predictors of poor vaccine response. HIV, cancer (particularly in persons receiving treatment with chemotherapy), chronic renal failure, and congestive heart failure all impair vaccine re-sponses in adults and have been widely recognized in case-control studies examining pneumococcal vaccine failure [9–12]. Despite limited vaccine ef-ficacy, patients with these comorbidities are precisely the ones who have the most to gain by immunization. This observation is particularly true for influenza, because much of the influenza-related morbidity and mortality is due to exacerbation of underlying disease. A recent study of over 140,000 older adults highlights the effects of influenza vaccine in reducing the exac-erbation of comorbid disease, demonstrating almost a twofold reduction in hospitalization and death owing to underlying disease [13].

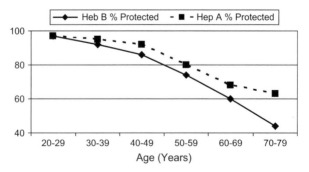

Fig. 3. Effect of age on response to hepatitis A and hepatitis B vaccine. Data summarized from [6–8].

Two additional comorbidities of epidemic proportion have received less attention but are discussed in greater detail herein—diabetes and obesity. Diabetes is associated with a well-known higher risk of bacterial infection than in the general population. Skin/soft tissue infection accounts for much of this risk and is believed to be related to poor blood flow and hyperglycemic effects on white blood cells. The efficacy of immunizations in diabetic patients has been a matter of debate for some time, but diabetes probably confers a greater risk of infection than vaccine failure. A recent publication indicates that, although diabetes may reduce efficacy for influenza vaccine to some degree, the vaccine remains effective in this population, significantly reducing death rates [14].

Obesity contributes to vaccine nonresponse not only by its association with many of the comorbidities identified previously but also because of the physical nature of obesity. The body mass index (BMI) and the width of subcutaneous fat increase with age. This physical reality means that longer needles are needed to deliver vaccines to the muscle for deltoid injections (Fig. 4) [15]. Ultrasound studies of the depth of injection required to reach muscle highly correlate with BMI [16,17], suggesting that longer needles (32 mm) are needed in women with a BMI greater than 35. Nevertheless, the shorter 25-mm needles typically used are adequate for women with a BMI of 35 or less and for most men. The CDC officially recommends needles of 25 mm (1 in) for women and men weighing less than 60 kg, needles of 25 to 38 mm (1–1.5 in) for women weighing 60 to 90 kg and men 60 to 118 kg, and needles of 38 mm (1.5 in) for women weighing greater than 90 kg and men greater than 118 kg. This recommendation and many other technical issues regarding vaccine administration have been reviewed in a valuable recent publication by the CDC [18].

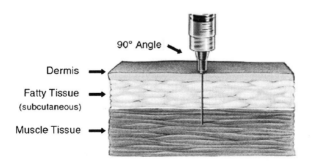

Adapted from California Immunization Branch

Fig. 4. The importance of needle length in achieving intramuscular delivery of vaccines. (*From* Kroger AT, Atkinson WL, Marcuse EK, et al. General recommendations on immunization. MMWR Morb Mortal Wkly Rep 2006;55(RR15):16.)

Efficacy and cost-effectiveness of currently recommended vaccines in older adults

Pneumococcal vaccine

The efficacy of the 23-valent pneumococcal polysaccharide vaccine (PPS) varies with the population studied and the endpoint used to determine efficacy. In immune competent older adults, PPS efficacy estimates range from 54% to 76% for the endpoint of preventing IPD (when IPD is defined as disease associated with a positive culture from blood or another sterile body site and not sputum or sinus cultures). Severe pneumococcal pneumonia [4] and death due to pneumonia [19] may also be reduced, but overall pneumonia rates and hospitalization for pneumonia are probably not significantly reduced [4,12]. A recent analysis suggests that if one is hospitalized for community-acquired pneumonia, complications and death are less likely if one has received PPS [20]. All-cause mortality has not been shown to be reduced by PPS in any one study, perhaps due to issues of statistical power. The largest cohort study of 47,365 subjects aged 65 years and over [12] showed an age-adjusted hazard ratio for all-cause mortality of 0.88 ($P < .001$) and a multivariate-adjusted ratio of 0.94 ($P = .08$).

Why is PPS not a more effective vaccine? One reason is the significant number of immunocompromised older adults in whom efficacy is attenuated. All of the major studies show markedly reduced estimates of PPS efficacy in immunocompromised hosts (21% to 50% for IPD), usually not reaching statistical significance [9–12]. A second reason for incomplete protection is IPD caused by serotypes not included in the PPS vaccine. Many pneumococcal serotypes have been identified from humans with disease, but only 23 of these serotypes are covered by current PPS vaccines. Even if one considers cross-reactivity to related strains, a significant number of pneumococcal strains remain unrepresented.

Probably the most important limitation of PPS vaccine in the elderly is the waning efficacy of PPS with advancing age. After blending efficacy rates for all adults aged 65 years and older, one recent study estimated that only 21% of all IPD is prevented by the current vaccine [21]. In adults aged 65 to 74 years, PPS is effective (70% to 80%), but the rate of IPD is only 29 cases per 100,000 population [9–12]. PPS efficacy falls to 53% to 67% in 75- to 84-year-old seniors who experience IPD at a rate of 47 cases per 100,000 population. The highest rates of IPD occur in seniors aged 85 years and above (85 cases per 100,000 population), yet PPS efficacy drops in this group to 0% to 22% [9–12]. A decrease in PPS efficacy occurs in precisely the age groups that need protection the most (Fig. 5), limiting the current vaccine and indicating that more effective pneumococcal vaccines are urgently needed to optimally protect older adults.

In no way should the limitations outlined herein dampen the enthusiasm for immunizing older adults with PPS, perhaps shifting the emphasis to

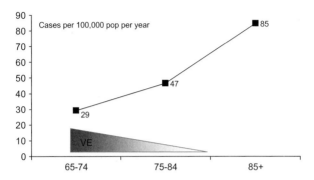

Fig. 5. Waning vaccine efficacy (VE) with age contrasted with incidence of IPD in older adults 65 to 74, 75 to 84, and 85+ years of age. (Figure courtesy of L. Jackson, MD, MPH, Durham, NC.)

immunizing "younger" old adults. Even if IPD is the only endpoint measured (ie, one assumes no reduction in pneumonia), PPS has been shown to be cost-effective, saving $8.27 per vaccination using typical assumptions and remaining cost-effective even if future health costs are included [22]. Under the most unfavorable assumptions, the cost was $35, 822/quality-adjusted life year gained for 65- to 74-year-olds. In a recent analysis from Australia, the number needed to vaccinate (NNV) for adults aged 65 years and over was 3333 (1429–12,500) to prevent one case of IPD and 14,493 (4762–83,333) to prevent one death at a cost of $11,494 and $49,972 (in Australian dollars), respectively [23]. This cost compares favorably with that of other medical interventions.

A common question in the care of older adults is whether pneumococcal vaccine is effective in nursing home residents, a group that is typically older, more likely to have multiple comorbidities, and afflicted by many of the conditions that predict vaccine failure. Limited data have addressed this issue [24,25], but a French study [26] showed an absolute risk reduction of 2.9% for all-cause pneumonia with a NNV of 35.1 to prevent one case of pneumonia. That older study was limited in that the 14-valent PPS vaccine was used, and 31% of subjects were lost to follow-up. Furthermore, a CDC study in New York City demonstrated that nonreceipt of PPS vaccine was a major risk factor for IPD in a recent outbreak [27], suggesting protection of PPS vaccine in older nursing home residents in outbreak situations. Given that PPS vaccine is an inexpensive and well-tolerated intervention, it is highly recommended that previously unvaccinated nursing home residents be immunized.

Influenza vaccine

Influenza vaccine is recommended for all adults aged 50 years and over, for anyone with underlying significant illness, and for anyone wishing to reduce their risk of serious influenza disease [28]. This recommendation is based on a large amount of data, yet controversy remains. Issues similar to those that have plagued pneumococcal vaccine studies (eg, observational and case-control rather than randomized/controlled studies and low event rates requiring a large number of subjects) contribute to the uncertainty regarding influenza vaccine efficacy. Other issues are how well the vaccine matches circulating viral strains in a given year, the vaccine shortages that have made administration spotty and mistimed versus the epidemic in some years, and the difficulty in identifying the most appropriate specific endpoints to be measured (eg, influenza-like illness versus confirmed influenza infection, exacerbation of underlying disease). Despite these difficulties, the bulk of the data suggest that influenza vaccine is highly efficacious, reducing all-cause mortality 39% to 69% (Table 2). Rates of hospitalization are also reduced by 20% to 50% in different series [28–30].

One of the major mechanisms through which influenza vaccine is thought to reduce mortality is by blunting influenza-triggered exacerbations of underlying disease. In a recent study, two cohorts of older adults numbering over 140,000 subjects were followed up in two different influenza seasons (1998–1999 and 1999–2000) [13]. The proportion immunized in each year was 55% to 60%, and the immunized group was sicker than the unvaccinated group in all categories measured (eg, more comorbidity, on more medications). Despite these differences, immunized subjects had a relative risk of death of 0.51 with a NNV of only 100 to prevent one death. Closer examination of the data indicates that influenza vaccine reduced the risk of death due to pneumonia as one would expect, but also reduced the risk of hospitalization and death due to cardiovascular disease. Importantly, this finding was consistent across age groups (65–74, 75–84, and ≥85 years),

Table 2
Estimated efficacy of influenza vaccine for preventing death in older adults during the 1990s

Influenza season	Estimated vaccine efficacy (95% confidence interval)
1990–1991	51% (30–65)
1991–1992	54% (39–65)
1992–1993	39% (19–53)
1993–1994	41% (25–53)
1994–1995	58% (44–67)
1995–1996	69% (56–79)
1996–1997	60% (55–65)
1997–1998	39% (33–44)
1998–1999	48% (43–53)
1999–2000	50% (45–54)

Efficacy varies based on, among other things, the match of the vaccine with circulating strains in a given year and the timing of immunization versus the period of epidemic of illness.

Data from McElhaney JE, Nichol KL. Influenza vaccines: crossing the transitional gap to improve outcomes in the elderly. Aging Health 2005;1:167–77.

indicating no waning of efficacy in the older age groups in contrast to the findings described for PPS.

Further support of influenza vaccine efficacy for older adults with comorbidity was demonstrated in a recent evaluation of how consistent influenza immunization annually influenced mortality. The risk of death was reduced in each year subjects received influenza vaccine for up to 6 years of successive immunization. If annual immunization was interrupted for some reason, the risk of death increased to 40% above baseline (Fig. 6) [30]. Re-initiating vaccine resulted in a reduction of risk back to that seen during the years of successive immunization.

Despite these impressive data, controversy remains regarding the effectiveness of influenza vaccine. A recent evaluation of data collected since 1980 concluded that because less than 10% of all winter-time deaths were attributable to influenza, observational studies overestimate the effect of influenza vaccine on mortality [31]. Another recent study supports the notion that there may be unmeasured differences between influenza-immunized versus unimmunized subjects that bias the data of case-control studies. In that study [32], reduced mortality during the 2001 to 2002 and 2004 to 2005 flu seasons was demonstrated in influenza vaccine recipients (relative risk of death, 0.56; 95% confidence interval [CI], 0.52–0.61); however, the database also allowed measurement of mortality during a 3-month period after immunization but before influenza began circulating in the community where subjects lived. Surprisingly, the relative risk of death for immunized subjects (0.39) was significantly lower even in this period of time (95% CI, 0.33–0.47), suggesting there may be something different between vaccine recipients and nonrecipients that is unmeasured in case-control and observational studies that use multivariate analyses in an attempt to control for bias. The

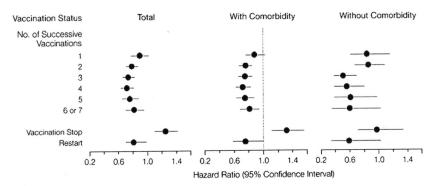

Fig. 6. Risk of death in older adults (with or without comorbidity) who received annual influenza vaccine in successive years. The risk of death if immunization was skipped in a given year (vaccination stop) shows an elevated risk of death in those with comorbidity that is again reduced below the expected risk if influenza immunization is restarted. (*Reprinted from* Voordouw AC, Sturkenboom MD, Dieleman JP, et al. Annual revaccination against influenza and mortality risk in community-dwelling elderly persons. JAMA 2004;292:2093; with permission.)

investigators in this study suggested this was a limitation of the data used and not an indictment of influenza vaccine, per se, but the estimate of its effect is difficult to determine from present studies.

Cost-effectiveness studies of influenza vaccine have used the estimates of efficacy previously described. In young adults, cost savings usually rely on the prevention of lost wages or work days. These issues are less relevant in older adults for whom the prevention of other medical costs must offset the cost of vaccine. Despite this more difficult hurdle, a series of studies have demonstrated that the vaccine is not only cost-effective but cost-saving in this population [33–35]. Estimates of cost-savings range from $171 per vaccinee in high-risk subjects likely to consume significant resources if they were to become ill to $7 per vaccinee for low-risk subjects [34]. Another study in a health maintenance organization (HMO), perhaps likely to enroll less ill older adults, influenza vaccine was cost-saving for the HMO in persons considered to be a high-risk vaccinee ($6.11 per vaccinee) but cost $4.82 per low-risk vaccinee. These numbers resulted in an overall cost-savings of $1.11 per vaccination provided to adults aged 65 years and over in the HMO [33].

Zoster vaccine

Zoster epidemiology, treatment, and prevention are covered in detail elsewhere in this issue. The reader is referred to that article for an extensive discussion of zoster vaccine, which was recently given provisional approval by the ACIP for all immunocompetent adults aged 60 years and over regardless of history of prior zoster [36].

Current strategies to maximize vaccine uptake and protection from vaccine-preventable diseases in older adults

Maximizing vaccine uptake

A variety of strategies have been investigated that are proven to enhance vaccine uptake, including standing orders, organized vaccine campaigns, provider reminders, mailings to patients, and immunization in non–health care settings [28]. Of these interventions, standing orders, a strategy that takes the physician out of the loop and allows nurses, pharmacists, or other health care professionals to order immunization after simple screening of all patients, is by far the most successful. This observation is true even in the inpatient setting where computerized order entry can facilitate physician reminders. In two recent studies comparing these strategies, standing orders were far superior [37,38].

Immunizing children to protect adults

Most respiratory infections circulate at much higher rates in children than in adults, and children are frequently the reservoir from which older adults contract disease. This observation is true for pneumococcal disease and influenza, and a growing body of data suggests that immunizing children, whose immune systems respond well to contemporary vaccines, is likely to translate into markedly reduced rates of illness in older adults.

The seven-valent conjugated pneumococcal vaccine (CPV) was introduced for widespread use in the early 1990s and has dramatically reduced rates of IPD in children. Although CPV is not usually administered to older adults, disease rates in adults aged 65 years and over have also declined since the introduction of CPV in children, particularly for the seven serotypes represented in the CPV (Fig. 7) [39]. The most likely explanation for this is a reduction in nasal carriage of these organisms in children and subsequent lower transmission from children to adults. Immunologic pressure exerted by widespread immunizations in children may be the best option for reducing IPD in adults. One particular caveat deserves mention. Currently, only seven serotypes are contained in the only CPV available. Concordant with a 55% decline in adult IPD caused by these seven serotypes, there was a 13% increase in the occurrence of pneumococcal serotypes not covered by the CPV or the 23-valent PPS vaccine given to older adults [39]. This finding demonstrates that sero-replacement can occur owing to immunologic pressure from vaccine use. The immune pressure created by the vaccine may provide a competitive advantage for those serotypes not contained in the vaccine. Often, these strains are somewhat less virulent and less likely to cause disease in healthy adults but are still likely to cause illness in debilitated hosts with multiple co-morbidities. Despite this finding, there has been a clear benefit for older adults by the practice of immunizing children for pneumococcal disease (Fig. 7).

A similar benefit with regard to influenza vaccine has been suggested by several studies [40]. A recent modeling study suggests that influenza

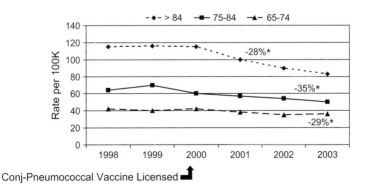

Fig. 7. Effect of use of the CPV on IPD rates in older adults aged 65 to 74, 75 to 84, or 85 years and over. Rates have fallen significantly in all three age groups over the period shown temporally associated with licensing of the CPV in children. (*Data from* Dexter PR, Perkins SM, Maharry KS, et al. Inpatient computer-based standing orders vs physician reminders to increase influenza and pneumococcal vaccination rates: a randomized trial. JAMA 2004;292(19):2366–71.)

vaccine coverage rates of 20% in children aged 6 months to 18 years could reduce influenza hospitalization and death by half (Fig. 8). This concept is further supported by a recent study in Russia in which one town in which school-aged children received mass immunization was compared with another town where immunization was not provided. Mass immunization in children resulted in greatly reduced rates of chronic disease exacerbation in adults (Table 3) [41]. As a comparator, rates in each town during the summer months (ie, not during influenza season) were evaluated and found to be similar. Influenza and pneumococcal vaccine use in children appears to decrease the risk of disease and complications of disease in older adults.

The immunization of children may also potentially lead to increased rates of illness in adults for some diseases. It is likely that many (most) adults were re-exposed to varicella virus via their children before widespread use of the varicella vaccine. This early/mid-adult exposure likely boosts immunity to varicella zoster virus, delaying the time to zoster occurrence. Adults who have lived in a household with young children experience an average zoster onset about 10 years later than adults who have never lived in a household with young children [42]. As varicella vaccine has been more commonly administered to children, the rate of varicella in the community has dropped dramatically. This decrease has been studied in observational data from Massachusetts. Varicella rates in children aged less than 20 years have dropped from 85% to less than 20% as varicella vaccine coverage rates have climbed above 90%. This decrease in childhood illness has been accompanied by a doubling in zoster incidence rates in adults [43]. For a disease such as zoster, immunization of children may decrease natural immunologic "boosting" of adults, resulting in increased rates of disease.

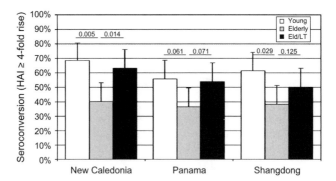

Fig. 8. Percent of young or elderly subjects who demonstrated a fourfold rise in hemagglutinin antibody titer after influenza immunization in young adults, and older adults immunized alone or immunized and treated with an *E coli* heat-labile toxin (LT) immunostimulant patch. (*Reprinted from* Frech SA, Kenney RT, Spyr CA, et al. Improved immune responses to influenza vaccination in the elderly using an immunostimulant patch. Vaccine 2005;23:948; with permission.)

Table 3
Relative risk (RR) and statistical significance of disease exacerbation in adults aged 60 years
and over in a Russian town in which school-aged children did not receive mass influenza immunization compared with disease rates in a similar town in which children were mass immunized

Disease	ILI	PNA	Asthma	COPD	CVD	DM
RR (winter)	3.4 (P<.01)	2.6 (P<.01)	2.6 (P<.01)	1.7 (P<.01)	3.4 (P<.01)	2.3 (P<.01)
RR (summer)	None	1	1	1	1.4 (P<.01)	1

Abbreviations: COPD, chronic obstructive pulmonary disease; CVD, cardiovascular disease;
DM, diabetes mellitus; ILI, influenza-like illness; PNA, pneumonia.
Data from Ghendon YZ, Kaira AN, Elshina GA. The effect of mass influenza immunization
in children on the morbidity of the unvaccinated elderly. Epidemiol Infect 2006;134(1):71–8.

Future promise for enhancing vaccine efficacy in older adults

Increased antigen dose

As stated previously, the causes for age-related declines in vaccine efficacy
have not been well defined at the basic level, but clinical observations suggest there may be some benefit to simply giving more antigen. The typical
influenza vaccine delivers 15 μg of each of three antigens. In a recent study
in older adults, increasing the dose to 60 μg/antigen improved neutralizing
antibody 54% to 79% for the three components of the vaccine [44]. In another study using baculovirus to produce antigen [45], increasing the dose to
even greater levels (135 μg of each antigen) increased hemagglutinin inhibition antibody titers almost fivefold. There were more local reactions in both
studies using higher antigen doses, but, overall, the vaccines were well tolerated. Although it might seem prudent to move forward with this strategy, it
would mean essentially quadrupling the influenza vaccine supply, which has
been stressed even to produce current levels, or would require a change to
mass production of specific proteins through different manufacturing processes and affect all of the toxicity and efficacy studies that would need to
follow. Certainly, this strategy deserves consideration for the future.

Conjugated vaccines

Conjugating polysaccharide to protein antigens has greatly enhanced the efficacy of pneumococcal and meningococcal vaccines in children. Although their
immune deficits clearly differ, could the same strategy work in older adults?
There are few studies of conjugated polysaccharide vaccines in older adults
[46–49], and most have enrolled relatively few subjects. Overall, there has
been little advantage over unconjugated polysaccharide vaccines in older adults.

Toll-like receptor adjuvants

Perhaps the most important development in vaccine basic science in the
last decade has been the realization that innate immune responses direct
the type and strength of the adaptive immune response. Toll-like receptors

---

Box 1. Toll-like receptors (TLR) and TLR-based adjuvants in development for specific vaccines [50,51]

TLR2
Heat-labile enterotoxin of *E coli*

TLR4
Monophosphoryl lipid A (MPL)
• Melanoma
AS02 (MPL + saponin QS-21)
• Malaria, hepatitis B, human papilloma virus, human immunodeficiency virus, cancers, *Mycobacterium tuberculosis*
AS04 (MPL + alum)
• Hepatitis B
RC-529 (MPL derivative)
• Hepatitis B

TLR9
CpG oligonucleotides
• Hepatitis B, influenza

Other TLR/ligands of interest and their primary agonists
TLR5–Flagellin
TLR7/8–Imidazoquinolines
TLR3–Poly I:C
TLR6-2, 6-1–Zymosan, lipoteichoic acid, peptidoglycan

(TLRs) recognize microbial substances and lead to the production of critical cytokines and the expression of co-stimulatory molecules on antigen-presenting cells. TLR agonists are being actively investigated as adjuvants (Box 1) [50,51]. A full review of this technology is beyond the scope of this article, and there are few data in older adults; however, as an example, one recent study investigated a TLR2 agonist, *Escherichia coli* heat-labile toxin, which was applied to the site of influenza immunization as a patch over the immunization site [52]. The older adults treated with the immunostimulant patch mounted serologic responses that were similar to those in young adults and significantly better than those in older adults who were not treated with the patch (Fig. 8). This study demonstrates the potential of TLR agonists to enhance vaccine responses even in older adults in whom immune senescence renders many vaccines less effective.

Summary

Although there are limitations of vaccine effectiveness in older adults, there remains strong evidence that PPS, influenza, and zoster vaccines significantly reduce the risk of severe disease and are cost-effective (or even cost-saving) in older adults when compared with many other preventive interventions. Standing orders remain the most important strategy for improving vaccine uptake in older adults, and provider support is essential to patient acceptance. Immunization of children, the vector through which many older adults acquire vaccine-preventable illnesses, may have an even bigger public health impact on disease in older adults than improved vaccine uptake in the aged. Increasing antigen dose or using new adjuvants such as TLR agonists holds promise for enhancing vaccine efficacy in older adults in the future.

References

[1] Available at: http://www.cdc.gov/nip/recs/adult-schedule.pdf. Accessed January 1, 2007.
[2] ACIP. Prevention and control of influenza. MMWR Morb Mortal Wkly Rep 2005; 54(RR08):1–40.
[3] Available at: http://www2.cdc.gov/nip/schoolsurv/nationalAvg.asp. Accessed January 1, 2007.
[4] Cornu C, Yzebe D, Leophonte P, et al. Efficacy of pneumococcal polysaccharide vaccine in immunocompetent adults: a meta-analysis of randomized trials. Vaccine 2001;19: 4780–90.
[5] CDC. Adult immunization: knowledge, attitudes, and practices—DeKalb and Fulton Counties, Georgia, 1988. MMWR 1988;37(43):657–61.
[6] Sjogren MH. Prevention of hepatitis B in nonresponders to initial hepatitis B virus vaccination. Am J Med 2005;118:34S–9S.
[7] Fisman D, Agrawal D, Leder K. The effect of age on immunologic response to recombinant hepatitis B vaccine: a meta-analysis. Clin Infect Dis 2002;35:1368–75.
[8] Wolters B, Junge U, Dzuiba S, et al. Immunogenicity of combined hepatitis A and B vaccine in elderly persons. Vaccine 2003;21:3623–8.
[9] Shapiro ED, Berg AT, Austrian R, et al. The protective efficacy of polyvalent pneumococcal polysaccharide vaccine. N Engl J Med 1991;325:1453–60.
[10] Butler JC, Breiman RF, Campbell JF, et al. Pneumococcal polysaccharide vaccine efficacy: an evaluation of current recommendations. JAMA 1993;270:1826–31.
[11] Jackson LA, Neuzil KM, Yu O, et al. Effectiveness of pneumococcal polysaccharide vaccine in older adults. N Engl J Med 2003;348:1747–55.
[12] Dominiquez A, Salleras L, Fedson DS, et al. Effectiveness of pneumococcal vaccination for elderly people in Catalonia, Spain: a case-control study. Clin Infect Dis 2005;40: 1250–7.
[13] Nichol K, Nordin J, Mulolly J, et al. Influenza vaccination and reduction in hospitalizations for cardiac disease and stroke among the elderly. N Engl J Med 2003;348:1322–32.
[14] Looijmans-Van den Akker I, Verheij TJ, Buskens E, et al. Clinical effectiveness of first and repeat influenza vaccination in adult and elderly diabetic patients. Diabetes Care 2006;29: 1771–6.
[15] Available at: http://www.cdc.gov/mmwr/preview/mmwrhtml/rr5515a1.htm. Accessed January 8, 2007.
[16] Poland GA, Borrud A, Jacobson RM, et al. Determination of deltoid fat pad thickness: implications for needle length in adult immunization. JAMA 1997;277:1709–11.
[17] Cook IF, Williamson M, Pond D. Definition of needle length required for intramuscular deltoid injection in elderly adults: an ultrasonographic study. Vaccine 2006;24:937–40.
[18] ACIP, Andrew T, Kroger AT, et al. General recommendations on immunization. MMWR 2006;55(RR15):1–48.

[19] Vila-Corcoles A, Ochoa-Gonder O, Hospital I, et al. Protective effects of the 23-valent pneumococcal polysaccharide vaccine in the elderly population: the EVAN-65 study. Clin Infect Dis 2006;43:860-8.

[20] Fisman D, Abrutyn E, Spaude KA, et al. Prior pneumococcal vaccination is associated with reduced death, complications, and length of stay among hospitalized adults with community-acquired pneumonia. Clin Infect Dis 2006;42:1093-101.

[21] Fry AM, Zell ER, Schuchat A, et al. Comparing potential benefits of new pneumococcal vaccines with the current polysaccharide vaccine in the elderly. Vaccine 2002;21:303-11.

[22] Sisk JE, Moskowitz AJ, Whang W, et al. Cost-effectiveness of vaccination against pneumococcal bacteremia among elderly people. JAMA 1997;278:1333-9 [erratum in: JAMA 2000;283:341].

[23] Kelly H, Attia J, Andrews R, et al. The number needed to vaccinate (NNV) and population extensions of the NNV: comparison of influenza and pneumococcal vaccine programmes for people aged 65 years and over. Vaccine 2004;22(17-18):2192-8.

[24] McCormack O, Meza J, Martin S, et al. Clinical inquiries. Is pneumococcal vaccine effective in nursing home patients? J Fam Pract 2003;52:150,152,154.

[25] Loeb M, Stevenson KB, for the SHEA Long-Term-Care Committee. Pneumococcal immunization in older adults: implications for the long-term-care setting. Infect Control Hosp Epidemiol 2004;25:985-94.

[26] Gaillet J, Zmirou D, Mallaret MR, et al. Essai clinique du vaccin antipneumococcoique chez des personnees agees vivant en institution [French]. [Clinical trial of an antipneumococcal vaccine in elderly subjects living in institutions]. Rev Epidemiol Sante Publique 1985;33: 437-44.

[27] CDC. Outbreak of pneumococcal pneumonia among unvaccinated residents of a nursing home–New Jersey. MMWR 2001;50:707-10.

[28] Advisory Committee on Immunization Practices, Smith NM, Bresee JS, et al. Prevention and control of influenza: recommendations of the advisory committee on immunization practices (ACIP). MMWR Recomm Rep 2006;55(RR-10):1-42 [erratum in: MMWR Morb Mortal Wkly Rep 2006;55(29):800].

[29] McElhaney JE, Nichol KL. Influenza vaccines: crossing the transitional gap to improve outcomes in the elderly. Aging Health 2005;1:167-77.

[30] Voordouw AC, Sturkenboom MD, Dieleman JP, et al. Annual revaccination against influenza and mortality risk in community-dwelling elderly persons. JAMA 2004;292: 2089-95.

[31] Simonsen L, Reichert TA, Viboud C, et al. Impact of influenza vaccination on seasonal mortality in the US elderly population. Arch Intern Med 2005;165:265-72.

[32] Jackson LA, Jackson ML, Nelson JC, et al. Evidence of bias in estimates of influenza vaccine effectiveness in seniors. Int J Epidemiol 2006;35:337-44.

[33] Mullooly JP, Bennett MD, Hornbrook MC, et al. Influenza vaccination programs for elderly persons: cost-effectiveness in a health maintenance organization. Ann Intern Med 1994;121: 947-52.

[34] Nichol KL, Wuorenma J, von Sternberg T. Benefits of influenza vaccination for low-, intermediate-, and high-risk senior citizens. Arch Intern Med 1998;158:1769-76.

[35] Riddiough MA, Sisk JE, Bell JC. Influenza vaccination. JAMA 1983;249:3189-95.

[36] Available at: http://www.cdc.gov/nip/recs/provisional_recs/zoster-11-20-06.pdf. Accessed January 17, 2007.

[37] Coyle CM, Currie BP. Improving the rates of inpatient pneumococcal vaccination: impact of standing orders versus computerized reminders to physicians. Infect Control Hosp Epidemiol 2004;25(11):904-7.

[38] Dexter PR, Perkins SM, Maharry KS, et al. Inpatient computer-based standing orders vs physician reminders to increase influenza and pneumococcal vaccination rates: a randomized trial. JAMA 2004;292(19):2366-71.

[39] Lexau CA, Lynfield R, Danila R, et al. Changing epidemiology of invasive pneumococcal disease among older adults in the era of pediatric pneumococcal conjugate vaccine. JAMA 2005;294:2043–51.

[40] Weycker D, Edelsberg J, Halloran E, et al. Population-wide benefits of routine vaccination of children against influenza. Vaccine 2005;23:1284–93.

[41] Ghendon YZ, Kaira AN, Elshina GA. The effect of mass influenza immunization in children on the morbidity of the unvaccinated elderly. Epidemiol Infect 2006;134(1):71–8.

[42] Brisson M, Gay NJ, Edmunds WJ, et al. Exposure to varicella boosts immunity to herpes-zoster: implications for mass vaccination against chickenpox. Vaccine 2002;20:2500–7.

[43] Yih WK, Brooks DR, Lett SM, et al. The incidence of varicella and herpes zoster in Massachusetts as measured by the behavioral risk factor surveillance system (BRFSS) during a period of increasing varicella vaccine coverage, 1998–2003. BMC Public Health 2005;5:68.

[44] Keitel WA, Atmar RL, Cate TR, et al. Safety of high doses of influenza vaccine and effect on antibody responses in elderly persons. Arch Intern Med 2006;166:1121–7.

[45] Treanor JJ, Schiff GM, Couch RB, et al. Dose-related safety and immunogenicity of a trivalent baculovirus-expressed influenza-virus hemagglutinin vaccine in elderly adults. J Infect Dis 2006;193:1223–8.

[46] Shelly MA, Jacoby H, Riley GJ, et al. Comparison of pneumococcal polysaccharide and CRM197-conjugated pneumococcal oligosaccharide vaccines in young and elderly adults. Infect Immun 1997;65(1):242–7.

[47] Gravenstein S, Drinka P, Duthie PH, et al. Efficacy of an influenza hemagglutinin-diphtheria toxoid conjugate vaccine in elderly nursing home subjects during an influenza outbreak. J Am Geriatr Soc 1994;42:245–51.

[48] Kantor E, Luxenburg JS, Lucas AH, et al. Phase I study of the immunogenicity and safety of conjugated *Haemophilus influenzae* type b vaccines in the elderly. Vaccine 1997;15:129–32.

[49] Powers DC, Anderson EL, Lottenbach K, et al. Reactogenicity and immunogenicity of a protein-conjugated pneumococcal oligosaccharide vaccine in older adults. J Infect Dis 1996;173:1014–8.

[50] Wack A, Rappuoli R. Vaccinology at the beginning of the 21st century. Curr Opin Immunol 2005;17:411–8.

[51] Pulendran B. Modulating vaccine responses with dendritic cells and Toll-like receptors. Immunol Rev 2004;199:227–50.

[52] Frech SA, Kenney RT, Spyr CA, et al. Improved immune responses to influenza vaccination in the elderly using an immunostimulant patch. Vaccine 2005;23:946–50.

ELSEVIER
SAUNDERS

Clin Geriatr Med 23 (2007) 687–713

CLINICS IN
GERIATRIC
MEDICINE

Travel Recommendations for Older Adults

Christie M. Reed, MD, MPH

*Travelers' Health Division of Global Migration and Quarantine, Centers for Disease Control
and Prevention, 1600 Clifton Road, MS E-03, Atlanta, GA 30333, USA*

Population-based estimates by age of the number of US residents traveling internationally are limited. According to the US Department of Commerce, 3 million US adults over the age of 65 years (9%) traveled abroad (excluding visits to Canada) in 2004 [1]. Eight million adults (25%) were 55 years or older, the leading edge of the 78 million baby boomers who began turning 60 in 2006 [2]. Nevertheless, for most nations including the United States, the 80 years and older age group is currently growing faster than any younger segment of the older population [3]. Persons aged 85 years and older represented 1.5% of the total US population in 2000. Their proportion is expected to grow to 5% in 2050 while still traveling [4]. Two surveys from US pre-travel clinic sites reported that the proportion of patients aged 65 years and older was 14% at one site, whereas at the other site one third were older than 60 years and 1.5% were older than 80 years [5,6]. The higher proportion of older travelers seen in the pre-travel clinic setting may reflect an increasing incidence of underlying medical conditions with age or increased disposable income, because pre-travel services are frequently not covered by insurance unless the travel is work related and is covered by the employer. Of persons aged 50 to 64 years, 24% to 32% have an underlying medical condition that places them at high risk for complications of influenza [7]. The percentage of US adults who self-rate their health status as fair or poor increases from 14.4% among 45- to 55-year-olds to 33.2% of those aged 75 or more years [8]. The oldest traveler to contact the Centers for Disease Control and Prevention (CDC) Travelers' Health Team in 2006 was aged 99 years.

E-mail address: creed@cdc.gov

0749-0690/07/$ - see front matter © 2007 Elsevier Inc. All rights reserved.
doi:10.1016/j.cger.2007.05.001   *geriatric.theclinics.com*

Who are older adult travelers and why do they travel?

Leisure travel is a frequent long-range goal for persons retired more than 5 years [9]. There are now ski clubs for the crowds aged 50 or more and 70 or more years, and ski boards (equipment that is shorter than the typical skis) are used with an emphasis on speed control [10]. The airline industry has also responded to the financial clout associated with this spending power and the fear of older Americans that they will not be able to travel on their own. Designers are experimenting with improved airplane interiors to make them more comfortable (easier latches, better signs, and roomier well-lit bathrooms) without making the passenger feel old [11]. People of all ages assess their subjective age as different from and usually younger than their chronologic age, and this gap widens as people grow older, with 60% to 75% of adults feeling younger than their chronologic age and more than half feeling 16 to 17 years younger. This subjective feeling is also coupled with a tendency in later years to search for self-fulfilling activities and experiences [12,13]. A total of 15,000 Muslim Americans went on Hajj in 2005 [14]. The entire spectrum of the older population is also better traveled than in prior generations. Family leisure international travel expanded in the 1960s, and the baby boomers backpacked around as students; "been there, done that" is a part of their lexicon. As a result of these economic and social forces, there is a concomitant boom in exotic travel and travel to learn [15–17]. Nevertheless, not all the "denture ventures," "SAGA louts," or "SKIers" (Spending the Kids Inheritance), as they have been referred to, take the luxury option; some older travelers prefer an adult "gap year" [18]. Lonely Planet Publications now has an "Older Travelers" chat room, and travelers aged more than 55 years make up 15% of Thailand's backpacker population compared with a token few only 10 years ago [19]. Other older travelers are either repeating their Peace Corps experience or, with their experience and maturity, being recruited for their "demonstrated ability." Six percent of the volunteers in 2006 were 50 years of age or older [20].

The older adult American traveler may also have been born in another country, often in a developing region of the world, and may be returning to visit friends and relatives. Between 1990 and 2003, the number of foreign-born US residents increased 69% from 19.8 million to 33.5 million, representing approximately 12% of the US population. The proportion of foreign-born residents aged 65 years or older was 11.1%, only slightly less than the 12.1% of the native population [21]. A visit to friends and relatives was listed as the main reason for travel for 46% of all international travelers in 2004 [22]. Travelers returning home to developing areas where travel-related infections are endemic may perceive that these infections do not cause serious illness or may believe that they are immune. Nevertheless, persons visiting friends and relatives experience a higher incidence of travel-related infectious diseases such as malaria, typhoid fever, tuberculosis, and hepatitis

A than do other groups of international travelers [23–28]. Suggested reasons are financial limitations, language barriers, and health beliefs that differ from those in the country of residence, which create barriers to obtaining and adhering to pre-travel health advice [29,30].

General considerations

Any international traveler should be advised to seek care at least 4 to 6 weeks before travel. The key elements to address at that time (Box 1) are the itinerary, duration of travel, style of travel, interval until travel, medical history, medications, allergies, immunocompetence, and age and sex of the traveler. Answers to these questions combined with current information about the risks at the destination are used to tailor specific recommendations regarding prophylactic immunizations, medications, and behaviors before, during, and after travel to decrease the risk of injury or illness.

Older age is an important factor to consider owing not only to physiologic changes and the increased probability of underlying medical conditions and prescription medications but also to immune status with regard to naturally acquired immunity versus immunization for vaccine-preventable diseases. Preparation of an older adult with a complex medical history may involve collaboration between the individual's primary health care and travel medicine providers and may include advice to defer travel or to consider alterations in the itinerary.

Travelers to the developed world (Canada, Western Europe, Japan, Australia, New Zealand) face health risks that are similar, but not identical, to those found in United States. Most deaths of Americans overseas occur in the developed countries of Western Europe where most Americans live or visit, and the patterns of death are similar to those in the United States. Deaths of Americans in less developed countries are not primarily from

---

Box 1. Elements of the pre-travel consultation

General recommendations
Immunizations
Gastrointestinal upset
    Food and water precautions
    Treatment
Avoidance of insect-transmitted diseases
    Insect repellent
    Barriers
    Malaria chemoprophylaxis
Itinerary-specific issues (eg, prevention of other infectious
    diseases, altitude, motion sickness, jet lag, sunburn)

infectious and tropical disease but are from chronic diseases, injuries, suicides, and homicides [31]. Cardiovascular events (including myocardial infarctions and cerebrovascular accidents) account for the majority of deaths (49%) abroad, followed by injuries (25%). Infectious diseases (other than pneumonia) account for 1% of the deaths [32].

General recommendations for travelers

Planning for healthy travel

Health Information for International Travel (The Yellow Book), which is published biennially by the CDC, remains the standard set of recommendations for health maintenance and prevention of illness among US travelers. The full content is available at the CDC Travelers' Health Web site (www.cdc.gov/travel), in addition to travel notices regarding the level of health risk, such as outbreaks of infectious diseases, and prevention information for travelers. All of the sites listed at this address are updated regularly and should be consulted periodically during planning for travel because situations are subject to change. The CDC site hosts a variety of other information for travelers and health care providers in addition to links to most of the sites listed in the following discussion.

Know Before You Go is the title of a US Customs and Border Protection travel brochure regarding regulations that affect returning US travelers. It may be downloaded at their Web site accessed at www.cbp.gov/xp/cgov/travel/. At this site travelers can also check the average wait times at the major airports and border crossings, which can be important when planning for supplemental oxygen or assistance such as wheelchairs. Current updates on departure security measures are available at the TSA Web site accessed at www.tsa.gov/travelers/. Information on what can be carried on board an aircraft in hand luggage and on special screening procedures for persons with disabilities can be found by clicking the hyperlink "What can I bring?" and then "Medications & Special Needs Devices." In general, prescription medications should be in their original containers and should be carried with the traveler, not in checked luggage. The traveler may ask to have these items hand checked. For example, materials such as insulin should not be frozen, and temperatures in the cargo compartment may not be controlled. The label on the prescription should match the passenger's name as it appears on the boarding pass to avoid further questioning. It may be useful to have a letter from the prescribing physician on letterhead, particularly for injectables.

Travelers with special needs, such as diabetics or those with prosthetics, may avoid removing their shoes if they alert the TSA agent but may be subject to additional procedures; therefore, they should allow plenty of time. Travelers should also be aware of regulations at their destinations, particularly regarding controlled substances such as pain medications, and should check with the embassy of their destination country to make sure any required medications are not considered illegal narcotics. The US Department of State has a valuable Web site for travelers (http://travel.state.gov) that contains information about visa requirements and security at the destination, as well as a link where travelers may register with the destination embassy or consulate or determine if their tour group has been registered. Travelers are reminded that, although the consulate can assist in locating health care abroad and notifying relatives at home, the fiscal responsibilities are those of the traveler. Travelers should check their medical insurance regarding coverage and should consider purchasing trip cancellation, supplemental medical, and medical evacuation coverage.

Travel Health Online (www.tripprep.com/scripts) provides a list of medical providers around the world. Travelers may also locate travel medicine clinics at the destination by consulting the Web site of the International Travel Medicine Society (http://www.istm.org). The traveler with an underlying medical condition should identify a possible source of care at the destination before travel. The International Association for Medical Assistance to Travelers (www.iamat.org) is a nonprofit organization established to, among other things, "make competent medical care available to travelers by western-trained doctors who speak English besides their mother tongue."

Supplemental oxygen

Travelers are in general responsible for their own arrangements throughout the travel experience and are not allowed to bring their own oxygen canisters on board an airplane. Arrangements are airline dependent in that some use an external supplier and some allow personal oxygen concentrators. Travelers should make these arrangements at least 48 to 72 hours before the flight. The Access-able Travel Source (www.access-able.com/tips/) provides information and resources for mature travelers and those with special needs, including traveling with oxygen.

Travel health kit

In addition to any prescription medications, travelers should prepare a travel health kit including any over-the-counter medications or supplies needed to treat minor health problems. A variety of kits can be found at commercial outfitters or online, but a kit can also be assembled at home (discussed in Chapter 3 of the publication *Health Information for International Travel* available in hard copy or online at www.cdc.gov/travel). A traveler with any pre-existing medical problems should carry a letter from his or her attending physician on letterhead describing the medical condition and any prescription medications, including the generic name of prescribed drugs. Travelers may also consider carrying copies of pertinent medical records such as a recent EKG and the contact information for their health care provider who manages the condition in question, an extra pair of glasses and a copy of the prescription, and any specific medications for the trip. Travelers are discouraged from purchasing over-the-counter or prescription medications abroad because they are not subject to the same controls as in the United States, and in many parts of the world there are concerns about counterfeit medications [33]. Travelers with diabetes should estimate the supply of insulin, syringes, test strips, insulin pens and cartridges, lancets, and alcohol wipes that will be needed and then bring twice the amount [34]. They should also include any other supplies such as glucagon, a sharps container, and glucose tablets and plan to wear a medical identification bracelet. Diabetic travelers should consider joining the American Diabetes Association if they have not already done so to take full advantage of their informative Web site and resources (accessible online at www.diabetes.org or by phone at 800-806-7801).

Injuries and accidents

According to US State Department data, road traffic crashes are the leading cause of injury death for US citizens while traveling internationally (34%), followed by homicide (17%) and drowning (13%). Approximately 13% of these road traffic deaths involve motorcycles, and 7% of victims are pedestrians. A study from Bermuda reported that tourists sustained a much higher rate of motorbike injuries than the local population; the highest rate (126.7 events per 1000 person years) was in persons aged 50 to 59 years, with a relative risk of 17 when compared with the local population of the same age. Loss of vehicular control, unfamiliar equipment, and inexperience with motorized two-wheelers contributed to crashes and injuries, even for travel at speeds less than 30 mph [35,36]. Road traffic crashes are also a leading cause of nonfatal injury among US citizens requiring emergency transport back to the United States [37]. Travelers should be alert when crossing the street, looking right, left, and then right again, and should follow the advice they would at home (ie, wear seat belts and helmets, avoid excessive alcohol, and consider hiring a driver familiar with the city and expert in maneuvering through local traffic). The Association for International Road Travel (www.asirt.org) has useful safety information for international travelers, including road safety checklists and country-specific driving risks.

Medical considerations

Underlying medical conditions and international travel

There is a trend toward lengthened intercontinental flight sectors, with the long-range variant of the Boeing 777 and Airbus 380 reportedly able to operate on 20-hour sectors. The US Federal Aviation Authority requires cabin pressure to be maintained no lower than the air pressure equivalent to an altitude of 8000 ft above mean sea level. All current guidelines reflect uncertainty in relation to the clinical circumstances when oxygen prescription during flight is essential; additional studies are in progress [38]. Cardiac, respiratory, and anemic patients should be evaluated, particularly if other comorbidities are present [39–41]. There are few recent data on the number of onboard medical incidents, but estimates from individual surveys have been low (eg, 0.1 to 0.3 deaths per million passengers year) [42,43]. The most common causes for the medical diversion of a flight are cardiac (28%), neurologic (20%), and gastrointestinal (20%) in origin [44,45]. Screening of elderly patients with memory or cognitive deficits may be warranted, because those with early dementia may be more prone to develop delirium in flight, particularly when combined with dehydration, alcohol, or the use of sleep aids (such as zolpidem) [46]. Preflight evaluation may lead to a recommendation that certain individuals be accompanied by a qualified escort [39].

Physicians or health educators should review with their patients and significant others any alterations to the existing maintenance plan that may be needed in association with travel, such as any modifications to medication dosing, particularly on the day of travel. For diabetics, travel over more than four to five time zones may require increases (traveling west) or decreases (traveling east) in insulin (http://ndep.nih.gov/diabetes/pubs/Diabetes_travel_article.pdf), just as decreased activity may require more insulin and increased activity may require less. The use of short-acting insulin that can be taken when meals are actually served is of great benefit; hypoglycemia was the main problem reported in a survey of Scottish travelers who used insulin [47]. Diabetic travelers should be reminded of the importance of well-fitting shoes and foot care, of the need to have medical insurance and to identify sources of health care in advance, and of the need to follow-up on any departure from the norm, such as the symptoms of a urinary tract infection or any soft-tissue wound [48].

Jet lag, motion sickness, and mental alertness

Older travelers do not differ from their younger counterparts in that they suffer more from phase advance (eastward travel) than from phase delay (westward travel) [49–52]. Phase advance is usually associated with truncated sleep, and there is some evidence that recovery from sleep deprivation takes longer in the elderly than in the young [53]. The baseline sleep hygiene of older persons (eg, early bedtime, sleeping more than 7 to 8 hours a night) may also contribute [54]. Although no results from rigorous studies of the safety or dosage of melatonin are available, limited evidence suggests that melatonin is safe and well tolerated. Doses of 0.5 to 5 mg may promote sleep and decrease jet lag symptoms in travelers crossing five or more time zones [55–57].

Motion sickness related to air flight can be minimized by flying at night, by sitting in a reclining position, by sitting away from the engines and over the wings near the center of gravity, or, if flying during daylight hours, by sitting near a window and focusing on the horizon to reduce vestibular stimulation [41–46]. Patients should be advised that medications for motion sickness, such as antihistamines, related to any form of travel should be taken with caution due to their sedating and anticholenergic effects, particularly in the elderly, who may be subject to urinary retention [46].

Air terminal stress has been described as the physical and mental stress the traveler encounters at the airport [58]. Flight delays, customs, baggage reclaim, and take off and landing were identified as stressors before the changes associated with 9/11 [59]. Expression of the psychologic stress on board the aircraft has been termed *air rage*, and reports from the airline industry indicate about 5000 episodes per year [60]. Also, there is an increasing trend toward self-direction and responsibility as ticket counters are replaced by kiosks, and passengers must frequently check the monitors for departure gate changes. Many of the potential sources of stress (eg, filling in forms, checking in at the correct gate, and locating the correct departure gate) may be exacerbated by poor eyesight, hearing impairments, and other disabilities in a crowded and noisy environment such as an airport [46].

Deep vein thrombosis, pulmonary embolism, and travel

Immobilization of the extremities, inherited abnormalities in components of the coagulation system, acquired conditions (eg, antiphospholipid syndrome and systemic lupus erythematosus), the use of oral contraceptives and hormone replacement therapy, pregnancy, cancer, recent surgery, increased age, obesity, and a history of previous blood clots are factors that increase the risk for deep vein thrombosis and pulmonary embolism. Travel by motor vehicle, train, and plane can be associated with periods of prolonged immobility. There are conflicting reports as to whether travel by air exacerbates the propensity to form clots, and there are no convincing data to suggest that using aspirin as a preventive measure before the immobility associated with travel will prevent abnormal clotting and pulmonary embolism [61]. The use of below-knee graduated compression stockings has been shown to reduce lower leg edema and the development of symptomless deep vein thrombosis [62]. Compression stockings may be prescribed or purchased online at sites such as www.travelsox.com/. All travelers should be advised to wear loose-fitting clothing, to make efforts to walk and stretch the legs and arms at regular intervals, and to stay hydrated as appropriate to their medical condition. Travelers with any of the risk factors for deep vein thrombosis and pulmonary embolism described previously should be advised to consult with their health care provider and may be advised to use prophylactic anticoagulant medication, such as low molecular weight heparin, during travel.

Immunizations

Routine. All travelers should be up to date on their routine immunizations (Box 2). Some adults incorrectly assume that the vaccines they received as

---

Box 2. Immunizations to consider

Routine
Influenza*
Diphtheria*
Pertussis*
Tetanus*
Measles-mumps-rubella*
Pneumococcal pneumonia*
Varicella*

Travel-related
Hepatitis A*
Hepatitis B*
Japanese encephalitis*
Meningococcal disease
Polio
Rabies*
Typhoid*
Yellow fever

---

* May require multiple doses.

---

children will protect them for the rest of their lives. Generally this is true, except for the following:

Some adults were never vaccinated as children.
Newer vaccines were not available when some adults were children.
Immunity can begin to fade over time.
As we age, we become more susceptible to serious disease caused by common infections (eg, flu, pneumococcus).

The CDC Adult Vaccine Preventable Diseases Web site page offers the adult vaccination schedule (www.cdc.gov/nip/recs/adult-schedule.htm) and is updated every year.

Although measles has been eliminated from the United States, immunization practices vary worldwide. In the last 2 years, there have been outbreaks of measles in many parts of the world, including Europe [63]. Adults born before 1957 can be considered immune to measles; however, adults born during 1957 (who will turn 50 this year) or afterward will need to be evaluated and may be asked to show proof of immunity by other countries attempting to control outbreaks [63,64]. Adults born before 1957 may also be considered to be immune to mumps but not rubella, and there have been recent international outbreaks of both [65]. There are no published data regarding the immunogenicity, protective efficacy, or side effects of measles-mumps-rubella vaccines in elderly recipients [66].

Diphtheria also poses a risk, sometimes fatal, to international travelers, particularly the elderly, who may either have waning or incomplete immunity [67–69]. The percentage of the US population with protective levels of antibody to diphtheria declines with increasing age to only 30% among men aged 60 to 69 years and even lower among women [70]. Even in developed countries, tetanus is primarily a disease of the elderly [71,72], and the pattern of protective antibody levels is similar. Levels decline to 45% in men at age 70 years, but the sex discrepancy is greater, with rates of only 21% among women in that age group. Although routine vaccination against tetanus and diphtheria began in the 1940s, the higher rate of cases of tetanus in the elderly and the lower level of protective antibody are thought to be related to the higher proportion of older adults, especially women, who have never received a primary series [70]. Vaccination during military service is thought to be one explanation for the higher rates in men; elderly persons who did not serve in the US military are unlikely to have been vaccinated during childhood and may be unprotected [73]. The Advisory Committee on Immunization Practices (ACIP) has recommended that adults receive a booster dose of tetanus toxoid-containing (Td) vaccine every 10 years or as indicated for wound care, and that adults with an uncertain history of primary vaccination receive a three-dose primary series with adult Td [74]. Pain at the site of injection and fatigue are the most commonly reported symptoms following booster vaccination against Td in all age groups, including those aged over 40 years, with a tendency toward higher rates if the interval since last vaccination was less than 10 years [75].

Waning immunity to pertussis, the widespread presence of the causative bacteria associated with community-wide outbreaks, and prolonged morbidity due to cough, which is of particular concern in the elderly population in whom it can rarely be associated with death, led to the 2006 recommendation by the ACIP that at least one decennial booster include acellular pertussis [74]. Nevertheless, the vaccine is only licensed for persons aged 11 to 64 years. To achieve protection in the older population, physicians need to be aware of and vaccinate vulnerable populations in middle age.

Td vaccine for elderly travelers is not only an opportunity to reach this vulnerable population with routine vaccination but is also important in preventing the possibility of unsafe injection practices abroad which may occur following acute injury. In many parts of the world, injections are still given with nonsterile equipment [76]. This practice raises concern not only about tetanus but also hepatitis B (HBV), hepatitis C, HIV, and even malaria or other blood-borne infections, particularly if the injection is associated with transfusion. Eight percent of travelers seek medical care while abroad, and 17% of those receive injections [5]. Twenty-four percent of travelers have baseline indications for HBV vaccine, and 8% report high-risk exposures during travel (higher risk in those aged <40 years), but only one third of travelers are vaccinated appropriately [77]. Hepatitis B vaccine should be considered based on the itinerary, the type of travel, and the frequency of travel, in addition to personal risk activities such as the likelihood of unprotected sex, especially in areas of high HBV prevalence. Arrest records reveal that older male travelers are among the most frequent patrons of commercial sex workers [78].

The most common vaccine-preventable disease in travelers to tropical or subtropical regions is influenza, and risk exists year round [79–85]. Influenza is a significant cause of morbidity in the elderly, yet US annual vaccination rates for persons aged 65 years or older were only 63.3% in 2005, similar to the rate of 63.7% for pneumococcal vaccine coverage [86]. Although the primary focus of influenza vaccine campaigns has been in the fall in the Northern Hemisphere, the vaccine does not expire until June and in many cases has significant crossover with the predominant Southern Hemisphere influenza viruses during that winter (April to October). Several summer outbreaks of influenza have occurred on cruises in both the Northern and Southern Hemispheres [87–91], prompting current recommendations for vaccination not only of persons aged 65 years and older but also for travel to the tropics, travel with organized tourist groups at any time of year, or travel to the Southern Hemisphere during April to September [92,93].

Hepatitis A virus (HAV) is also a common cause of vaccine-preventable morbidity in travelers. The risk among persons who do not receive immune globulin or vaccine before departure has been estimated to be 4 to 30 cases per 100,000 months of stay in developing countries [94]. Complications including death occur more frequently in populations older than 40 years [95]. Individuals over 40 years of age have been thought to have high levels of acquired immunity through prior infection; however, the Third National Health and Nutrition Examination Survey (NHANES-III) conducted during 1988 to 1994 showed that the rate of HAV seropositivity decreased significantly with age from 75% among those aged greater than 70 years to 33% for persons aged 40 to 49 years. The seroprevalence rate was lowest among non-Hispanic whites in all adult age groups, reaching only 37% among 50- to 59-year-olds. Since the completion of NHANES-III in 1994, HAV vaccination of children has become the norm in the United States, with a concomitant decline in the incidence of disease in the entire population [96]. Increasing segments of the adult population will not have natural immunity or immunity associated with childhood vaccines for several decades and will remain vulnerable, and the risk appears to be increased even among travelers who reported observing protective measures and staying in urban areas or luxury hotels (CDC, unpublished data, 2005). Mexican Americans and persons born outside the United States had a 3.0- and 2.7-fold higher age-adjusted prevalence in NHANES, respectively, when compared with persons born in the United States; therefore, it may be cost-effective to screen persons born outside the United States for serologic evidence of protection when considering vaccination for travel [97].

The antibody response to HAV after vaccination tends to be slower in older people, with significantly lower titers after the first dose; however, the clinical significance is unclear, because titers still exceed those required for seroprotection [66]. In another study, seroprotection after a booster dose in the population over 50 years of age reached 98% [98]. Hepatitis A has a long incubation period, and there have been no confirmed reports of infection after HAV vaccination in elderly people [99]. The response to a combined HA/BV vaccine appears to be as immunogenic as either monovalent vaccine [100]. In a trial comparing a combined HA/BV vaccine with HBV alone in a population that included persons through 80 years of age, the immune response to HBV in the combined vaccine appeared to be less influenced by age [101].

Aging appears to be associated with a reduced response to vaccines, described as immunosenescence. It has been postulated that this observation is associated with thymic atrophy, with resultant decreased output of naïve T cells and their associated cytokines as the most important factor [102–104]. The role of chronic mild inflammation in the elderly, as evidenced by mild increased levels of acute-phase reactants and the deregulation of cytokine production after vaccination, has also been proposed to affect the activation of lymphocytes by antigen-presenting cells of the monocyte/macrophage system [105]. In booster studies of tetanus, diphtheria, pertussis, and polio vaccines, immune responses to all antigens in terms of antibody titers tended to be lower in subjects aged more than 40 years but protective; serologic status before vaccination was also significant and was related to the time since last vaccination for diphtheria and tetanus. In this study, almost 70% of subjects aged more than 40 years were seronegative for diphtheria at baseline despite a history of prior vaccination, and 20% remained unprotected 1 month after the booster. Conversely, the incidence of both local and systemic post-vaccination symptoms was lower for the over-40 age group across all vaccine groups [75,106].

The anamnestic response seems to be intact in older travelers who may need to have a booster dose to some inactivated vaccines [66], such as HAV [98] and diphtheria [75], sooner to achieve protective levels before travel and then may require reboosting. These recommendations are all areas of research, but they have specific implications for vaccine strategies for the older traveler with an incomplete vaccination history. Travelers should be encouraged to schedule a pre-travel consultation 4 to 6 weeks before travel in the event that multiple doses are needed.

The route of delivery is also important. For adults and adolescents, the deltoid muscle is recommended for routine intramuscular vaccinations. The anterolateral thigh also can be used. For men and women weighing less than 130 lbs (<60 kg), a 5/8- to 1-inch needle is sufficient to ensure intramuscular injection. For women weighing 130 to 200 lbs (60–90 kg) and men 130 to 260 lbs (60–118 kg), a 1- to 1.5-inch needle is needed. For women weighing more than 200 lbs (>90 kg) or men weighing more than 260 lbs

(> 118 kg), a 1.5-inch needle is required [107]. Although there is general loss of muscle mass with increasing age, the body mass index has been increasing over the last 5 decades. Health care professionals delivering intramuscular and subcutaneous vaccines to the elderly should make sure that the correct needle length is used to ensure delivery to the correct tissue space [108,109].

Travel specific. Eradication efforts have dramatically reduced the number of countries where travelers are at risk for polio. As of January 2007, these areas included Africa, South Asia, Southeast Asia, and the Middle East. For current information on the status of polio eradication efforts and vaccine recommendations, one should consult the CDC travel notices at www.cdc.gov/travel or the Global Polio Eradication Initiative (www.polioeradiation.org). Vaccination is recommended for all travelers to polio-endemic or epidemic areas. Unvaccinated adults who are at increased risk should receive a primary vaccination series with inactivated polio vaccine. Adult travelers without documentation of vaccination status should be considered unvaccinated. If three doses of inactivated polio vaccine cannot be administered within the recommended intervals before protection is needed, an accelerated schedule is suggested. Travelers who have had a primary series of oral polio vaccine or inactivated polio vaccine can receive another dose of inactivated polio vaccine. Available data do not indicate the need for more than a single lifetime booster dose for adults [109].

Rabies vaccination might be considered pre-travel in certain situations, such as possible occupational exposure, but would be considered as part of post-exposure management of an animal bite in much of the world. There are a limited number of studies in which the age of the recipient has been compared or in which the age was greater than 50 or 60 years. Although antibody levels are discussed in relation to vaccination, they are imperfect measures of protection. In two prospective studies, titers post vaccination were lower in older groups, but participants of all ages developed protective titers [66]. In a subsequent study of antibody titers in persons seen at a travel clinic in Nepal who had been previously vaccinated in 14 different countries, all but one had acceptable titers, and there was no statistically significant association with age, although the oldest person was only 60 years [110]. Similar results were found in an Australian study that included persons aged 9 to 74 years and that used an intradermal route of injection instead of the usual intramuscular route [111]. Intradermal injections may be difficult in elderly patients, and this route is not recommended for post-exposure therapy.

Similarly, travelers are generally considered to be at low risk for Japanese encephalitis unless they will be staying for prolonged periods in rural areas. The currently available (in the United States) Japanese encephalitis vaccine is inactivated and derived from mouse brain. As is true for rabies, it is unclear how the antibody level relates to protection, and few studies have included elderly individuals, particularly in areas of non-endemicity. In a study by Nothdurft and colleagues [112], 54% of the vaccinees (which

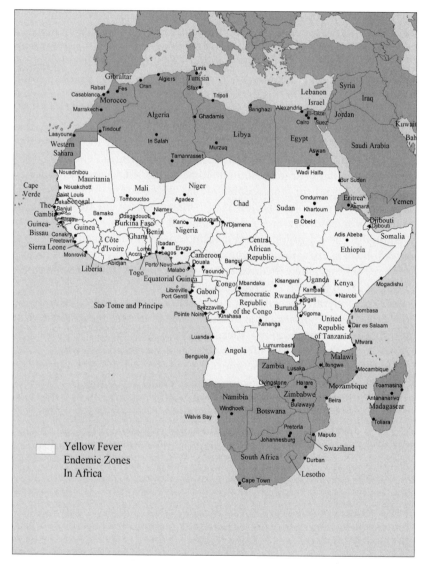

Fig. 1. Yellow fever–endemic zones in Africa, 2007. (Source: *Health Information for International Travel*, 2008. Available at: www.cdc.gov/travel.)

included persons to age 72 years) reported mild constitutional side effects such as mild-to-moderate edema at the injection site similar to that seen with HAV. There were none of the serious anaphylactic side effects that have been reported in some travelers.

Although rare, most typhoid cases in the United States are related to travel, primarily involving the Indian subcontinent [28] Infection does not induce immunity, and there is no clear immunologic response that correlates with protection after vaccination. Two forms of vaccine are available in the United States—the purified polysaccharide and the oral live attenuated Ty21. Most efficacy studies have been done in young populations in endemic countries [66]. Mortality due to *Salmonella typhi* is higher in persons aged more than 50 years when compared with persons younger than 50 years; therefore, vaccine is recommended for adults traveling to areas of the world where typhoid is endemic, even for short trips [28].

Meningococcal vaccination is recommended for persons traveling to sub-Saharan Africa ("the meningitis belt") during the dry season (December to June). Vaccination is also required by the government of Saudi Arabia for all travelers to Mecca during the annual Hajj. Two vaccines are available—a polysaccharide form and a conjugate. The conjugate is not licensed for persons aged older than 55 years [113]. In their review of travel vaccinations in the elderly, Leder and colleagues [66] noted only one study of meningococcal vaccine in the elderly; that study showed no significant difference in 1-month post-vaccination titers in persons aged 6 to 25, 26 to 45, and 46 to 65 years.

Yellow fever virus is endemic in sub-Saharan Africa (Fig. 1) and tropical South America (Fig. 2). Based on data for US travelers during 1996 to 2004, the overall risk for serious illness and death due to yellow fever in travelers has been estimated to be 0.05 to 0.5 cases per 100,000 travelers to yellow fever endemic areas. Because of recent reports of deaths due to yellow fever among unvaccinated travelers to endemic areas, vaccination of travelers to high-risk areas should be encouraged as a key prevention strategy. Nevertheless, within the last 10 years, two serious adverse reaction syndromes have been described among recipients of yellow fever vaccines produced by different manufacturers: yellow fever vaccine–associated viscerotropic disease (YEL-AVD) and yellow fever vaccine–associated neurologic disease (YEL-AND) [114] YEL-AVD cases have been reported worldwide; 7 (58%) of the 12 US cases have been fatal. Reported US cases of YEL-AND have consisted of encephalitis and autoimmune neurologic disease, including Guillain-Barré syndrome and acute disseminated encephalomyelitis. All cases of these severe adverse events have occurred in primary vaccinees. Crude estimates of the reported incidence of YEL-AVD in the United States indicate an overall rate of 0.3 to 0.5 cases per 100,000 doses of vaccine distributed. This frequency appears to be higher for persons older than 60 years of age; the estimated reporting rate in this group is approximately 1.8 cases per 100,000 doses distributed [115]. The risk of any serious adverse event following yellow fever vaccination has been estimated at about 4 events per 100,000 doses for persons aged 60 to 69 years and 7.5 events per 100,000 doses for persons aged 70 years and older [116], but there was a lower incidence of common minor side effects [117].

A history of thymus disease has also been identified as a contraindication to yellow fever vaccine [118]. As noted previously, age-associated thymic involution is thought to have a role in the reduced response to vaccination.

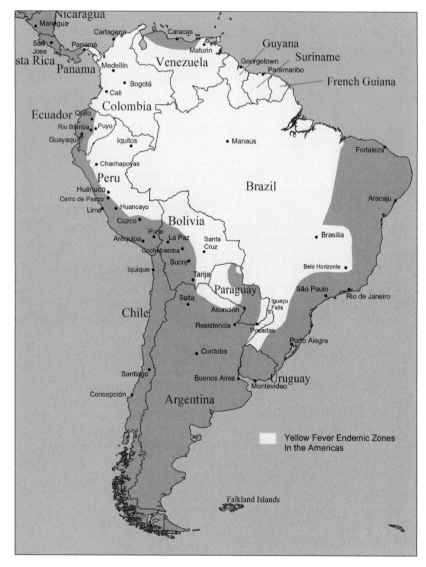

Fig. 2. Yellow fever–endemic zones in South America, 2007. (Source: *Health Information for International Travel*, 2008. Available at: www.cdc.gov/travel.)

Health care providers should be careful to ask about a history of thymus disorder, including myasthenia gravis, thymoma, or prior thymectomy, when screening a patient before administering yellow fever vaccine [116]. Health care providers should discuss with all travelers, particularly those older than 60 years, the risks described herein versus the benefits of vaccination in the context of the destination-specific risk for exposure to yellow fever virus.

INTERNATIONAL CERTIFICATE OF VACCINATION OR REVACCINATION AGAINST YELLOW FEVER

CERTIFICAT INTERNATIONAL DE VACCINATION DU DE REVACCINATION CONTRE LA FIEVRE JAUNE

This is to certify that   sex
Je soussigné(e) certifie que   sexe

whose signature follows   date of birth
dont la signature suit   né(e)

has on the date indicated been vaccinated or revaccinated against yellow fever.
A été vacciné(e) ou revacciné (e) contre la fièvre jaune è la date indiquée.

Date	Signature and professional status of vaccinator Signature et titre du vaccinateur	Manufacturer & Batch number of vaccine Fabricant du vaccine Et numero du lot	Official stamp of Vaccinating center Cachet official du Centre de vaccination
1.			
2.			

Fig. 3. International Certificate of Vaccination. (Source: *Health Information for International Travel*, 2008. Available at: www.cdc.gov/travel.)

The International Health Regulations (IHR) (www.who.int/csr/ihr/en) allow countries to require proof of vaccination for entry or from travelers arriving from certain countries. For the purposes of international travel, yellow fever vaccine produced by different manufacturers worldwide must be approved by the World Health Organization and administered at an approved yellow fever vaccination center. Vaccinees should receive a completed International Certificate of Vaccination (ICV) (Fig. 3) signed and validated with the center's stamp where the vaccine was given. This certificate is valid 10 days after vaccination and for a subsequent period of 10 years. Travelers who lack a completed ICV and who arrive in a country that requires proof of vaccination may be quarantined or refused entry unless they submit to on-site vaccination. (Note: The IHR (2005) which goes into effect June 15, 2007 revised the ICV to become an International Certificate of Vaccination and Prophylaxis (ICV&P). At the time of publication the new format was not available. It is recommended that the current form be used until the new ICV&P are available. In the past, previous versions of ICVs have been acceptable to other countries.)

If a physician concludes that a yellow fever vaccine should not be administered for medical reasons, the traveler should be given a signed and dated exemption letter on the physician's letterhead stationery that bears the official stamp used to validate the ICV. Waivers of requirements obtained from

---

MEDICAL CONTRAINDICATION TO VACCINATION
Contre-indication médicale á la vaccination

This is to certify that immunization against
Je soussigné(e) certifie que la vaccination contre

_____ for
(Name of disease — Nom de la maladie)   pour

                                                     is medically
_____ est
(Name of traveler — Nom du voyageur)   médicalement

contraindicated because of the following conditions:
contre-indiquée pour les raisons suivantes:

_____

_____

_____

_____

                        _____
                        (Signature and address of physician)
                        (Signature et adresse du medecin)

Fig. 4. Yellow Fever Vaccination Waiver. (Source: *Health Information for International Travel*, 2008. Available at: www.cdc.gov/travel.)

embassies or consulates should be documented by appropriate letters and retained for presentation with the completed Medical Contraindication to Vaccination section of the ICV (Fig. 4). Reasons other than medical contraindications are not acceptable for exemption from vaccination. The traveler should be advised that issuance of a waiver does not guarantee that the destination country will accept it; on arrival at the destination, the traveler may be faced with quarantine, refusal of entry, or vaccination on site.

Gastrointestinal issues

Approximately 6% to 50% of travelers will be affected by diarrhea during international travel, with the rate depending on the destination and the origin of the traveler. Travelers from developed areas to developing areas have the highest rates. Increasing age appears to be protective, even when the data are controlled for the type of travel and length of stay. Postulated reasons are differences in food selection, the quantity of food, and immunity [119]. Illness is primarily associated with ingestion of contaminated food or water. Travelers with achlorhydria due to diabetes, medications, or gastric surgery may be at increased risk of some enteric infections [120,121]. The ability of patients with cardiac disease or those taking diuretics to tolerate diarrhea and electrolyte imbalance should also be taken into consideration when advising prospective travelers [122].

Travelers, particularly to the developing world, are advised to eat only food that is served piping hot or that the traveler can peel, to drink only liquids that are bottled and sealed or served hot, and to avoid food from street vendors. Water can be rendered safe by boiling or adding chemicals such as iodine, but ice should be avoided because it may be prepared with local water. Travelers should also be reminded to wash their hands with soap and water before eating or to use a hand gel containing greater than 60% alcohol if soap and water are not available [123,124].

The typical course of traveler's diarrhea is characterized by the sudden onset of abdominal discomfort, followed by frequent watery stools and a sense of fecal urgency. Bacteria are the most common cause (80% to 85%), followed by parasites (10%) and viruses (5%) [125]. Travelers with fever or blood in the stool should seek medical care, but most cases are self-limited and respond to a short course of antibiotic therapy. Fluoroquinolones are the first line, with azithromycin as an alternative. Over-the-counter agents such as bismuth subsalicylate (Pepto-Bismol) and loperamide have been shown to bring symptomatic relief. Bismuth subsalicylate should be used with caution in travelers with renal insufficiency or in those receiving aspirin or anticoagulant therapy, and antimotility agents may cause rebound constipation.

In otherwise healthy adult travelers, severe dehydration from traveler's diarrhea is unusual unless vomiting is present. Vomiting may be the result of toxic gastroenteritis caused by the ingestion of a preformed toxin or viral pathogens such as norovirus. Older travelers would not be at decreased risk; in fact, they may frequent the scenarios, such as cruise ships and group travel and the types of food settings such as buffets, where these agents may be more likely. These agents are found in developed and developing areas, and hand gels in which alcohol is the active ingredient may not be effective against them. Travelers should be reminded to use only sealed or carbonated beverages for fluid replacement and, in the event of severe fluid loss, to reconstitute oral rehydration solutions. Packets of oral rehydration solutions can be included in the travel kit described previously. World Health Organization packets of oral rehydration solutions are also commonly available in pharmacies and markets in developing areas.

Alterations in diet associated with travel, such as a reduction in fresh fruits and vegetables, or a reduction in fluid consumption may contribute to constipation and should be considered when preparing a travel kit [120].

Diseases transmitted by mosquitoes, ticks, fleas, and other insects and arthropods

The primary method to prevent vector-borne diseases is to prevent the initial bite. Vaccines exist for yellow fever and Japanese encephalitis viruses, and medications can be taken for malaria prevention, but these methods do not exist for most entities that pose a risk to travelers to the tropics such as dengue and emerging infections such as chikungunya, two viruses transmitted by the bite of infected mosquitos. Repellents such as DEET for exposed skin and permethrin-based products for clothing, shoes, tents, and so on are effective if properly applied for use against some vectors. Repellents should be combined with other behavioral measures, such as wearing loose clothing with long sleeves and long pants and limiting exposure during active periods for the vector. Physical measures such as wearing close-toed shoes are necessary to prevent tungiasis, the nodular lesions associated with the bite of some sand flies. To prevent cutaneous larva migrans, a towel should be used if sitting or lying on a beach where animals defecate.

Recommendations for appropriate antimalarial agents need to be tailored to the itinerary, medical history of the client, and side-effect profile of the drug. Depending on the destination, atovaquone/proguanil, chloroquine, doxycycline, mefloquine, or primaquine may be recommended. Chloroquine and mefloquine resistance limit their use in some parts of the world. Drug interactions are a major consideration because more than 80% of US adults report taking at least one medication during the previous week, and drug use increases with age; 23% of women aged more than 65 years take at least five prescription medications [126]. Dosages may also need to be adjusted for decreased renal or hepatic function. Persons with a history of epilepsy or psychiatric disorders, including depression, which may affect 15% of the ambulatory elderly [127], should not use mefloquine [128]. The most common adverse events associated with doxycycline are gastrointestinal effects, photosensitivity, and *Candida* vaginitis; the esophagitis and nausea can be reduced by taking the pill with food and plenty of water in the morning and remaining upright. All travelers to the tropics should be advised to use sunscreen on exposed skin [61,121,128,129]. To be effective, an antimalarial agent should be taken as prescribed before, during, and after travel in the malarious area. Travelers should also be advised to have any fever that occurs for 12 months after travel evaluated immediately and should inform their health care provider where they have traveled. Deaths continue to occur in the United States due to delays in recognition, diagnosis, and appropriate treatment of malaria in returned travelers [130].

Role of the primary health care provider

There is a dichotomy among older travelers; some continue to be fit and active while the percent of the population that is obese and sustaining diabetes and hypertension is also at an all-time high. All travelers are impacted to some degree by the biologic aspects of aging in terms of changes in the immune system, body composition, hearing, and vision. Advances in medical care have contributed to increased numbers of persons surviving cancer treatment, living with transplants, or receiving immunosuppressive drugs for rheumatologic conditions that allow them to have enhanced mobility and the desire to accomplish life-long dreams such as safaris in Africa; however, these therapies also raise concerns for vaccination and susceptibility to infections. The primary health care provider has a key role in optimizing medical management, assessing whether the patient is medically fit to travel, and providing documentation as necessary for the patient to carry or for the travel health care consultant.

Ensuring that all patients are current in routine immunizations is a key step, as is inquiring about the travel history of patients being seen for acute illness and the role of travel in the patient's future, particularly among immigrant populations. Travel medicine is a dynamic field because conditions worldwide are subject to rapid change. The patient's itinerary is listed first among the key elements, because it is the destination that determines much of the specific travel advice. Clinicians must maintain a current base of knowledge if they will be regularly advising travelers in pre-travel consultations. A threshold should be set for when a referral might be made to a travel medicine specialist, considering the traveler's best interest and the need to provide the most complete and up-to-date information.

Acknowledgments

The author extends sincere thanks to Mary-Christine Sullivan and Susan Graham for their contribution to the preparation of this manuscript.

References

[1] US Department of Commerce. Office of Travel and Tourism Industries, Survey of International Air Travelers US to Overseas and Mexico by Birth, Citizenship 2004 Report. January-December, 2004. Banner 1, Table 30.

[2] USCensus Bureau. Oldest baby boomers turn 60! 2006. Available at: http://www.census.gov/PressRelease/www/releases/archives/facts_for_featuresspecial_editions/006105.html. Accessed February 2, 2007.

[3] Popuiation Division, Department of Education and Social Affairs, United Nations. IV. Demographic profile of the older population 1950-2050. 2006, 23–27. Available at: http://www.un.org/esa/population/publications/worldageing19502050/. Accessed November 7, 2006.

[4] US Census Bureau. 2004. US interim projections by age, sex, race, and Hispanic origin. Available at: http://www.census.gov/ipc/www/usinterimproj/. Accessed November 7, 2006.

[5] Hill DR. Health problems in a large cohort of Americans traveling to developing countries. J Travel Med 2000;7:259–66.

[6] Scoville SL, Bryan JP, Tribble D, et al. Epidemiology, preventive services, and illnesses of international travelers. Mil Med 1997;162:172–8.

[7] Centers for Disease Control and Prevention. Prevention and control of influenza: recommendations of the Advisory Committee on Immunization Practices (ACIP). MMWR Recomm Rep 2005;54:1–40.

[8] Zahran HS, Kobau R, Moriarty DG, et al. Health-related quality of life surveillance–United States, 1993-2002. MMWR Surveill Summ 2005;54:1–35.

[9] Staats S, Pierfelice L. Travel: a long-range goal of retired women. J Psychol 2003;137:483–94.

[10] Ryst S. Winter games: ski resorts are designing more programs and services for the 50-plus crowd. Wall St J (East Ed) 2004;R12.

[11] Pinto B. Getting air travel ready for baby boom generation. ABC News Original Report. 2005. Available at: http://abcnews.go.com/WNT/LivingLonger/story?id=125695. Accessed November 8, 2006.

[12] Cleaver M, Muller TE. I want to pretend I'm eleven years younger: subjective age and seniors' motives for vacation travel. Soc Indic Res 2002;60:227–41.

[13] Muller TE, O'Cass A. Targeting the young at heart: seeing senior vacationers the way they see themselves. Journal of Vacation Marketing 2001;7:285–301.

[14] Terhune L. American Muslims go on Hajj. USINFO StateGov. 2006. Available at: http://usinfo.state.gov/xarchives/display.html?p=washfile-english&y=2006&m=December&x=20061222104002mlenuhret0.876919. Accessed January 10, 2007.

[15] Francese P. The exotic travel boom. Am Demogr 2002;24:48–9.

[16] Ruffenach G. Road scholars: a new travel program tries to take some of the 'elder' out of elderhostel. Wall St J (East Ed) 2004;R.6.

[17] Osborne L. Never too old to learn. NY Times (Print) [Late Edition (East Coast)]. February 18, 2005: F1.

[18] Campbell S. The denture venturers. The Spectator. August 12, 2006. Available at: http://www.findarticles.com/p/articles/mi_qa3724/is_200608/ai_n17189064. Accessed October 25, 2006.

[19] Prystay C. Backpacking in the golden years; more retirees take to road for exotic, no-frills travel; skip talk about colonoscopy. Wall St J (East Ed) 2004;B1.

[20] Schlesinger R. Giving peace a chance. American Association of Retired Persons (AARP) Bulletin Online. 2006. Available at: http://www.aarp.org/bulletin/yourlife/peacecorps.html. Accessed November 1, 2006.

[21] US Census Bureau. The foreign-born population in the United States: 2003. 2004. Available at: http://www.census.gov/population/www/socdemo/foreign/cps2003.html. Accessed December 5, 2006.

[22] US Department of Commerce, International Trade Administration, Office of Travel and Tourism Industries, Survey of International Travelers. 2005 profile of US resident travelers visiting overseas destinations–outbound. 2006. Available at: http://tinet.ita.doc.gov/cat/f-2005-101-002.html. Accessed November 1, 2006.

[23] Behrens RH, Collins M, Botto B, et al. Risk for British travellers of acquiring hepatitis A. BMJ 1995;311:193.

[24] Leder K, Tong S, Weld L, et al. Illness in travelers visiting friends and relatives: a review of the GeoSentinel Surveillance Network. Clin Infect Dis 2006;43:1185–93.

[25] Lynch M, Bulens S, Polyak C, et al. Multi-drug resistance among Salmonella typhi isolates in the United States, 1999-2003. Presented at the Sixth International Conference on Typhoid Fever and Other Salmonelloses. Guilin, China; November 12, 2005.

[26] Scolari C, Tedoldi S, Casalini C, et al. Practices on malaria preventive measures of migrants attending a public health clinic in northern Italy. J Travel Med 2002;9:160–2.

[27] Skarbinski J, James EM, Causer LM, et al. Malaria surveillance–United States, 2004. MMWR Surveill Summ 2006;55:23–37.

[28] Steinberg EB, Bishop R, Haber P, et al. Typhoid fever in travelers: who should be targeted for prevention? Clin Infect Dis 2004;39:186–91.

[29] Angell SY, Cetron MS. Health disparities among travelers visiting friends and relatives abroad. Ann Intern Med 2005;142:67–72.

[30] Bacaner N, Stauffer B, Boulware DR, et al. Travel medicine considerations for North American immigrants visiting friends and relatives. JAMA 2004;291:2856–64.

[31] Baker TD, Hargarten SW, Guptill KS. The uncounted dead–American civilians dying overseas. Public Health Rep 1992;107:155–9.

[32] Hargarten SW, Baker TD, Guptill K. Overseas fatalities of United States citizen travelers: an analysis of deaths related to international travel. Ann Emerg Med 1991;20:622–6.

[33] Chen LH, Wilson ME, Schlagenhauf P. Prevention of malaria in long-term travelers [review]. JAMA 2006;296:2234–44.

[34] Lumber T, Strainic PA. Have insulin, will travel: planning ahead will make traveling with insulin smooth sailing. Diabetes Forecast 2005;58(8):50–4.

[35] Carey MJ, Aitken ME. Motorbike injuries in Bermuda: a risk for tourists. Ann Emerg Med 1996;28:424–9.

[36] Petridou E, Dessypris N, Skalkidou A, et al. Struggling with incomplete data. Accid Anal Prev 1999;31:611–5.

[37] Hargarten SW, Bouc GT. Emergency air medical transport of US citizen tourists: 1988 to 1990. Air Med J 1993;12:398–402.

[38] Seccombe LM, Peters MJ. Oxygen supplementation for chronic obstructive pulmonary disease patients during air travel [review]. Curr Opin Pulm Med 2006;12:140–4.

[39] Jorge A, Pombal R, Peixoto H, et al. Preflight medical clearance of ill and incapacitated passengers: 3-year retrospective study of experience with a European airline. J Travel Med 2005;12:306–11.

[40] American Thoracic Society. Air travel. Standards for the diagnosis and treatment of patients with chronic obstructive pulmonary disease. 2007. Available at: http://www.thoracic.org/sections/copd/for- health-professionals/management-of-stable-copd/air-travel/index.html. Accessed January 12, 2007.

[41] Aerospace Medical Association Medical Guidelines Task Force. Medical guidelines for airline travel. 2nd edition. Aviat Space Environ Med 2003;74:A1–19.

[42] Chan SB, Hogan TM, Silva JC. Medical emergencies at a major international airport: inflight symptoms and ground based follow-up. Aviat Space Environ Med 2002;73:1021–4.

[43] Delaune EF III, Lucas RH, Illig P. In-flight medical events and aircraft diversions: one airline's experience. Aviat Space Environ Med 2003;74:62–8.

[44] Goodwin T. In-flight medical emergencies: an overview [review]. BMJ 2000;321:1338–41.

[45] Dowdall N. "Is there a doctor on the aircraft?" Top 10 in-flight medical emergencies [review]. BMJ 2000;321:1336–7.

[46] Low JA, Chan DKY. Air travel in older people. Age Ageing 2002;31:17–22.

[47] Burnett JC. Long- and short-haul travel by air: issues for people with diabetes on insulin. J Travel Med 2006;13:255–60.

[48] Mileno MD, Bia FJ. The compromised traveler. Infect Dis Clin North Am 1998;12:369–412.

[49] Monk TH, Buysse DJ, Carrier J, et al. Inducing jet-lag in older people: directional asymmetry. J Sleep Res 2000;9:101–16.

[50] Monk TH. Aging human circadian rhythms: conventional wisdom may not always be right. J Biol Rhythms 2005;20:366–74.

[51] Monk TH, Buysse DJ, Reynolds CF III, et al. Inducing jet lag in an older person: directional asymmetry. Exp Gerontol 1995;30:137–45.

[52] Monk TH, Buysse DJ, Reynolds CF III, et al. Inducing jet lag in older people: adjusting to a 6-hour phase advance in routine. Exp Gerontol 1993;28:119–33.

[53] Brendel DH, Reynolds CF III, Jennings JR, et al. Sleep stage physiology, mood, and vigilance responses to total sleep deprivation in healthy 80-year-olds and 20-year-olds. Psychophysiology 1990;27:677–85.

[54] Adams PF, Schoenborn CA. Health behaviors of adults: United States, 2002-04. Vital Health Stat 10 2006;10(230):1–140.

[55] Parry BL. Jet lag: minimizing its effects with critically timed bright light and melatonin administration. J Mol Microbiol Biotechnol 2002;4:463–6.

[56] Herxheimer A. Jet lag. Clin Evid 2005;13:2178–83.

[57] Buscemi N, Vandermeer B, Hooton N, et al. Efficacy and safety of exogenous melatonin for secondary sleep disorders and sleep disorders accompanying sleep restriction: meta-analysis. BMJ 2006;332:385–93.

[58] Cox ID, Blight A, Lyons JP. Air-terminal stress and the older traveller. Age Ageing 1999;28:236–7.

[59] McIntosh IB, Swanson V, Power KG, et al. Anxiety and health problems related to air travel. J Travel Med 1998;5:198–204.

[60] DeHart RL. Health issues of air travel. Annu Rev Public Health 2003;24:133–51.

[61] Centers for Disease Control and Prevention. Health information for international travel 2008. Atlanta (GA): US Department of Health and Human Services, Public Health Services; 2007. p. 487–92.

[62] Sajid MS, Tai NR, Goli G, et al. Knee versus thigh length graduated compression stockings for prevention of deep venous thrombosis: a systematic review. Eur J Vasc Endovasc Surg 2006;32:730–6.

[63] van Treeck U. Measles outbreak in Germany: update. Eurosurveillance Weekly Report. 2006;11(4). Available at: http://www.eurosurveillance.org/ew/2006/060413.asp. Accessed November 1, 2006.

[64] Consular Information Sheet. Venezuela. US Department of State. 2006. Available at: http://travel.state.gov/travel/cis_pa_tw/cis/cis_1059.html. Accessed December 12, 2006.

[65] Centers for Disease Control and Prevention. Notice to readers: updated recommendations of the Advisory Committee on Immunization Practices (ACIP) for the control and elimination of mumps. MMWR Morb Mortal Wkly Rep 2006;55:629–30.

[66] Leder K, Weller PF, Wilson ME. Travel vaccines and elderly persons: review of vaccines available in the United States. Clin Infect Dis 2001;33:1553–66.

[67] Centers for Disease Control and Prevention. Fatal respiratory diphtheria in a US traveler to Haiti—Pennsylvania, 2003. MMWR Morb Mortal Wkly Rep 2004;52:1285–6.

[68] Galazka AM, Robertson SE. Diphtheria: changing patterns in the developing world and the industrialized world. Eur J Epidemiol 1995;11:107–17.

[69] Galazka A. The changing epidemiology of diphtheria in the vaccine era. J Infect Dis 2000; 181(Suppl 1):S2–9.

[70] McQuillan GM, Kruszon-Moran D, Deforest A, et al. Serologic immunity to diphtheria and tetanus in the United States. Ann Intern Med 2002;136:660–6.

[71] Quinn HE, McIntyre PB. Tetanus in the elderly: an important preventable disease in Australia. Vaccine 2007;25:1304–9.

[72] Volzke H, Kloker KM, Kramer A, et al. Susceptibility to diphtheria in adults: prevalence and relationship to gender and social variables. Clin Microbiol Infect 2006;12:961–7.

[73] Santibanez TA, Zimmerman RK. Immunizations in adulthood. Prim Care 2002;29:649–65.

[74] Kretsinger K, Broder KR, Cortese MM, et al. Preventing tetanus, diphtheria, and pertussis among adults: use of tetanus toxoid, reduced diphtheria toxoid and acellular pertussis vaccine recommendations of the Advisory Committee on Immunization Practices (ACIP) and recommendation of ACIP, supported by the Healthcare Infection Control Practices Advisory Committee (HICPAC), for use of Tdap among health-care personnel. MMWR Recomm Rep 2006;55:1–37.

[75] Grimprel E, Von Sonnenburg F, Sanger R, et al. Combined reduced-antigen-content diphtheria-tetanus-acellular pertussis and polio vaccine (dTpa-IPV) for booster vaccination of adults. Vaccine 2005;23:3657–67.

[76] Hutin YL, Hauri YM, Husson B, Armstrong GL. Use of injections in healthcare settings worldwide, 2000: literature review and regional estimates. BMJ 2003;327(1075):1075.

[77] Conner GA, Jacobs RJ. Hepatitis B risk and immunization coverage among US travelers. Presented at the Proceedings of the 9th Conference of the International Society of Travel Medicine. Lisbon (Portugal): May 1–5, 2005. p. 107.

[78] Wright ER. Travel, tourism, and HIV risk among older adults. J Acquir Immune Defic Syndr 2003;33(Suppl 2):S233–7.

[79] Wong CM, Chan KP, Hedley AJ, et al. Influenza-associated mortality in Hong Kong. Clin Infect Dis 2004;39:1611–7.

[80] Leder K, Sundararajan V, Weld L, et al. Respiratory tract infections in travelers: a review of the GeoSentinel surveillance network. Clin Infect Dis 2003;36:399–406.

[81] Dosseh A, Ndiaye K, Spiegel A, et al. Epidemiological and virological influenza survey in Dakar, Senegal: 1996-1998. Am J Trop Med Hyg 2000;62:639–43.

[82] Chew FT, Doraisingham S, Ling AE, et al. Seasonal trends of viral respiratory tract infections in the tropics. Epidemiol Infect 1998;121:121–8.

[83] Mutsch M, Tavernini M, Marx A, et al. Influenza virus infection in travelers to tropical and subtropical countries. Clin Infect Dis 2005;40:1282–7.

[84] Reed C, Cox C, Weld L, et al, and the GeoSentinel Surveillance Group. Influenza morbidity among travelers to the tropics: a review of the GeoSentinel Network, January 1998-June 2004. Presented at the Proceedings of the 9th Conference of the International Society of Travel Medicine. Lisbon (Portugal): May 1–5, 2005. p. 74.

[85] Ferson MJ, Morgan K, Robertson PW, et al. Concurrent summer influenza and pertussis outbreaks in a nursing home in Sydney, Australia. Infect Control Hosp Epidemiol 2004;25: 962–6.

[86] Centers for Disease Control and Prevention. Influenza and pneumococcal vaccination coverage among persons aged ≥ 65 years—United States, 2004–2005. MMWR Morb Mortal Wkly Rep 2006;55:1065–8.

[87] Ferson M, Paraskevopoulos P, Hatzi S, et al. Presumptive summer influenza A: an outbreak on a trans-Tasman cruise. Commun Dis Intell 2000;24:45–7.

[88] Public Health Agency of Canada. Influenza in travellers to Alaska, the Yukon Territory, and on west coast cruise ships, summer of 1999. Can Commun Dis Rep 1999;25: 137–9.

[89] Miller JM, Tam TW, Maloney S, et al. Cruise ships: high-risk passengers and the global spread of new influenza viruses. Clin Infect Dis 2000;31:433–8.

[90] Brotherton JM, Delpech VC, Gilbert GL, et al. A large outbreak of influenza A and B on a cruise ship causing widespread morbidity. Epidemiol Infect 2003;130:263–71.

[91] Centers for Disease Control and Prevention. Influenza B virus outbreak on a cruise ship—Northern Europe, 2000. Morb Mortal Wkly Rep 2001;50:137–40.

[92] Freedman DO, Leder K. Influenza: changing approaches to prevention and treatment in travelers [review]. J Travel Med 2005;12:36–44.

[93] Smith NM, Bresee JS, Shay DK, et al. Prevention and control of influenza: recommendations of the Advisory Committee on Immunization Practices (ACIP). Morb Mortal Wkly Rep Recomm Rep 2006;55:1–42.

[94] Mutsch M, Spicher VM, Gut C, et al. Hepatitis A virus infections in travelers, 1988-2004. Clin Infect Dis 2006;42:490–7.

[95] Steffen R, Kane MA, Shapiro CN, et al. Epidemiology and prevention of hepatitis A in travelers. JAMA 1994;272:885–9.

[96] Fiore AE, Wasley A, Bell BP. Prevention of hepatitis A through active or passive immunization: recommendations of the Advisory Committee on Immunization Practices (ACIP). Morb Mortal Wkly Rep Recomm Rep 2006;55:1–23.

[97] Fishbain JT, Eckart RE, Harner KC, et al. Empiric immunization versus serologic screening: developing a cost-effective strategy for the use of hepatitis A immunization in travelers. J Travel Med 2002;9:71–5.

[98] Genton B, D'Acremont V, Furrer HJ, et al. Hepatitis A vaccines and the elderly. Travel Med Infect Dis 2006;4:303–12.

[99] D'Acremont V, Herzog C, Genton B. Immunogenicity and safety of a virosomal hepatitis A vaccine (Epaxal) in the elderly. J Travel Med 2006;13:78–83.

[100] Van der WM, Van Damme P, Chlibek R, et al. Hepatitis A/B vaccination of adults over 40 years old: comparison of three vaccine regimens and effect of influencing factors. Vaccine 2006;24:5509–15.

[101] Rendi-Wagner P, Kundi M, Stemberger H, et al. Antibody response to three recombinant hepatitis B vaccines: comparative evaluation of multicenter travel-clinic based experience. Vaccine 2001;19:2055–60.

[102] Gruver AL, Hudson LL, Sempowski GD. Immunosenescence of ageing. J Pathol 2007;211: 144–56.

[103] Effros RB. Role of T lymphocyte replicative senescence in vaccine efficacy. Vaccine 2007;25: 599–604.

[104] Haynes L. How vaccines work on the background of the aging immune system. Exp Gerontol 2007;42(5):438–40.

[105] El Yousafi M, Mercier S, Breuille D, et al. The inflammatory response to vaccination is altered in the elderly. Mech Ageing Dev 2005;126:874–81.

[106] Kaml M, Weiskirchner I, Keller M, et al. Booster vaccinations in the elderly: their success depends on the vaccine type applied earlier in life as well as on pre-vaccination antibody titers. Vaccine 2006;24:6808–11.

[107] Kroger AT, Atkinson WL, Marcuse EK, et al. General recommendations on immunization: recommendations of the Advisory Committee on Immunization Practices (ACIP). Morb Mortal Wkly Rep Recomm Rep 2006;55:1–48.

[108] Cook IF, Williamson M, Pond D. Definition of needle length required for intramuscular deltoid injection in elderly adults: an ultrasonographic study. Vaccine 2006;24:937–40.

[109] Prevots DR, Burr RK, Sutter RW, et al. Poliomyelitis prevention in the United States: updated recommendations of the Advisory Committee on Immunization Practices (ACIP). Morb Mortal Wkly Rep Recomm Rep 2000;49:1–22.

[110] Ranney M, Partridge R, Jay GD, et al. Rabies antibody seroprotection rates among travelers in Nepal: "rabies seroprotection in travelers.". J Travel Med 2006;13:329–33.

[111] Lau C, Sisson J. The effectiveness of intradermal pre-exposure rabies vaccination in an Australian travel medicine clinic. J Travel Med 2002;9:285–8.

[112] Nothdurft HD, Jelinek T, Marschang A, et al. Adverse reactions to Japanese encephalitis vaccine in travellers. J Infect 1996;32:119–22.

[113] Bilukha OO, Rosenstein N. Prevention and control of meningococcal disease: recommendations of the Advisory Committee on Immunization Practices (ACIP). Morb Mortal Wkly Rep Recomm Rep 2005;54:1–21.

[114] Centers for Disease Control and Prevention. Adverse events associated with 17D-derived yellow fever vaccination–United States, 2001-2002. Morb Mortal Wkly Rep 2002;51(44):989–93.

[115] Centers for Disease Control and Prevention. Health Information for International Travel 2008. Atlanta (GA): US Department of Health and Human Services, Public Health Services; 2007. p. 362–79.

[116] Khromava AY, Eidex RB, Weld LH, et al. Yellow fever vaccine: an updated assessment of advanced age as a risk factor for serious adverse events. Vaccine 2005;3256–63.

[117] Monath TP, Cetron MS, McCarthy K, et al. Yellow fever 17D vaccine safety and immunogenicity in the elderly. Hum Vaccin 2005;1:207–14.

[118] Barwick R. History of thymoma and yellow fever vaccination. Lancet 2004;364:936.

[119] Brewster SJ, Taylor DN. Epidemiology of travelers' diarrhea. Travel Medicine. In: Keystone JS, Kozarsky PE, Freedman DO, editors. London: Elsevier; 2004. p. 175–84.

[120] Cooper MC. The elderly travellers. Travel Med Infect Dis 2006;4:218–22.

[121] Gordon ME. Gastrointestinal and other vulnerabilities for geriatric globetrotters. Clin Geriatr Med 1991;7:321–30.

[122] Albrecht CR, Cumbo TA, Gambert SR. Health issues, travel, and the elderly. Clin Geriatr 2003;11:24–33.

[123] Sattar SA, Abebe M, Bueti AJ, et al. Activity of an alcohol-based hand gel against human adeno-, rhino-, and rotaviruses using the fingerpad method. Infect Control Hosp Epidemiol 2000;21:516–9.

[124] Morton JL, Schultz AA. Healthy hands: use of alcohol gel as an adjunct to handwashing in elementary school children. J Sch Nurs 2004;20:161–7.

[125] Black RE. Epidemiology of travelers' diarrhea and relative importance of various pathogens. Rev Infect Dis 1990;12(Suppl 1):S73–9.

[126] Kaufman DW, Kelly JP, Rosenberg L, et al. Recent patterns of medication use in the ambulatory adult population of the United States: the Slone survey. JAMA 2002;287:337–44.

[127] VanItallie TB. Subsyndromal depression in the elderly: underdiagnosed and undertreated. Metabolism 2005;54:39–44.

[128] Schlagenhauf P, Beallor C, Kain KC. Malaria. Travel Medicine. In: Keystone JS, Kozarsky PE, Freedman DO, editors. London: Elsevier; 2004. p. 137–67.

[129] Wallace MR, Sharp TW, Smoak B, et al. Malaria among United States troops in Somalia. Am J Med 1996;100:49–55.

[130] Newman RD, Parise ME, Barber AM, et al. Malaria-related deaths among US travelers, 1963-2001. Ann Intern Med 2004;141:547–55.

ELSEVIER
SAUNDERS

Clin Geriatr Med 23 (2007) 715–720

CLINICS IN
GERIATRIC
MEDICINE

Index

Note: Page numbers of article titles are in **boldface** type.

A

Abscesses, intra-abdominal, as cause of fever, 652–653

Adenoviruses, 548

Age, chronologic, subjective age assessed as younger, 688

AIDS, in United States, 567, 568, 569

Amantadine, 540

Amitriptyline, in herpes zoster pain management, 623

Amoxicillin-clavulanate, 489

Analgesics, in herpes zoster pain management, 622

Antibacterials, in community-acquired pneumonia, 528–529
in pneumonia, 523–527

Antibiotics, cumulative exposure to, 484
in bacteremia and sepsis, 642
in fever of unknown origin, 663, 664
in nursing-home acquired pneumonia, 557–560
resistance to, infection control practitioners and, 507–508

Antigen dose, increased, in vaccines, 680–681

Antigen presentation, changes with aging, 468

Antimalarial agents, 706

Antimicrobials, de-escalation of use of, after pathogen identification, 482
dosing with, effects of physiologic changes and pharmacodynamics on, 485–488
guiding use of, by older adults, 482
in urinary tract infection, 590, 592
principles of use, in older adults, **481–497**

Antiretroviral therapy, in HIV infection, 572–577

Antiviral therapy, in varicella-zoster virus infections, 619–622

Antivirals, influenza, 540–542

B

B cells, changes in healthy older adults, 472

Bacteremia, and sepsis in older patients, **633–647**
definition of, 633
diagnostic challenges in, 638–639
epidemiology of, 634–636
management in, 641–644
prognosis in, age as factor in, 639–641
risk factors for, 636–637

Bacteriuria, asymptomatic, and urinary tract infection, in older adults, **585–594**
diagnosis of, 585
management of, 586–587
microbiology of, 586
prevalence of, 586
prevention of, 587–588

Beta-lactams, in pneumonia, 523, 524–525, 526

Bocavirus, human, 548

Boils, 599–600

Bone marrow biopsy, to investigate fever of unknown origin, 663

C

Carbuncles, 599–600

Cellulitis, 595–697

Chest radiography, in pneumonia, 520

Cognitive dysfunction, HIV-associated, 579

Colonoscopy, to investigate fever of unknown origin, 662

Community-acquired pneumonia. See *Pneumonia, community-acquired.*

Coronaviruses, 545–547

doi:10.1016/S0749-0690(07)00050-X

Moving?

Make sure your subscription moves with you!

To notify us of your new address, find your **Clinics Account Number** (located on your mailing label above your name), and contact customer service at:

E-mail: elspcs@elsevier.com

800-654-2452 (subscribers in the U.S. & Canada)
407-345-4000 (subscribers outside of the U.S. & Canada)

Fax number: 407-363-9661

Elsevier Periodicals Customer Service
6277 Sea Harbor Drive
Orlando, FL 32887-4800

*To ensure uninterrupted delivery of your subscription, please notify us at least 4 weeks in advance of move.